PATHWAYS OF ADDICTION

OPPORTUNITIES IN DRUG ABUSE RESEARCH

Committee on Opportunities in Drug Abuse Research

Division of Neuroscience and Behavioral Health

INSTITUTE OF MEDICINE

NATIONAL ACADEMY PRESS
Washington, D.C. 1996

NATIONAL ACADEMY PRESS • 2101 Constitution Avenue, NW • Washington, DC 20418

Support for this study was provided by the National Institute on Drug Abuse (contract no. N01DA-3-8000).

Library of Congress Cataloging-in-Publication Data

Pathways of addiction : opportunities in drug abuse research / Committee on Opportunities in Drug Abuse Research, Division of Neuroscience and Behavioral Health, Institute of Medicine.
p. cm.
Includes bibliographical references and index.
ISBN 0-309-05533-4
1. Substance abuse—Research—United States. 2. Substance abuse—Research—Government policy—United States. I. Committee on Opportunities in Drug Abuse Research.
RC564.P365 1996
362.29′072073—dc20 96-30998
CIP

Pathways of Addiction: Opportunities in Drug Abuse Research is available for sale from the National Academy Press, 2101 Constitution Avenue, NW, Box 285, Washington, DC 20055. 800-624-6242 or 202-334-3313 (in the Washington metropolitan area). **http://www.nap.edu.**

Cover: Gloria Monteiro Rall, "Overlapping," with permission of the artist.

Printed in the United States of America.

The serpent has been a symbol of long life, healing, and knowledge among almost all cultures and religions since the beginning of recorded history. The image adopted as a logotype by the Institute of Medicine is based on a relief carving from ancient Greece, now held by the Staalichemusseen in Berlin.

COMMITTEE ON OPPORTUNITIES IN DRUG ABUSE RESEARCH

RICHARD J. BONNIE,* *Chair*, John S. Battle Professor of Law, University of Virginia School of Law, Charlottesville, Virginia

JUDITH S. BROOK, Professor of Community Medicine, Mount Sinai School of Medicine, New York, New York

RICHARD CLAYTON, Director, Center for Prevention Research, University of Kentucky, Lexington, Kentucky

JOHN E. DONOVAN, Scientific Director, Pittsburgh Adolescent Alcohol Research Center, Western Psychiatric Institute and Clinic, and Associate Professor, Department of Psychiatry, University of Pittsburgh School of Medicine, Pittsburgh, Pennsylvania

MARIAN W. FISCHMAN, Professor of Behavioral Biology, College of Physicians and Surgeons of Columbia University, and Research Scientist, New York State Psychiatric Institute, New York, New York

ROBERT E. FULLILOVE, III, Associate Dean for Community and Minority Affairs, Columbia University School of Public Health, New York, New York

JAMES G. HAUGHTON,* Medical Director, Division of Public Health Programs and Services, Los Angeles County Department of Health Services, Los Angeles, California

JAMES A. INCIARDI, Director, Center for Drug and Alcohol Studies, University of Delaware, Newark, Delaware

GEORGE F. KOOB, Director, Division of Psychopharmacology, and Professor, Department of Neuropharmacology, The Scripps Research Institute, La Jolla, California

MITCHELL B. MAX, Chief, Clinical Trials Unit, Neurobiology and Anesthesiology Branch, National Institute of Dental Research, National Institutes of Health, Bethesda, Maryland

ERIC J. NESTLER, Elizabeth Mears and House Jameson Professor, Departments of Psychiatry and Pharmacology, Yale University School of Medicine, New Haven, Connecticut

PATRICK M. O'MALLEY, Program Director, Survey Research Center, Institute for Social Research, University of Michigan, Ann Arbor, Michigan

PETER SELWYN, Associate Professor, Department of Internal Medicine, Epidemiology, and Public Health, Yale University School of Medicine, New Haven, Connecticut

*Member, Institute of Medicine.

BARBARA R. WILLIAMS, Vice President Emeritus, RAND, Washington, D.C.

GEORGE E. WOODY, Clinical Professor of Psychiatry, University of Pennsylvania, and Chief, Substance Abuse Treatment Unit, Philadelphia Veterans Affairs Medical Center, Philadelphia, Pennsylvania

BARRY ZUCKERMAN, Professor and Chairman, Department of Pediatrics, Boston University School of Medicine, Boston, Massachusetts

Special Advisors to the Committee

LAURIE CHASSIN, Professor, Department of Psychology, Arizona State University, Tempe, Arizona

MIRIAM DAVIS, Science and Health Policy Consultant, Silver Spring, Maryland

JEFFREY FAGAN, Associate Professor, School of Criminal Justice, Rutgers University, New York, New York

LINDA MAYES, Arnold Gesell Associate Professor of Child Development and Pediatrics, Yale Child Study Center, Yale University School of Medicine, New Haven, Connecticut

KATHLEEN MERIKANGAS, Director, Genetic Epidemiology Research Unit, Yale University School of Medicine, New Haven, Connecticut

DAVID MUSTO, Professor of Psychiatry and the History of Medicine, Yale University School of Medicine, New Haven, Connecticut

JEFFREY SWANSON, Associate Professor, Psychiatric Epidemiology and Health Services Research Program, Duke University Medical Center, Durham, North Carolina

STAFF

CAROLYN E. FULCO, Study Director

CATHARYN LIVERMAN, Program Officer

CARRIE INGALLS, Research Assistant

TERRI SCANLAN, Project Assistant

CONSTANCE PECHURA, Director, Division of Neuroscience and Behavioral Health

Preface

Drug abuse can be viewed from many perspectives. At different times and in different contexts, each of us uses multiple vocabularies to describe and discuss drug abuse. Sometimes we use the vocabulary of choice and responsibility. Sometimes we use the vocabulary of health and disease. Sometimes we use the marketplace vocabulary of supply and demand. Sometimes we use the vocabulary of crime and punishment. The list goes on.

Scientific study cannot be expected to erase or reconcile fully our multiple understandings and interpretations of drug abuse. Were it not for scientific research, however, we would be unable to understand drug abuse from any of those perspectives. Were it not for scientific research, we would be unable to harness the social and political energy needed to respond to drug abuse in a rational manner.

When the National Institute on Drug Abuse (NIDA) was established in 1974, the nation was grappling with a major epidemic of illicit drug use. As part of a multipronged national response to this problem, Congress made a significant investment in drug abuse research. Over the ensuing two decades, substantial advances have been made along numerous scientific paths, ranging from the discovery of endogenous opioids to an assessment of the impact of needle sharing on the transmission of HIV (human immunodeficiency virus) disease. As the primary federal funding agency for drug abuse research, NIDA deserves credit for stimulating and supporting the talented scientists who have moved the field forward,[1] for maintaining a coherent scientific agenda in the face of shifting political winds, and for building a strong foundation for continuing scientific progress in the years ahead.

In January 1995, at NIDA's request, the Institute of Medicine (IOM) formed the Committee on Opportunities in Drug Abuse Research to assess current knowledge and accomplishments and to propose a research agenda for the next decade. The committee was asked to take a broad perspective, considering not only NIDA's research portfolio but any opportunity for increasing knowledge about drug abuse through research, for promoting effective prevention and treatment strategies, and for ameliorating the consequences of drug abuse and dependence. In order to fulfill this charge, the IOM selected for membership on the committee individuals with expertise in a variety of scientific disciplines who have conducted research on many fields of inquiry bearing on drug abuse, including neuroscience, clinical research and treatment, psychopharmacology, epidemiology, etiology, prevention, AIDS/HIV research, fetal and child development, public health, and law and public policy.

During the course of the study, the committee met four times and solicited written suggestions and opinions from experts in a variety of fields. In conjunction with its meetings, the committee invited presentations from treatment experts, criminologists, individuals associated with community prevention programs and treatment centers, neuroscientists, behavioral scientists, and other interested persons (see Appendix A).

The committee's primary charge was to identify directions for future research. The committee recognized, however, that the setting of research priorities is not a purely scientific task. Priorities must reflect a compound assessment of scientific opportunity and social significance. Scientific hunches must be filtered through social aspirations. In the end, judgments about research in the multiplicity of fields relating to drug abuse must be based on a shared conception of the *goals* of the nation's investment in drug abuse research. In light of the diverse perspectives and values that shape this field of research, it seems appropriate to set forth the committee's own perspective on its task.

In the committee's view, scientific research pertaining to drug abuse is most usefully organized and evaluated within a public health framework. The ultimate aim of the nation's investment in drug abuse research is to enable society to take more effective measures to prevent abuse of and dependence on harmful drugs (e.g., alcohol, nicotine, cocaine, opi-

[1]Other sources of research support include the National Institute on Mental Health, the National Institute on Alcohol Abuse and Alcoholism, the Substance Abuse and Mental Health Services Administration (SAMHSA), and the Department of Justice. However, NIDA supports 85 percent of the world's research on drug abuse and addiction.

ates) and to reduce the harmful individual and social consequences associated with abuse and dependence. The menu of potentially useful societal interventions encompasses those available for any public health problem, including actions focused on the host (user), agent (drug), and environment (setting). This is not to say that the public health perspective is the only way to think about drug abuse, for as noted, drug abuse can be interpreted and understood from many perspectives. However, a public health framework is well suited to the task because it is comprehensive enough to incorporate many diverse fields of scientific inquiry and supple enough to embrace almost all policy positions that people hold about drug abuse control.

Another virtue of the public health paradigm is that it encompasses and integrates strategies of "demand reduction" and "supply reduction" that are too often used to bifurcate drug abuse prevention programs. At first glance, those categories seem to fit well within a public health paradigm: supply reduction strategies aim to reduce the availability of abusable drugs (the agent), whereas demand reduction strategies aim to reduce the "host's" drug-using behavior. From an empirical perspective, however, the usefulness of this dichotomy is limited. Most importantly, it fails to encompass strategies explicitly designed to ameliorate the *consequences* of abuse and dependence. Also, in practice, those terms are usually defined to put all "law enforcement" research in the supply reduction category and all "health" research in the demand reduction category. That misleading practice creates fiscal and conceptual impediments to a comprehensive research agenda because it signals a division of effort between the research-sponsoring agencies in the Departments of Justice and of Health and Human Services. For example, even though legal sanctions aimed at users are a key part of the societal effort to reduce demand for illicit drugs, the behavioral effects of legal sanctions are rarely included in a research agenda for "prevention" or demand reduction. Similarly, because efforts to suppress the availability of controlled substances are seen as supply reduction, the actual effects of those efforts on the prevalence and social consequences of drug abuse tend to be ignored, as do the effects of controlled substance regulation on legitimate medical practice.

A public health perspective provides criteria of relevance and a framework for assessing priorities. Drawing on that perspective, the committee decided to include within its vision any fields of inquiry that, if productive, could enable the nation to reduce the individual and social costs of drug abuse. More specifically, the "field" of drug abuse research encompasses research designed to enhance our understanding of (1) the nature and scope of drug abuse and dependence; (2) the causes and consequences of drug abuse and dependence; and (3) the efficacy and costs of interventions aimed at reducing drug abuse and dependence and ameliorating its adverse consequences.

The nation's drug abuse policy has been subject to persistent debate for 75 years. Awareness of the continuing controversy led the committee to think about the relationship between drug abuse research and drug abuse policy. History teaches that the drug abuse research agenda is inevitably shaped by prevailing assumptions and values, especially those embedded in existing public policies and laws (see Appendix B). At one level, this is altogether appropriate; after all, drug abuse research is primarily a public investment, and the social value of proposed research is properly influenced by public opinion and judged by politically accountable decisionmakers.

At the same time, open mindedness is a sine qua non of scientific progress. In all value-charged areas of scientific research, including drug abuse, scientists must always be prepared to ask whether important and potentially fruitful avenues of inquiry are being foreclosed because they are not "politically correct." In this spirit of critical reflection, the committee has asked whether and to what extent the goals of drug abuse research are circumscribed by existing social policies. Use of unprescribed opiates, cocaine, and other "controlled substances" is prohibited by law. In common parlance, the term "drug abuse" typically refers to any use of those drugs, whereas nicotine and alcohol are generally not regarded as drugs at all, much less drugs of abuse. However, the committee questioned whether the objectives of drug abuse research differ from the objectives of research concerning nicotine and alcohol. In the committee's view, the answer is no. Differences in the legal status of these substances do not require or entail separate research agendas; to the contrary, differences in legal controls present specific researchable issues within the framework of a common public health research agenda.

The ultimate goal of social policy for alcohol, nicotine, and controlled substances is to reduce the adverse health and social consequences associated with abuse of, or dependence on, these harmful drugs and thereby to reduce the staggering social costs associated with their use. The controversial *policy* question is whether and to what extent society should aim to discourage or suppress use as a means of reducing abuse and dependence. In the context of alcohol, prevailing policy aims to suppress consumption by minors but does not aim to discourage "responsible use" by adults. In the context of nicotine, national policy aims to suppress use by minors and is moving toward a policy of regulatory discouragement for adults. In the context of prohibited drugs, prevailing policy aims to suppress use by everyone as a means of preventing abuse. In all three contexts, however, the aim of scientific *research* is the same: to advance our knowledge regarding the causes and consequences of using these drugs; to determine the best methods (including prevention of both initiation and escalation of use) for minimizing adverse consequences; and to determine the benefits and costs of alternative strategies for reducing abuse and dependence.

During the course of its deliberations, the committee also discussed the issue of so-called root causes that repeatedly surfaces in contemporary public debate about crime, drug abuse, and other social problems. Some members believe that a major national commitment to improve the social and economic conditions of the disintegrating and impoverished communities of this country—to enhance educational opportunities, to create jobs, to protect children, and generally, to nurture hope where there is now despair—would substantially reduce drug abuse and other symptoms of social distress. Other committee members are not so sanguine about the preventive impact of such an investment, pointing out that the existing etiological research does not provide strong scientific support for the root cause hypothesis.

In the end, the debate about root cause turns as much on political philosophy as it does on empirical evidence, and definitive answers are unlikely to be produced by scientific investigation. However, reflection on this issue enriched the committee's understanding of the factors that should be taken into account in the design of a research agenda that is at once ambitious and realistic. No one thinks that drug abuse research can reasonably be expected to yield the "magic bullet"—a vaccine or a pharmacological cure—that would eliminate drug abuse and dependence in all individuals. Drug abuse is an endemic public health problem in modern societies, and it is a mistake, in the committee's opinion, for either policymakers or research scientists to promise more than they can achieve. At the same time, committee members are confident that a comprehensive research strategy, proceeding on all fronts of basic and applied research described in this report, can reasonably be expected to enable our nation to reduce drug abuse and dependence and to ameliorate its adverse social consequences.

In the final analysis, the value of the investment in drug abuse research is measured in lives saved and reclaimed, in the success of each young person who stays in school and joins the work force, and in the happiness of each child nurtured by his or her parents rather than abused or abandoned by them. On the surface, this report is about the pursuit of opportunities in science; however, its real meaning can be seen in the faces of people who suffer, and cause others to suffer, because they use drugs. They are the beneficiaries of drug abuse research and of the recommendations presented in this report.

Richard J. Bonnie, LL.B., *Chair*
Committee on Opportunities in Drug Abuse Research

Acknowledgments

The committee appreciates the expert support of the IOM project staff, division director, Division of Neuroscience and Behavioral Health, Constance Pechura, for her negotiating skills, practical comments, and guidance during the committee's deliberations. We thank study director, Carolyn Fulco, and program officer, Catharyn Liverman, for their contributions to the structure and substance of the report and in the editing of this document. We are indebted to Carrie Ingalls for her excellent research skills in collecting, analyzing, and presenting a range of information, in addition to verifying all committee references; and project assistant, Terri Scanlan for providing logistical assistance for the workshop and all committee meetings, overseeing report production; and preparing the camera-ready copy of the report.

The committee benefitted from the expertise of Deborah Beck, Laurie Chassin, Miriam Davis, Jeffrey Fagan, Linda Mayes, Kathleen Merikangas, Klaus Miczek, David Musto, and Jeffrey Swanson for their input into the committee's deliberations. The committee wishes to acknowledge the input of Douglas Anglin, Guardia Bannister, Thomas Crowley, Loretta Finnegan, Barry Glick, Elizabeth Griffin, Yifrah Kaminer, Herbert Kleber, Thomas Kosten, Nancy McLaughlin, Peter Reuter, and David Rosenbloom.

The committee appreciates the copy editing by Paul Phelps and Florence Poillon; the assistance of Claudia Carl in guiding the report through review; and Mike Edington's assistance in report production.

The IOM staff and the committee appreciate the thoughtful input and contributions of Timothy Condon, Jean Comolli, and the staff at NIDA. We are also indebted to the reviewers whose comments greatly improved the quality of this document. We also wish to thank the many representatives of federal agencies, congressional staff, academia, advocacy groups, and professional organizations who shared their expertise with the committee. Those individuals are acknowledged in Appendix A.

Contents

PATHWAYS OF ADDICTION

Executive Summary

Drug abuse research is an important public investment that has yielded substantial advances in scientific understanding about all facets of drug abuse and important discoveries in basic neurobiology, psychiatry, pain research, and other adjacent fields of inquiry. A sustained research effort will strengthen society's capacity to reduce drug abuse and ameliorate its adverse consequences. Drug abuse research, however, must compete for funding with research in other fields of public health, research in other scientific domains, and other pressing public needs. Recognizing the scarcity of resources, mechanisms are identified to effectively increase the yield per dollar invested in research. Those mechanisms include: stable funding; use of a comprehensive public health framework; wider acceptance of a medical model of drug dependence; better translation of research findings into practice; raising the status of drug abuse research; and facilitating interdisciplinary research.

The ultimate aim of the nation's investment in drug abuse research is to enable society to take effective measures to prevent drug use, abuse, and dependence, and thereby reduce adverse individual and social consequences and associated costs. Health consequences of drug abuse include increased rates of human immunodeficiency virus (HIV) transmission , increased spread of tuberculosis; adverse developmental consequences to children of drug-abusing parents; and increased violence. The extent of the impact of drug use, abuse, and dependence on society is evidenced by its enormous economic burden. When the cost of illicit drug use, abuse, and dependence is tallied with that of alcohol and nicotine, the collective costs of drug use and abuse (approximately $257 billion) exceeds the estimated annual $117 billion cost of heart disease and the estimated annual $104 billion cost of cancer (AHA, 1992; ACS, 1993; D. Rice, University of California at San Francisco, personal communication, 1995). The federal government investment in drug abuse research and development (in FY 1995) was $542.2 million, which represents 4 percent of the $13.3 billion spent by the federal government on drug abuse (ONDCP, 1996). By comparison, $8.5 billion (64 percent of the FY 1995 budget) was spent on criminal justice programs; $2.7 billion (20 percent) on treatment of drug abuse, and $1.6 billion (12 percent) on prevention efforts.

The widespread prevalence of illicit drug use in the United States presents another indication of the need for continued research. It was estimated that in 1994, 12.6 million people had used illicit drugs (primarily marijuana) in the past month (SAMHSA, 1995). The number of heavy drug users, using at least once a week, is difficult to determine. It has been estimated that in 1993 there were 2.1 million heavy cocaine users and 444,000 to 600,000 heavy heroin users (Rhodes et al., 1995).

In light of the magnitude of the drug abuse problem in the United States and the adverse health and social consequences, the National Institute on Drug Abuse (NIDA) requested that the Institute of Medicine (IOM) examine accomplishments in drug abuse research and provide guidance for future research. The IOM Committee on Opportunities in Drug Abuse Research (formed in January 1995) is convinced that the field is on the threshold of significant advances, and that a sustained research effort will strengthen society's capacity to reduce drug abuse and ameliorate its adverse consequences. The committee's report focuses broadly on opportunities and priorities for future scientific research in drug abuse.

VOCABULARY

In the committee's view, the term drug should be understood, in its generic sense, to encompass alcohol and nicotine as well as illicit drugs. It is very important for the general public to recognize that alcohol and nicotine constitute, by far, the nation's two largest drug problems, whether measured in terms of morbidity, mortality, or social cost. Continued separation of alcohol, nicotine, and illicit drugs in everyday speech is an impediment to public education, prevention, and therapeutic progress.

Although the committee uses the term drug in its generic sense, to encompass alcohol and nicotine, the report focuses, at NIDA's request, on research opportunities relating to illicit drugs; research on alcohol and nicotine is discussed only when the scientific inquiries are intertwined. Because the report sometimes ranges more broadly than illicit drugs, however, the committee has adopted several semantic conventions to promote clarity and avoid redundancy. First, the term drug, unmodified, refers to all psychoactive drugs, including alcohol and nicotine. When reference is intended to refer solely to illicit drugs such as heroin, cocaine, and other drugs regulated by the Controlled Substances Act, the committee says so explicitly. Occasionally, to ensure that the intended meaning is clear, the report refers to "illicit drugs and nicotine" or to "illicit drugs and alcohol," as the case may be.

The report employs the standard three-stage conceptualization of drug-taking behavior that applies to all psychoactive drugs, whether licit or illicit. Each stage—use, abuse, dependence—is marked by higher levels of use and increasingly serious consequences. Thus, when the report refers to the "use" of drugs, the term is usually employed in a narrow sense to distinguish it from intensified patterns of use. Conversely, the term "abuse" is used to refer to any harmful use, irrespective of whether the behavior constitutes a "disorder" in the DSM-IV diagnostic nomenclature. When the intent is to emphasize the clinical categories of abuse and dependence, that is made clear.

The committee also draws a clear distinction between patterns of drug-taking behavior, however described, and the harmful consequences of that behavior for the individual and for society. These consequences include the direct, acute effects of drug taking such as a drug-induced toxic psychosis or impaired driving, the effects of repeated drug taking on the user's health and social functioning, and the effects of drug-seeking behavior on the individual and society. It bears emphasizing that adverse consequences can be associated with patterns of drug use that do not amount to abuse or dependence in a clinical sense.

BEHAVIORAL RESEARCH

Behavioral research has contributed to our understanding of many of the factors involved in drug abuse, including initiation, maintenance, cessation, and relapse. The major contribution of behavioral research to the study of drug abuse has been the development of the drug self-administration model, which has been augmented by the development of additional complementary models. Behavioral models are useful for developing drug abuse pharmacotherapies; improving treatment engagement and compliance; developing novel procedures for both strengthening weak positive behaviors and attenuating strong drug-related behaviors; addressing questions related to mechanisms of craving and relapse; and promoting better understanding of drug use over the life span of drug users. Increased understanding of various drugs' mechanisms of action can also lead to better understanding of behavior and of vulnerability to drug abuse, which may not be elucidated with familial and drug use histories. The continued development of behavioral models is necessary to improve integration of data and variables being studied.

The committee recommends the use of behavioral models (involving both humans and nonhumans) to further our understanding of the various aspects of drug use, abuse, and dependence (such as initiation, relapse, prolonged abstinence, craving, and transitions from drug use to abuse); to develop improved behavioral and pharmacological interventions for the treatment of drug abuse and dependence; and to inform prevention efforts.

NEUROSCIENCE

Drug dependence has long been associated with some perturbation of the brain reward systems. At the system level, specific neural circuits have been identified that mediate the acute reinforcing effects of drugs. Cellular studies have identified specific changes in the function of different components of the midbrain-forebrain system and are beginning to provide a framework for understanding the adaptive changes within neurons that are associated with withdrawal and sensitization. Molecular studies not only have identified the specific neurotransmitter receptors and receptor subtypes important for mediating those acute reinforcing effects of drugs, but also have begun to provide a molecular basis for the long-term plasticity associated with relapse and vulnerability. Additionally, in the past decade, enormous technological advances in the field of functional brain imaging present the possibility of eliminating the gap between basic neurosciences and clinical research.

Significant progress has been made in understanding the neural substrates of drug dependence, and yet—due to the complexity of the brain and the difficulties inherent in studying the pathogenesis of any brain disease—there is still much more work to be done. Although physical withdrawal from drugs can now be managed with the aid of pharmacotherapies, currently available treatments for the behavioral aspects of dependence remain inadequate for most people. By utilizing increasingly sophisticated research techniques and methods, future neurobiological studies at all levels of inquiry—molecular, cellular, and system—will provide essential information for developing drug abuse treatment and prevention measures.

Advances in neuroscience have shown that pain and addiction research have more in common than a shared clinical pharmacology. Molecular, cellular, and behavioral analyses of animal models of pain and drug abuse provide complementary insights into the brain systems for reward and aversion.

The committee recommends continued support for fundamental investigations in neuroscience on the molecular, cellular, and systems levels. Research should be supported in the following areas: developing better animal models of the motivational aspects of drug dependence (with particular emphasis on protracted abstinence and propensity to relapse); genetics research; brain imaging; the neurobiology of co-occurring psychiatric disorders and drug abuse; animal models of the effects of HIV infection on the brain; the neurotoxicity of drug dependence; immunological approaches to drug abuse treatment; and pain and analgesia.

EPIDEMIOLOGY

Epidemiological research provides information essential for defining the scope of the drug abuse problem by identifying populations at risk. This research also provides insights into the etiology of drug initiation and use. A major accomplishment of epidemiological research has been the establishment of a variety of data systems that measure different aspects of drug use and abuse. Two major data systems provide broad-based statistics on trends in drug use in the general population: the National Household Survey on Drug Abuse, and the Monitoring the Future study. Although these two major systems provide reasonably accurate epidemiologic data on drug use among the general population, they are limited in assessing the extent of drug abuse or dependence.

The committee recommends continued epidemiological research to allow for the assessment of a broader range of issues. Those issues may include the extent of drug abuse and dependence; the nature and extent of drug use and abuse among youth; the nature and extent of co-occurring drug abuse and psychiatric disorders; and improvement in the reliability and validity of the methods for collecting and analyzing the data.

ETIOLOGY

Etiologic research has identified many factors that affect drug use, although no single variable or set of variables explains drug use by an individual. Further, there is no reason to believe that the same factor will affect all individuals in the same way, nor is there any reason to believe that the factors responsible for initiation of drug use are of equal importance in continuation or escalation of use. There appears to be no consensus as to what factors are involved in all cases of drug use and abuse. Generally, etiological studies conducted on population samples have focused on drug use; those conducted on clinical samples, especially those concerned with familial factors, have tended to focus on the etiology of drug abuse and dependence.

Two general categories of variables have been examined—risk factors and protective factors—although research, to date, has been focused primarily on risk factors associated with drug use rather than on abuse and dependence. There are biological, psychosocial, and contextual risk factors associated with drug use and abuse. Risk factors are related to the probability of an individual's developing a disease or to vulnerability which is a predisposition to a specific disease process. Protective factors are variables that are statistically associated with reduced likelihood of drug use. In statistical terms, a protective factor moderates the relationship between a risk factor and drug use and abuse, or it buffers the impact of risk factors on the individual. When the protective factor is present, it is assumed that there will be considerably less drug use and abuse than would otherwise be expected, given the risk factors that are also present.

The committee recommends multidisciplinary research to investigate the combined effects of biological, psychosocial, and contextual factors as they relate to the development of drug use, abuse, and dependence. The committee further recommends that studies be of long enough duration to enable follow-up of participants in determining the role of risk and protective factors related to the transition from use to abuse and dependence. Research areas should include the role of the following: family factors in the etiology of drug use and abuse; psychopathology as a precursor to drug use and abuse in adolescents and adults; risk and protective factors related to drug use and abuse, especially during discrete developmental stages; and childhood risk and protective factors that are associated with adult drug abuse and dependence.

PREVENTION

Drug abuse prevention research parallels recent trends in mental and physical health promotion and the emerging new discipline of prevention science. This enterprise requires the integration of epidemiological, etiological, and preventive intervention research. As applied to drug abuse, prevention science began in the mid- to late 1970s with attempts to prevent cigarette smoking among adolescents. The early focus was on changing the individual rather than the environment, and interventions usually occurred in schools.

Public health officials categorize preventive interventions based on when the intervention occurs: primary prevention involves intervening before the behavior appears; secondary prevention involves intervening after the onset of the behavior but before it becomes habitual; tertiary prevention involves intervening after the behavior has become habitual, with the goal of reducing or eliminating the behavior. Since 1990, a second model has been used increasingly to supplement these public health categories for preventive interventions: universal (delivered to the general population); selective (targeted at those presumed to be most "at risk"); and indicated (targeted at those who are exhibiting some clinically demonstrable abnormality, though perhaps not the "disease" itself).

Although there has been a debate about the relative value of universal and selective interventions, they do not have to be viewed as mutually exclusive. In fact, it is more fruitful to view them as mutually supportive rather than competing alternatives. For example, universal interventions can promote antidrug norms in the larger society, and selective interventions can then build on universal preventive messages. Moreover, preventive intervention messages designed specifically for high-risk youth can be delivered within the context of universal prevention programs, avoiding the risk of harmful labeling. Both universal and targeted interventions have promise for prevention science but require more careful examination.

The committee recommends rigorous evaluation of universal versus targeted prevention intervention programs with regard to effectiveness and cost-effectiveness, with particular focus on the initiation of use and on the transition from use to abuse and dependence. Emphasis should be placed on school-, family-, media-, and community-based interventions; interventions appropriate for high-risk populations; interventions aimed at ethnic subgroups; and multicomponent interventions especially at the community level.

CONSEQUENCES

The ramifications of drug abuse extend far beyond the individual drug abuser, because the health and social consequences of drug abuse—HIV/AIDS, violence, tuberculosis, fetal effects, crime, and disruptions in family, workplace, and educational environments—have devastating impacts on society and exact a cost of billions of dollars annually. The committee focused on three areas that involve pronounced social consequences and where the need for strategic preventive interventions are greatest: (1) the transmission and course of HIV infection; (2) fetal and child development; and (3) violent behavior.

HIV/AIDS

It now appears that injection drug use is the leading risk factor for new HIV infection in the United States (Holmberg, 1996). More than one-third (35 percent) of AIDS cases reported through December 1995 were related to injection of illicit drugs through three mechanisms: the sharing of contaminated injection equipment, heterosexual contact with an injection drug user (IDU), or through maternal injection of illicit drugs (CDC, 1995).

The committee recommends continued and expanded research efforts regarding noninjecting and injecting drug use and HIV transmission. Specifically, epidemiological studies of the prevalence and correlates of HIV infection in vulnerable populations of drug users and IDUs; and studies of effective risk reduction strategies for changing sexual risk behaviors and drug injection behaviors are needed.

Fetal and Child Development

Drug abuse can have a significant impact on the health of children who either are exposed to nicotine, alcohol, or illicit drugs, prenatally through maternal drug abuse or grow up in a drug-abusing household. Nicotine, alcohol, heroin, marijuana, and cocaine readily cross the placenta and the blood-brain barrier, creating a potentially increased risk of adverse biologic consequences to overall fetal development and specifically to fetal brain development. Further, the majority of women who use heroin, marijuana, or crack cocaine also use varying amounts of alcohol and/or nicotine and may use one or more illicit drugs in combination. Children without prenatal exposure may also suffer collateral health effects due to growing up in a drug-abusing household.

The committee recommends continued research on the magnitude and extent of the effects of maternal drug abuse on the prenatally exposed infant and child over time and the effects on children of growing up in a drug-abusing household.

Violence

Drugs may act as a cause, response, moderator, and/or mediator of violent behavior. Additionally, there is evidence of a complex linkage between violence, drug abuse, and co-occurring psychiatric disorders. Illicit drug and alcohol abuse are significantly more prevalent among persons who suffer from psychiatric disorders (e.g., schizophrenia, bipolar disorder, and depression) than among persons without psychiatric disorders and are particularly common among those with personality disorders. Those individuals with co-occurring disorders (who are also at risk for violent behavior) tend to manifest poor outcomes in standard treatment programs and often receive no treatment at all; thus, they pose a special challenge to the treatment and criminal justice systems.

The committee recommends research on violence, drug abuse, and co-occurring psychiatric disorders. Particular emphasis should be placed on the mechanisms underlying comorbidity and violent behavior and on developing effective prevention and treatment interventions.

TREATMENT

Treatment is clearly indicated for individuals diagnosed with drug dependence, the most serious of the three levels of drug consumption—use, abuse, and dependence. As a consequence of compulsive drug-seeking behavior and loss of control over consumption, drug dependence is usually a chronically relapsing disorder (i.e., one that may persist indefinitely and is prone to recur even after periods of remission).

Research has shown that drug abuse treatment is both effective and cost-effective in reducing not only drug consumption but also the associated health and social consequences. Structured treatment programs are generally classified according to four major treatment modalities—methadone maintenance, outpatient drug-free programs, therapeutic communities, and chemical dependency programs. Treatment gains are typically found in reduced intravenous and other drug use, reduced criminality, and enhanced health and productivity. Treatment research has greatly expanded the range of pharmacotherapeutic and psychosocial treatment approaches available, and most clinical settings utilize both treatment approaches.

The continued research challenge will be to develop more effective and cost-effective pharmacotherapeutic and psychosocial treatments that address the specific needs of individual patients and to refine the tools and techniques for clinical assessment and diagnostic differentiation.

The committee recommends that the appropriate federal and private agencies continue to support research to improve and evaluate the effectiveness of drug abuse treatment. This includes studies on optimal strategies for matching patients to the most appropriate treatment modalities; development of medications for the treatment of drug abuse and dependence; the efficacy of pharmacotherapies and psychosocial therapies to treat individuals with co-occurring

psychiatric disorders and drug abuse; the natural history of HIV infection among drug users and effective models of health care delivery for HIV-infected drug abusers; and the efficacy of treatment programs designed toward addressing the needs of special populations (i.e., women, adolescents, and prisoners).

MANAGED CARE

Managed care has become an important trend in drug abuse treatment. In response to the escalating costs of treatment, managed drug abuse care proposes to contain costs, increase access, and ensure quality. It entails many changes from traditional fee-for-service coverage, including changes in the organization, financing, and delivery of services—most recognizably through case management which seeks to match patients to the most appropriate, yet least restrictive, treatment setting.

Despite its enormous growth, there is a dearth of peer-reviewed research about whether managed drug abuse care is achieving those goals. The only definitive conclusion to be reached on the pivotal claims of managed care—that it enhances access, lowers cost, and ensures quality—is that there are insufficient data. The modest body of research does point to lower costs and less reliance on inpatient care. However, treatment outcomes are still unknown due to the current lack of research on the effectiveness and cost-effectiveness of managed care treatment. Additionally, there is no research on what could potentially be inadequacies in managed drug abuse care: denial of treatment; undertreatment; and cost-shifting to other providers, public health and welfare agencies, and the criminal justice system.

The committee recommends that the appropriate federal agencies (e.g., the Substance Abuse and Mental Health Services Administration [SAMHSA], the Health Care Financing Administration [HCFA], the National Institute on Drug Abuse [NIDA], and the National Institute on Alcohol Abuse and Alcoholism [NIAAA]) and private organizations undertake studies of the organization, financing, and characteristics of drug abuse treatment in the managed care setting, including variations in the content, intensity, continuum of care, and duration of treatment as they relate to patient needs.

DRUG CONTROL

The effects of drug control are usually not included within the ambit of "drug abuse research" and are assumed to lie instead within the purview of criminal justice research. In the committee's view, however, the effects of legal controls, and of different strategies for implementing and enforcing them, should be seen as an important component of a comprehensive drug abuse research strategy. Conceived broadly, policy-relevant effects encompass all the benefits of legal controls (in reducing use, abuse, and dependence on illicit drugs and the associated adverse consequences) and the costs, or side-effects, of those controls (ranging from violence associated with the illicit drug trade to the costs of imprisonment). On many of these questions, there is no dearth of opinion but little in the way of systematic, rigorous research.

An integrated perspective that encompasses interventions aimed at both supply and demand can yield important advances by overcoming disciplinary and bureaucratic boundaries. Four specific opportunities for research on the public health effects of drug control are identified in the report: (1) the effects of controlled substance regulation on legitimate medical use and scientific research; (2) the effects of supply reduction on drug consumption; (3) the effects of criminal sanctions (including coerced treatment) on drug use; and (4) the effects of confidentiality on participation in treatment.

The committee encourages NIDA, the National Institute of Justice (NIJ), and other public and private sponsors of drug abuse research to incorporate policy-relevant studies of drug control within a comprehensive scientific agenda.

This report sets forth drug abuse research initiatives for the next decade based on an assessment of what is now known and a calculated judgment about what initiatives are most likely to advance our knowledge in useful ways. This report is not meant to be a road map or tactical battle plan, but is best regarded as a strategic outline. Prudent research planning must respond to newly emerging opportunities and needs while maintaining a steady commitment to the achievement of long-term objectives.

REFERENCES

ACS (American Cancer Society). 1993. *Cancer Facts and Figures, 1993*. Washington, DC: American Cancer Society.

AHA (American Heart Association). 1992. *1993 Heart and Stroke Fact Statistics*. Dallas, TX: American Heart Association.

CDC (Centers for Disease Control and Prevention). 1995. *HIV/AIDS Surveillance Report* 7(2).

Holmberg SD. 1996. The estimated prevalence and incidence of HIV in 96 large U.S. metropolitan areas. *American Journal of Public Health* 86(5):642–654.

ONDCP (Office of National Drug Control Policy). 1996. *National Drug Control Strategy*. Washington, DC: ONDCP.

Rhodes W, Scheiman P, Pittayathikhun T, Collins L, Tsarfaty V. 1995. *What America's Users Spend on Illegal Drugs, 1988–1993*. Prepared for the Office of National Drug Control Policy, Washington, DC.

SAMHSA (Substance Abuse and Mental Health Services Administration). 1995. *National Household Survey on Drug Abuse: Population Estimates 1994*. Washington, DC: U.S. Department of Health and Human Services.

1

Introduction

Drug abuse research became a subject of sustained scientific interest by a small number of investigators in the late nineteenth and early twentieth centuries. Despite their creative efforts to understand drug abuse in terms of general advances in biomedical science, the medical literature of the early twentieth century is littered with now-discarded theories of drug dependence, such as autointoxication and antibody toxins, and with failed approaches to treatment. Eventually, escalating social concern about the use of addictive drugs and the emergence of the biobehavioral sciences during the post-World War II era led to a substantial investment in drug abuse research by the federal government (see Appendix B). That investment has yielded substantial advances in scientific understanding about all facets of drug abuse and has also resulted in important discoveries in basic neurobiology, psychiatry, pain research, and other related fields of inquiry. In light of how little was understood about drug abuse such a short time ago, the advances of the past 25 years represent a remarkable scientific accomplishment. Yet there remains a disconnect between what is now known scientifically about drug abuse and addiction, the public's understanding of and beliefs about abuse and addiction, and the extent to which what is known is actually applied in public health settings.

During its brief history, drug abuse research has been supported mainly by the federal government, with occasional investments by major private foundations. At the federal level, the lead agency for drug abuse research is the National Institute on Drug Abuse (NIDA), which supports

85 percent of the world's research on drug abuse and addiction. Other sponsoring agencies include the National Institute of Mental Health (NIMH), the National Institute on Alcohol Abuse and Alcoholism (NIAAA), and the Substance Abuse and Mental Health Services Administration (SAMHSA), all in the Department of Health and Human Services; as well as the Office of Justice Programs (OJP) in the Department of Justice. Throughout the federal government, the FY 1995 investment in drug abuse research and development was $542.2 million, which represents 4 percent of the $13.3 billion spent by the federal government on drug abuse (ONDCP, 1996). By comparison, $8.5 billion (64 percent of the FY 1995 budget) was spent on criminal justice programs,[1] $2.7 billion (20 percent) on treatment of drug abuse, and $1.6 billion (12 percent) on prevention efforts.

In 1992, the General Accounting Office (GAO) released a report *Drug Abuse Research: Federal Funding and Future Needs*, which recommended that Congress review the place of research in drug control policy and its modest 4 percent share of the drug control budget. The report questioned whether the federal commitment to research was adequate, given the enormity of research needs (GAO, 1992), and whether adequate evaluation research was being conducted to determine the efficacy of various drug control programs. In FY 1995, drug abuse research was still little more than 4 percent of the entire drug control budget.

In January 1995, NIDA requested the Institute of Medicine (IOM) to examine accomplishments in drug abuse research and provide guidance for future research opportunities. This report by the IOM Committee on Opportunities in Drug Abuse Research focuses broadly on opportunities and priorities for future scientific research in drug abuse. After a brief review of major accomplishments in drug abuse research, the remainder of this chapter discusses the vocabulary and basic concepts used in the report, highlights the importance of the nation's investment in drug abuse research, and explores some of the factors that could improve the yield from that investment.

MAJOR ACHIEVEMENTS IN DRUG ABUSE RESEARCH

There have been remarkable achievements in drug abuse research over the past quarter of a century as researchers have learned more about the biological and psychosocial aspects of drug use, abuse, and dependence. Behavioral researchers have developed animal and human mod-

[1] Criminal justice programs include interdiction, investigation, international efforts, prosecution, correction efforts, and intelligence programs.

els of drug-seeking behavior, that have, for example, yielded objective measures of initiation and repeated administration of drugs, thereby providing the scientific foundation for assessments of "abuse liability" (i.e., the potential for abuse) of specific drugs (see Chapter 2). This information is an essential predicate for informed regulatory decisions under the Food, Drug and Cosmetic Act and the Controlled Substances Act. Taking advantage of technological advances in molecular biology, neuroscientists have identified receptors or receptor types in the brain for opioids, cocaine, benzodiazepines, and marijuana and have described the ways in which the brain adapts to, and changes after, exposure to drugs. Those alterations, which may persist long after the termination of drug use, appear to involve changes in gene expression. They may explain enhanced susceptibility to future drug exposure, thereby shedding light on the enigmas of withdrawal and relapse at the molecular level (see Chapter 3). Epidemiologists have designed and implemented epidemiological surveillance systems that enable policymakers to monitor patterns of drug use in the population (Chapter 4) and that enable researchers to investigate the causes and consequences of drug use and abuse (Chapters 5 and 7, respectively). Paralleling broader trends in health promotion and disease prevention in the past 20 years, the field of drug abuse prevention has made significant progress in evaluating the effectiveness of interventions implemented in a range of settings including communities, schools, and families (see Chapter 6).

Marked gains have also been made in treatment research, including improvements in diagnostic criteria; development of a wide range of treatment interventions and sophisticated methods to assess treatment outcome; and development and approval of *levo*-alpha-acetylmethadol (LAAM), a medication for the treatment of opioid dependence. Pharmacological and psychosocial treatments, alone or in combination, have been shown to be effective for drug dependencies, and treatment has been shown to reduce drug use, HIV (human immunodeficiency virus) infection rates, health care costs, and criminal activity (see Chapter 8).

Drug abuse researchers have also made major contributions to knowledge in adjacent fields of scientific inquiry. For example, NIDA-sponsored research was the driving force in the identification of morphine-like substances that serve as neurotransmitters in specific neurons located throughout the central and peripheral nervous systems (Olson et al., 1994). Identification of these substances represents a dramatic breakthrough in understanding the mechanisms of pain, reinforcement, and stress. Additionally, the discovery of opioid peptides as neurotransmitters played a key role in the identification of numerous other peptide neurotransmitters (Cooper et al., 1991; Goldstein, 1994; Hokfelt et al., 1995). These discoveries have broadened the understanding of brain function and now form the basis of many current strategies in the design of new drug treatments for neuropsychiatric disorders. Additionally, drug abuse research has contributed to the development of brain imaging techniques.

Drug abuse research has also provided a major impetus for neuropharmacological research in psychiatry since the late 1950s, when it was discovered that LSD (lysergic acid diethylamide; a hallucinogen that produces psychotic symptoms) affected the brain's serotonin systems (Cooper et al., 1991). That seminal discovery stimulated decades of research in the neuropharmacological basis of behavior and psychiatric disorders. The impact on antipsychotic research has been dramatic. In addition, stimulants (e.g., cocaine and amphetamine) were found to produce a state of paranoid psychosis, resembling schizophrenia, in some people. The actions of stimulants on the brain's dopamine pathways continue to inform researchers of the potential role of those pathways in the treatment, and perhaps the pathophysiology, of schizophrenia (Kahn and Davis, 1995). Drug abuse research also has had an impact on antidepressant research (e.g., the actions of drugs of abuse on the brain's serotonin systems have provided useful models with which to investigate the role of those systems in depression and mania). Depression is a risk factor for treatment failure in smoking cessation (Glassman et al., 1993) and depression-like symptoms are dominant during cocaine withdrawal (DiGregorio, 1990). Consequently, treatment of depression in nicotine- and cocaine-dependent individuals has been an area of interest for drug abuse research.

Some drugs that are abused, most notably the opioid analgesics, have essential medical uses. Since its founding, NIDA has been the major supporter of research into brain mechanisms of pain and analgesia, analgesic tolerance, and analgesic pharmacology. The resulting discoveries have led to an understanding of which brain circuits are required to generate pain and pain relief (Wall and Melzack, 1994), have revolutionized the treatment of postoperative and cancer pain (Foley and Inturrisi, 1986; Carr et al., 1992; Jacox et al., 1994), and have led to improved treatments for many other conditions that result in chronic pain (see Chapter 3).

VOCABULARY OF DRUG ABUSE

Ordinarily, scientific vocabulary evolves toward greater clarity and precision in response to new empirical discoveries and reconceptualizations. That creative process is evident within each of the disciplines of drug abuse research covered in various chapters of this report. Interestingly, however, the words describing the field as a whole, and connecting each chapter to the next, seem to defy the search for clarity and precision. Does "drug" include alcohol and tobacco? What is "abuse"? Are use and abuse mutually exclusive categories? Are abuse and dependence mutually exclusive categories? Does use of illicit drugs per se amount to abuse? Does abuse include underage use of nicotine? Is addiction synonymous with dependence?

These ambiguities have persisted for decades because the vocabulary of drug abuse is inevitably influenced by peoples' attitudes and values. If the task were solely a scientific one, precise terminology would have emerged long before now. However, because the choice of words in this field always carries a nonscientific message, scientists themselves cannot always agree on a common vocabulary.

Consider the case of nicotine; from a pharmacological standpoint, nicotine is functionally similar to other psychoactive drugs. However, many researchers and policymakers choose to exclude nicotine from the category of drug. The same is true of alcohol; for example, other terms, such as "chemical dependency" or "substance abuse," are often used as generic terms encompassing the abuse of nicotine and alcohol as well as abuse of illicit drugs. This semantic strategy is chosen to signify the difference in legal status among alcohol, nicotine, and illicit drugs. In recent years, however, a growing number of researchers have adopted a more inclusive use of the term drug. In the case of nicotine, this move tends to reflect a policy judgment that nicotine should be classified as a drug under the federal Food, Drug and Cosmetic Act.

In the committee's view, the term drug should be understood, in its generic sense, to encompass alcohol and nicotine as well as illicit drugs. It is very important for the general public to recognize that alcohol and nicotine constitute, by far, the nation's two largest drug problems, whether measured in terms of morbidity, mortality, or social cost. Abuse of and dependence on those drugs have serious individual and societal consequences. Continued separation of alcohol, nicotine, and illicit drugs in everyday speech is an impediment to public education, prevention, and therapeutic progress.

Although the committee uses the term drug, in its generic sense, to encompass alcohol and nicotine, the report focuses, at NIDA's request, on research opportunities relating to illicit drugs; research on alcohol and nicotine is discussed only when the scientific inquiries are intertwined. Because the report sometimes ranges more broadly than illicit drugs, however, the committee has adopted several semantic conventions to promote clarity and avoid redundancy. First, the term drug, unmodified, refers to all psychoactive drugs, including alcohol and nicotine. When reference is intended solely to illicit drugs such as heroin, cocaine, and other drugs regulated by the Controlled Substances Act, the committee says so explicitly. Occasionally, to ensure that the intended meaning is clear, the report refers to "illicit drugs and nicotine" or to "illicit drugs and alcohol," as the case may be. Additionally, the words opiate and opioid are used interchangeably, although opiates are derivative of morphine and opioids are all compounds with morphine-like properties (they may be synthetic and not resemble morphine chemically).

The report employs the standard three-stage conceptualization of drug-taking behavior that applies to all psychoactive drugs, whether licit or illicit. Each stage—use, abuse, dependence—is marked by higher levels of use and increasingly serious consequences. Thus, when the report refers to the "use" of drugs, the term is usually employed in a narrow sense to distinguish it from intensified patterns of use. Conversely, the term "abuse" is used to refer to any harmful use, irrespective of whether the behavior constitutes a "disorder" in the DSM-IV diagnostic nomenclature (see Appendix C). When the intent is to emphasize the clinical categories of abuse and dependence, that is made clear.

The committee also draws a clear distinction between patterns of drug-taking behavior, however described, and the harmful consequences of that behavior for the individual and for society. These consequences include the direct, acute effects of drug taking such as a drug-induced toxic psychosis or impaired driving, the effects of repeated drug taking on the user's health and social functioning, and the effects of drug-seeking behavior on the individual and society. It bears emphasizing that adverse consequences can be associated with patterns of drug use that do not amount to abuse or dependence in a clinical sense, although the focus of this report and the committee's recommendations is on the more intensified patterns of use (i.e., abuse and dependence) since they cause the majority of the serious consequences.

DEFINITIONS AND BASIC CONCEPTS

Drug use may be defined as occasional use strongly influenced by environmental factors. Drug use is not a medical disorder and is not listed as such in either of the two most important diagnostic manuals—the *Diagnostic and Statistical Manual of Mental Disorders*, Fourth Edition (DSM-IV; APA, 1994); or the International Classification of Diseases (ICD-10; WHO, 1992). (See Appendix C for DSM-IV and ICD-10 diagnostic criteria.) Drug use implies intake for nonmedical purposes; it may or may not be accompanied by clinically significant impairment or distress on a given occasion.

Drug abuse is characterized in DSM-IV as including regular, sporadic, or intensive use of higher doses of drugs leading to social, legal, or interpersonal problems. Like DSM-IV, ICD-10 identifies a nondependent but problematic syndrome of drug use but calls it "harmful use" instead of abuse. This syndrome is defined by ICD-10 as use resulting in actual physical or psychological harm.

Drug dependence (or addiction) is characterized in both DSM-IV and ICD-10 as drug-seeking behavior involving compulsive use of high doses of one or more drugs, either licit or illicit, for no clear medical indication, resulting in substantial impairment of health and social functioning. Dependence is usually accompanied by tolerance and withdrawal[2] and (like abuse) is generally associated with a wide range of social, legal, psychiatric, and medical problems. Unlike patients with chronic pain or persistent anxiety, who take medication over long periods of time to obtain relief from a specific medical or psychiatric disorder (often with resulting tolerance and withdrawal), persons with dependence seek out the drug and take it compulsively for nonmedical effects.

Tolerance occurs when certain medications are taken repeatedly. With opiates for example, it can be detected after only a few days of use for medical purposes such as the treatment of pain. If the patient suddenly stops taking the drug, a withdrawal syndrome may ensue. Physicians often confuse this phenomenon, referred to as physical dependence, with true addiction. That can lead to withholding adequate medication for the treatment of pain because of the very small risk that addiction with drug-seeking behavior may occur.

As a consequence of its compulsive nature involving the loss of control over drug use, dependence (or addiction) is typically a chronically relapsing disorder (IOM, 1990, 1995; Meyer, 1996; O'Brien and McLellan, 1996; McLellan et al., in press). Although individuals with drug dependence can often complete detoxification and achieve temporary abstinence, they find it very difficult to sustain that condition and avoid relapse over time. Most persons who achieve sustained remission do so only after a number of cycles of detoxification and relapse (Daley and Marlatt, 1992). Relapse is caused by a constellation of biological, family, social, psychological, and treatment factors and is demonstrated by the fact that at least half of former cigarette smokers quit three or more times before they successfully achieve stable remission from nicotine addiction (Schelling, 1992). Similarly, within one year of treatment, relapse occurs in 30–50 percent of those treated for drug dependence, although the level

[2]Tolerance refers to the situation in which repeated administration of a drug at the same dose elicits a diminishing effect or involves the need for an increasing dose to produce the same effect. Withdrawal syndrome is characterized by physical or motivational disturbances when the drug is withdrawn. It is important to emphasize that the phenomena of tolerance, dependence, and withdrawal are not associated uniquely with drugs of abuse, since many medications used clinically that are not addicting (e.g., clonidine, propranolol, tricyclic antidepressants) can produce these types of effects.

of drug use may not be as high as before treatment (Daley and Marlatt, 1992; McLellan et al., in press). Unlike those who use (or even abuse) drugs, individuals with addiction have a substantially diminished ability to control drug consumption, a factor that contributes to their tendency to relapse.

Another terminological issue arises in relation to the terms addiction and dependence. For some scientists, the proper terms for compulsive drug seeking is addiction, rather than dependence. In their view, addiction more clearly signifies the essential behavioral differences between compulsive use of drugs for their nonmedical effects and the syndrome of "physical dependence" that can develop in connection with repeated medical use. In response, many scientists argue that dependence has been defined in both ICD-10 and DSM-IV to encompass the behavioral features of the disorder and has become the generally accepted term in the diagnostic nomenclature. Moreover, some scientists object to the term addiction on the grounds that it is associated with stigmatizing social images and that a less pejorative term would help to promote public understanding of the medical nature of the condition. The committee has not attempted to resolve this controversy. For purposes of this report, the terms addiction and dependence are used interchangeably.

An inherent aspect of drug addiction is the propensity to relapse. Relapse should not be viewed as treatment failure; addiction itself should be considered a brain disease similar to other chronic and relapsing conditions such as hypertension, diabetes, and asthma (IOM, 1995; O'Brien and McLellan, 1996). In the latter, significant improvement is considered successful treatment even though complete remission or cure is not achieved. In the area of drug abuse, however, many individuals (both lay and professional) expect treatment programs to perform like vaccine programs, where one episode of treatment offers lifetime immunity. Not surprisingly, because of that expectation, people are inevitably disappointed in the relatively high relapse rates associated with most treatments. If, however, addiction is understood as a chronically relapsing brain disease, then—for any one treatment episode—evidence of treatment efficacy would include reduced consumption, longer abstention periods, reduced psychiatric symptoms, improved health, continued employment, and improved family relations. Most of those results are demonstrated regularly in treatment outcome studies.

The idea that drug addiction is a chronic relapsing condition, requiring long-term attention, has been resisted in the United States and in some other countries (Brewley, 1995). Many lay people view drug addiction as a character defect requiring punishment or incarceration. Proponents of the medical model, however, point to the fact that addiction is a distinct morbid process that has characteristics and identifiable signs and symptoms that affect organ systems (Miller, 1991; Meyer, 1996). Characterization of addiction as a brain disease is bolstered by evidence of genetic vulnerability to addiction, physical correlates of its clinical course, physiological changes as a result of repeated drug use, and fundamental changes in brain chemistry as evidenced by brain imaging (Volkow et al., 1993). This is not to say that behavioral, social, and environmental factors are immaterial—they all play a role in onset and outcome, just as they do in heart disease, kidney disease, tuberculosis, or other infectious diseases. Thus, the contemporary understanding of disease fully incorporates the voluntary behavioral elements that lead many people to be skeptical about the applicability of the medical model to drug addiction. In any case, the committee embraces the disease concept, not because it is indisputable but because this paradigm facilitates scientific investigation in many important areas of knowledge, without inhibiting or distorting scientific inquiry in other parts of the field.

IMPORTANCE OF DRUG ABUSE RESEARCH

The widespread prevalence of illicit drug use in the United States is well documented in surveys of households, students, and prison and jail inmates (Chapter 4). Based on the National Household Survey on Drug Abuse (NHSDA), an annual survey presently sponsored by SAMHSA, it was estimated that in 1994, 12.6 million people had used illicit drugs (primarily marijuana) in the past month (SAMHSA, 1995). That figure represents 6 percent of the population 12 years of age or older.[3] The number of heavy drug users, using drugs at least once a week, is difficult to determine. It has been estimated that in 1993 there were 2.1 million heavy cocaine users and 444,000–600,000 heavy heroin users (Rhodes et al., 1995). This population represents a significant burden to society, not only in terms of federal expenditures but also in terms of costs related to the multiple consequences of drug abuse (see Chapter 7).

The ultimate aim of the nation's investment in drug abuse research is to enable society to take effective measures to prevent drug use, abuse, and dependence, and thereby reduce its adverse individual and social consequences and associated costs. The adverse consequences of drug abuse are numerous and profound and affect the individual's physical health and psychological and social functioning. Consequences of drug abuse include increased rates of HIV infection and tuberculosis (TB); education and vocational impairment; developmental harms to children of

[3]It is important to note that the total number of users results from the rates of use in different age groups in the population and from the demographic structure of the population. The actual number of users may increase while the rates of use are declining.

drug-using parents associated with fetal exposure or maltreatment and neglect; and increased violence (see Chapter 7). It now appears that injection drug use is the leading risk factor for new HIV infection in the United States (Holmberg, 1996). Most (80 percent) HIV-infected heterosexual men and women who do not use injection drugs have been infected through sexual contact with HIV-infected injection drug users (IDUs). Thus, it is not surprising that the geographic distribution of heterosexual AIDS cases has been essentially the same as the distribution of male injection drug users' AIDS cases (Holmberg, 1996) Further, the IDUs-associated HIV epidemic in men is reflected in the heterosexual epidemic in women, which is reflected in HIV infection in children (CDC, 1995). Nearly all children who acquire HIV infection do so perinatally (see Chapter 7).

The extent of the impact of drug use and abuse on society is evidenced by its enormous economic burden. In 1990, illicit drug abuse is estimated to have cost the United States more than $66 billion. When the cost of illicit drug use and abuse is tallied with that of alcohol and nicotine (Table 1.1), the collective cost of drug use and abuse exceeds the estimated annual $117 billion cost of heart disease and the estimated annual $104 billion cost of cancer (AHA, 1992; ACS, 1993; D. Rice, University of California at San Francisco, personal communication, 1995).

As noted above, the federal government accounts for a large segment of the societal expenditure on illicit drug abuse control—spending more than $13.3 billion in FY 1995 (ONDCP, 1996). About two-thirds was devoted to interdiction, intelligence, incarceration, and other law enforcement activities. Research, however, accounts for only 4 percent of federal outlays, a percentage that has remained virtually unchanged since 1981 (ONDCP, 1996) (Figure 1.1). Given the social costs of illicit drug abuse and the enormity of the federal investment in prevention and control, research into the causes, consequences, treatment, and prevention of drug abuse should have a higher priority. Enhanced support for drug abuse research would be a socially sound investment, because scientific research can be expected to generate new and improved treatments, as well as prevention and control strategies that can help reduce the enormous social burden associated with drug abuse.

THE CONTEXT OF DRUG ABUSE RESEARCH

In the chapters that follow, the committee identifies research initiatives that seem most promising and most likely to lead to successful efforts to reduce drug abuse and its associated social costs. Although the yield from these initiatives will depend largely on the creativity and skill of scientists, the many contextual factors that will also have a major bear-

TABLE 1.1 Estimated Economic Costs (million dollars) of Drug Abuse, 1990

Type of Cost	Illicit Drugs	Alcohol	Nicotine
Total	$66,873	$98,623	$91,269
Core Costs	14,602	80,763	91,269
Direct	3,197	10,512	39,130
Mental health/specialty organizations	867	3,469	—
Short-stay hospitals	1,889	4,589	21,072
Office-based physicians	88	240	12,251
Other professional services	32	329	—[a]
Prescription drugs	—	—	1,469
Nursing homes	—	1,095	3,858
Home health services	—	—	480
Support costs	321	790	—
Indirect	11,405	70,251	52,139
Morbidity[b]	7,997	36,627	6,603
Mortality[c]	3,408	33,624	45,536
Other Related Costs	45,989	15,771	—
Direct	18,043	10,436	—
Crime	18,035	5,807	—
Motor vehicle crashes	—	3,876	—
Fire destruction	—	633	—
Social welfare administration	8	120	—
Indirect	27,946	5,335	—
Victims of crime	1,042	576	—
Incarceration	7,813	4,75	—
Crime careers	19,091	—	—
AIDS	6,282	—	—
Fetal Alcohol Syndrome		2,089	—

NOTE: 1990 costs for illicit drugs and alcohol abuse are based on socioeconomic indexes applied to 1985 estimates (Rice et al., 1990; cigarette direct smoking costs are deflated from 1993 direct cost estimates (MMWR, 1994); cigarette indirect costs are from Rice et al., 1992.

[a]Amounts spent for other professional services are included in office-based physicians' costs.

[b]Value of goods and services lost by individuals unable to perform their usual activities because of drug abuse or unable to perform them at a level of full effectiveness (Rice et al., 1990).

[c]Present value of future earnings lost, illicit drugs and alcohol discounted at 6 percent, nicotine discounted at 4 percent.

SOURCE: D. Rice, University of California at San Francisco, personal communication (1995).

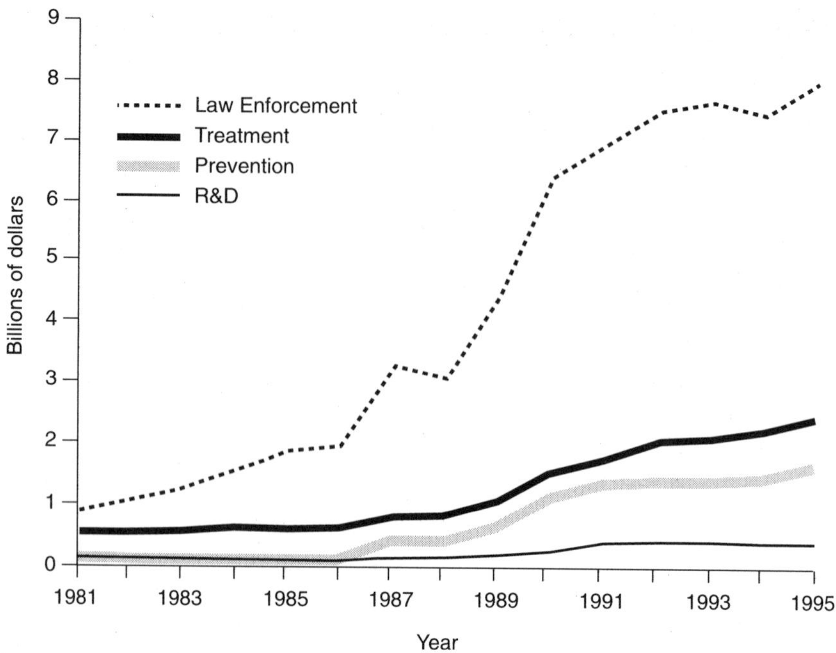

FIGURE 1.1 Federal drug control budget trends (1981–1995). NOTE: Figures are in current dollars. SOURCE: ONDCP (1996).

ing on the payoff from scientific inquiry cannot be ignored. The committee has identified six major factors that, if successfully addressed, could optimize the gains made in each area of drug abuse research: stable funding; use of a comprehensive public health framework; wider acceptance of a medical model of drug dependence; better translation of research findings into practice; raising the status of drug abuse research; and facilitating interdisciplinary research.

Stable Funding

A stable level of funding in any area of biomedical research is needed to sustain and build on research accomplishments, to retain a cadre of experts in a field, and to attract young investigators. Drug abuse research, in comparison with many other research venues, has not enjoyed consistent federal support (IOM, 1990, 1995; see also Appendix B). The field has suffered from difficulties in recruiting and retaining young researchers and clinicians and in maintaining a stable research infrastructure (IOM, 1995). Society's capacity to contain and manage drug abuse depends upon a stable, long-term investment in research. The vicissitudes in federal research funding often reflect changing currents in public opinion toward drugs and drug users (Appendix B). However, drug abuse will not disappear; it is an endemic social and public health problem. The nation must commit itself to a sustained effort. The social investment in research is an investment in "human capital" that must be sustained over the long term in order to reap the expected gains. An investment in this field is squandered if researchers who have been recruited and trained in drug abuse research are drawn to other fields because of uncertainty about the stability of future funding.

Adoption of a Comprehensive Public Health Framework

The social impact of drug abuse research can be enhanced significantly by conceptualizing goals and priorities within a comprehensive public health framework (Goldstein, 1994). All too often, public discourse about drug abuse is characterized by such unnecessary and fruitless disputes as whether drug abuse should be viewed as a social and moral problem or a health problem, whether the drug problem can best be solved by law enforcement or by medicine, whether priority should be placed on reducing supply or reducing demand, and so on. The truth is that these dichotomies oversimplify a brain disease impacted by a complex set of behaviors and a diverse array of potentially useful social responses. Forced choices of this nature also tend to inhibit or foreclose potentially useful research strategies. Confusion about social goals can lead to confusion about research priorities and can obscure the links between investigations viewing the subject through different lenses.

Some issues tend to recur. A prominent dispute centers on whether preventing drug use is important in itself or whether society should be more concerned with abuse or with the harmful consequences of use. The answer, of course, is that such a forced choice obscures, rather than clarifies, the issues. From a public health standpoint, drug use is a risk factor; the significance of use (whether of alcohol, nicotine, or illicit drugs) lies in the risk of harm associated with it (e.g., fires from smoking, impaired driving from alcohol or illicit drugs, or developmental setbacks) and in the risk that use will intensify, escalating to abuse or dependence. Those risks vary widely in relation to drug, user characteristics, social context, etc. Attention to the consequences of use and to the risk of escalation helps to set priorities (for research and policy) and provides a framework for assessing the impact of different interventions.

From a public policy standpoint, arguments about goals and priorities are fraught with controversy. From the standpoint of research strategy, however, the key lies in asking the right questions (e.g., What influences the pathways from use, to abuse, to dependence? What are the effects of needle exchange programs on illicit drug use and on HIV disease?) and in generating the knowledge required to facilitate informed policy debate. The main virtues of a comprehensive public health approach are that it helps to disentangle scientific questions from policy questions and that it encompasses all of the pertinent empirical questions, including the causes and consequences of use, abuse, and dependence, as well as the efficacy and cost of all types of interventions. In sum, the social payoff from drug abuse research can be enhanced substantially by integrating diverse strands of inquiry within a public health framework.

Acceptance of a Medical Model of Drug Dependence

Drug dependence is a chronic, relapsing brain disease that, like other diseases, can be evaluated and treated with the standard tools of medicine, including efforts in prevention, diagnosis, and treatment with medications and behavioral or psychosocial therapies. Unfortunately, the medical model of dependence is not universally accepted by health professionals and others in the treatment community; it is widely rejected within the law enforcement community and often by the public at large, which tends to view the complex and varied patterns of use, abuse, and dependence as an undifferentiated behavior rather than a medical problem.

Resistance to the medical model takes many forms. One is resistance to pharmacotherapies, such as methadone, that are seen as substituting licit drugs for illicit drugs without changing drug-taking behavior. Conversely, treatment approaches that adopt a rigid drug-free strategy preclude the use of medications for patients with other psychiatric disorders that are easily treated by pharmacotherapeutic approaches. On a subtler level, resistance to the use of pharmacotherapies is evidenced by the routine use of inadequate doses of methadone (D'Aunno and Vaughn, 1992). Finally, for others, all forms of drug abuse signify a failure of willpower or a moral weakness requiring punishment, incarceration, or moral education rather than treatment (Anglin and Hser, 1992).

Resistance to the medical model of drug dependence presents numerous barriers to research. Clinical researchers experience difficulty in soliciting participation by both treatment program administrators and patients, who are sometimes mistrustful of researchers' motives. If research involves a medication that is itself prone to abuse, there are additional regulatory requirements for drug scheduling, storage, and record keeping that act to discourage investigation (see Chapter 10; IOM, 1995). The ever-present threat of inappropriate intrusion by law enforcement agents has a chilling effect on treatment research (McDuff et al., 1993). All barriers to inquiry, irrespective of whether they are legal or social in origin, raise the cost of research and discourage researchers from entering the field. Additionally, those barriers diminish the likelihood that a pharmaceutical company will invest in the development of antiaddiction medications (IOM, 1995).[4] Broader acceptance of the medical model of drug dependence would provide an incentive for researchers and clinicians to enter this field of research. Over time, a developing consensus in support of the medical model could facilitate common discourse, help to shape a shared research agenda within a public health framework, and diminish tensions between the research and treatment communities and the criminal justice system.

Better Translation of Research Findings into Practice and Policy

To benefit society, new research findings must be disseminated adequately to treatment providers, educators, law enforcement officials, and community leaders. In the case of prevention practices, it is often difficult for communities to change entrenched policies, particularly when combined with political imperatives for action to counteract drug abuse. In the case of treatment, technology transfer is impeded by the heterogeneity of providers and their marginalization at the outskirts of the medical community (see IOM, 1990, 1995; see also Chapter 8). Physicians and psychiatrists are seldom employed by specialized drug treatment facilities (approximately one-quarter employ medical doctors), and treatment is delivered by counselors whose training and supervision vary greatly and who have little access to and understanding of research results (Ball and Ross, 1991; Batten et al., 1993). These factors not only impede the transfer of research findings to the field but also impede communication from the field to the laboratory so that research designs can be modified in response to clinical realities (Pentz, 1994). Thus, there is a real need for bidirectional communication, from bench to bedside and back to the basic scientist (IOM, 1994).

The committee is aware, however, of recent technology transfer efforts in the field such as the Treatment Improvement Protocol Series, an initiative to establish guidelines for drug abuse treatment with an emphasis on incorporating research findings (SAMHSA, 1993), and the Prevention Enhancement Protocol System, a process implemented by the Center

---

[4]In recognition of the barriers to pharmaceutical company investment in this area of drug development, Congress in 1990 created NIDA's Medications Development Division (IOM, 1990) to stimulate the discovery and development of new medications for the treatment of drug abuse.

for Substance Abuse Prevention in which scientists and practitioners develop protocols to identify and evaluate the strength of evidence on topics related to prevention interventions. Similar efforts will be invaluable for communicating and integrating research results to the treatment community.

Research frequently results in product development leading to changes in operations and an overall enhancement of the value of the enterprise. For example, in the pharmaceutical industry research often leads to the development of new medications or devices. In the public sector, however, research is often divorced from the implementation of findings and development. Research is often more basic than applied, and the fruits of research are not realized by the government, but by the private sector. Although that approach may be appropriate, it is unfortunately not always the most productive strategy for advancing research, knowledge, and product development. That is particularly true in the development of medications for opiate and cocaine addictions, where there is a great need for commitment from the private sector. However, many obstacles prevent active involvement of the pharmaceutical industry in this area of research and development (IOM, 1995).

A similar problem arises in relation to policymaking. Because debates about drug policy tend to be so highly polarized and politicized, research findings are often distorted, or selectively deployed, for rhetorical purposes. Researchers cannot prevent this practice, which is a common feature of political debate in a democratic society. However, researchers and their sponsors should not be indifferent to the disconnect between policy discourse and science. Researchers should establish and support institutional mechanisms for communicating an important message to policymakers and to the general public. Scientific research has produced a solid, and growing, body of knowledge about drug abuse and about the efficacy of various interventions that aim to prevent and control it. As long as drug abuse remains a poorly understood social problem, policy will be based mainly on wish and supposition; steps should be taken to educate policymakers about the scientific and technological advances in addiction research. Only then will it be possible for policymaking to support legislation that adequately funds new research and applies research findings. To some extent, persisting failure to reap the fruits of drug abuse research is attributable to the low visibility of the field—a problem to which the discussion now turns.

Raising the Status of Drug Abuse Research

Drug abuse research is often an undervalued area of inquiry, and most scientists and clinicians choose other disciplines in which to develop their careers. Compared with other fields of research, investigators in drug abuse are often paid less, have less prestige among their peers, and must contend with the unique complexities of performing research in this area (e.g., regulations on controlled substances) (see IOM, 1995). The overall result is an insufficient number of basic and clinical researchers. IOM has recently begun a study, funded by the W. M. Keck Foundation of Los Angeles, to develop strategies to raise the status of drug abuse research.[5]

Weak public support for this field of study is evident in unstable federal funding (see above), a lack of pharmaceutical industry investment in the development of antiaddiction medications (IOM, 1995), and inadequate funding for research training (IOM, 1995). NIDA's FY 1994 training budget, which is crucial to the flow of young researchers into the field, was about 2 percent of its extramural research budget, a percentage substantially lower than the overall National Institutes of Health (NIH) training budget, which averages 4.8 percent of its extramural research budget.

Beyond funding problems, investigators face a host of barriers to research: research subjects may pose health risks (e.g., TB, HIV/AIDS, and other infectious diseases), may be noncompliant, may deny their drug abuse problems, and may be involved in the criminal justice system. Even when research is successful and points to improvements in service delivery, the positive outcome may not be translated into practice or policy. For example, more than a year after the Food and Drug Administration's (FDA's) approval of *levo*-alpha-acetylmethadol (LAAM) as the first new medication for the treatment of opiate dependence in over 20 years, fewer than 1,000 patients nationwide actually had received the medication (IOM, 1995). More recently, scientific evidence regarding the beneficial effects of needle exchange programs (NRC, 1995) has received inadequate attention. Continuing indifference to scientific progress in drug abuse research inevitably depresses the status of the field, leading in turn to difficulties in recruiting new investigators.

Increasing Interdisciplinary Research

The breadth of expertise needed in drug abuse research spans many disciplines, including the behavioral sciences, pharmacology, medicine, and the neurosciences, and many fields of inquiry, including etiology, epidemiology, prevention, treatment, and health services research. Aspects of research relating to drug use tend to draw on developmental perspectives and to focus on general population samples in community settings, especially schools. Aspects of research relating to abuse and de-

---

[5] The report on raising the profile of drug abuse will be published in the Fall of 1996.

pendence tend to be more clinical in nature, drawing on psychopathological perspectives. Additionally, a full account of any aspect of drug-taking behavior must also reflect an understanding of social context. The rich interplay between neuroscience and behavioral research and between basic and clinical research poses distinct challenges and opportunities.

Unfortunately, research tends to be fragmented within disciplinary boundaries. The difficulties in conducting successful interdisciplinary research are well known. Funds for research come from many separate agencies, such as the NIDA, NIMH, and SAMHSA. These agencies all have different programmatic emphases as they attempt to shape the direction of research in their respective fields. In times of funding constraints, agencies may be less inclined to fund projects at the periphery of their interests.

Additionally, NIH study sections, which rank grant proposals, are discipline specific, making it difficult for interdisciplinary proposals to "qualify" (i.e., receive a high rank) for funding. Another problem is that the most advanced scientific literature tends to be compartmentalized within discipline or subject matter categories, making it difficult for scientists to see the whole field. The problem is exacerbated by what Tonry (1990) has called "fugitive literatures," studies carried out by private sector research firms or independent research agencies and available only in reports submitted to the sponsoring agency.

In light of lost opportunities for collaboration and interdisciplinary research, IOM (1995) previously recommended the creation and expansion of comprehensive drug abuse centers to coordinate all aspects of drug abuse research, training, and treatment. The field of drug abuse research presents a real opportunity to bridge the intellectual divide between the behavioral and neuroscience communities and to overcome the logistical impediments to interdisciplinary research.

INVESTING WISELY IN DRUG ABUSE RESEARCH

This report sets forth drug abuse research initiatives for the next decade based on a thorough assessment of what is now known and a calculated judgment about what initiatives are most likely to advance our knowledge in useful ways. This report is not meant to be a road map or tactical battle plan, but is best regarded as a strategic outline. Within each discipline of drug abuse research, the committee has highlighted priorities for future research. However, the committee did not make any attempt to prioritize recommendations across varied disciplines and fields of research. Prudent research planning must respond to newly emerging opportunities and needs while maintaining a steady commitment to the achievement of long-term objectives. The ability to respond to new goals and needs may be the real challenge for the field of drug abuse research.

Drug abuse research is an important public investment. The ultimate aim of that investment is to reduce the enormous social costs attributable to drug abuse and dependence. Of course, drug abuse research must also compete for funding with research in other fields of public health, research in other scientific domains, and other pressing public needs. Recognizing the scarcity of resources, the committee has also considered ways in which the research effort can be harnessed most effectively to increase the yield per dollar invested. These include stable funding, use of a comprehensive public health framework, wider acceptance of a medical model of drug dependence, better translation of research findings into practice and policy, raising the status of drug abuse research, and facilitating interdisciplinary research.

The committee notes that there have been major accomplishments in drug abuse research over the past 25 years and commends NIDA for leading that effort. The committee is convinced that the field is on the threshold of significant advances, and that a sustained research effort will strengthen society's capacity to reduce drug abuse and to ameliorate its adverse consequences.

ORGANIZATION OF THE REPORT

This report sets forth a series of initiatives in drug abuse research.[6] Each chapter of the report covers a segment of the field, describes selected accomplishments, and highlights areas that seem ripe for future research. As noted, the committee has not prioritized areas for future research but, instead, has identified those areas that most warrant further exploration.

Chapter 2 describes behavioral models of drug abuse and demonstrates how the use of behavioral procedures has given researchers the ability to measure drug-taking objectively and to study the development, maintenance, and consequences of that behavior. Chapter 3 discusses drug abuse within the context of neurotransmission; it describes neurobiological advances in drug abuse research and provides the foundation for the current understanding of addiction as a brain disease. The epidemiological information systems designed to gather information on drug use in the United States are identified in Chapter 4. The data collected from the systems provide an essential foundation for systematic study of

[6]As noted earlier, the primary focus of the report is research on illicit drugs, such as heroin and cocaine. Research on alcohol and nicotine is cited in the text where it has illuminated our knowledge of illicit drug abuse.

the etiology and consequences of drug abuse, which are addressed, respectively, in Chapters 5 and 7. Chapter 6 addresses the efficacy of interventions designed to prevent drug abuse. The effectiveness of drug abuse treatment and the difficulties in treating special populations of drug users are discussed in Chapter 8, while the impact of managed care on access, costs, utilization, and outcomes of treatment is addressed in Chapter 9. Finally, Chapter 10 discusses the effects of drug control on public health and identifies areas for policy-relevant research.

Specific recommendations appear in each chapter. Although these recommendations reflect the committee's best judgment regarding priorities within the specific domains of research, the committee did not identify priorities or rank recommendations for the entire field of drug abuse research. Opportunities for advancing knowledge exist in all domains. It would be a mistake to invest too narrowly in a few fields of inquiry. At the present time, soundly conceived research should be pursued in all domains along the lines outlined in this report.

REFERENCES

ACS (American Cancer Society). 1993. *Cancer Facts and Figures, 1993*. Washington, DC: ACS.

AHA (American Heart Association). 1992. *1993 Heart and Stroke Fact Statistics*. Dallas, TX: AHA.

Anglin MD, Hser Y. 1992. Treatment of drug abuse. In: Watson RR, ed. *Drug Abuse Treatment. Vol. 3, Drug and Alcohol Abuse Reviews*. New York: Humana Press.

APA (American Psychiatric Association). 1994. *Diagnostic and Statistical Manual of Mental Disorders*. 4th ed. Washington, DC: APA.

Ball JC, Ross A. 1991. *The Effectiveness of Methadone Maintenance Treatment*. New York: Springer-Verlag.

Batten H, Horgan CM, Prottas J, Simon LJ, Larson MJ, Elliott EA, Bowden ML, Lee M. 1993. *Drug Services Research Survey Final Report: Phase I*. Contract number 271-90-8319/1. Submitted to the National Institute of Drug Abuse. Waltham, MA: Bigel Institute for Health Policy, Brandeis University.

Brewley T. 1995. Conversation with Thomas Brewley. *Addiction* 90:883–892.

Carr DB, Jacox AK, Chapman CR, et al. 1992. *Acute Pain Management: Operative or Medical Procedures and Trauma. Clinical Practice Guidelines*. AHCPR Publication No. 92-0032. Rockville, MD: U.S. Public Health Service, Agency for Health Care Policy and Research.

CDC (Centers for Disease Control and Prevention). 1995. *HIV/AIDS Surveillance Report* 7(2).

Cooper JR, Bloom FE, Roth RH. 1991. *The Biochemical Basis of Neuropharmacology*. 6th ed. New York: Oxford University Press.

Daley DC, Marlatt GA. 1992. Relapse prevention: Cognitive and behavioral interventions. In: Lowinson JH, Ruiz P, Millman RB, Langrod JG, eds. *Substance Abuse: A Comprehensive Textbook*. Baltimore: Williams and Wilkins.

D'Aunno T, Vaughn TE. 1992. Variation in methadone treatment practices. *Journal of the American Medical Association* 267:253–258.

DiGregorio GJ. 1990. Cocaine update: Abuse and therapy. *American Family Physician* 41(1):247–250.

Foley KM, Inturrisi CE, eds. 1986. *Opioid Analgesics in the Management of Clinical Pain. Advances in Pain Research and Therapy. Vol. 8.* New York: Raven Press.

GAO (General Accounting Office). 1992. *Drug Abuse Research: Federal Funding and Future Needs.* GAO/PEMD-92-5. Washington, DC: GAO.

Glassman AH, Covey LS, Dalack GW, Stetner F, Rivelli SK, Fleiss J, Cooper TB. 1993. Smoking cessation, clonidine, and vulnerability to nicotine among dependent smokers. *Clinical Pharmacology and Therapeutics* 54(6):670–679.

Goldstein A. 1994. *Addiction: From Biology to Drug Policy.* New York: W.H. Freeman.

Hokfelt TGM, Castel MN, Morino P, Zhang X, Dagerlind A. 1995. General overview of neuropeptides. In: Bloom FE, Kupfer DJ, eds. *Psychopharmacology: Fourth Generation of Progress.* New York: Raven Press. Pp. 483–492.

Holmberg SD. 1996. The estimated prevalence and incidence of HIV in 96 large U.S. metropolitan areas. *American Journal of Public Health* 86(5):642–654.

IOM (Institute of Medicine). 1990. *Treating Drug Problems.* Washington, DC: National Academy Press.

IOM (Institute of Medicine). 1994. *AIDS and Behavior: An Integrated Approach.* Washington, DC: National Academy Press.

IOM (Institute of Medicine). 1995. *The Development of Medications for the Treatment of Opiate and Cocaine Addictions.* Washington, DC: National Academy Press.

Jacox A, Carr DB, Payne R, et al. 1994. *Management of Cancer Pain. Clinical Practice Guideline.* AHCPR Publication No. 94-0592. Rockville, MD: U.S. Public Health Service, Agency for Health Care Policy and Research.

Kahn RS, Davis KL. 1995. New developments in dopamine and schizophrenia. In: Bloom FE, Kupfer DJ, eds. *Psychopharmacology: Fourth Generation of Progress.* New York: Raven Press. Pp. 1193–1204.

McDuff DR, Schwartz RP, Tommasello A, Tiegel S, Donovan T, Johnson JL. 1993. Outpatient benzodiazepine detoxification procedure for methadone patients. *Journal of Substance Abuse Treatment* 10:297–302.

McLellan AT, Metzger DS, Alterman AI, Woody GE, Durell J, O'Brien CP. In press. Is addiction treatment "worth it"? Public health expectations, policy-based comparisons. *Milbank Quarterly.*

Meyer R. 1996. The disease called addiction: Emerging evidence in a 200-year debate. *Lancet* 347:162–166.

Miller NS. 1991. Drug and alcohol addiction as a disease. In: Miller NS, ed. *Comprehensive Handbook of Drug and Alcohol Addiction.* New York: Marcel Dekker.

MMWR (Morbidity and Mortality Weekly Report). 1994. Medical care expenditures attributable to cigarette smoking, United States, 1993. *Morbidity and Mortality Weekly Report* 43(26):469–472.

NRC (National Research Council). 1995. *Preventing HIV Transmission: The Role of Sterile Needles and Bleach.* Washington, DC: National Academy Press.

O'Brien CP, McLellan AT. 1996. Myths about the treatment of addiction. *Lancet* 347:237–240.

Olson GA, Olson RD, Kastin AJ. 1994. Endogenous opiates, 1993. *Peptides* 15:1513–1556.

ONDCP (Office of National Drug Control Policy). 1996. *National Drug Control Strategy.* Washington, DC: ONDCP.

Pentz M. 1994. Directions for future research in drug abuse prevention. *Preventive Medicine* 23:646–652.

Rhodes W, Scheiman P, Pittayathikhun T, Collins L, Tsarfaty V. 1995. *What America's Users Spend on Illegal Drugs, 1988–1993.* Prepared for the Office of National Drug Control Policy, Washington, DC.

Rice DP, Kelman S, Miller LS, Dunmeyer S. 1990. *The Economic Costs of Alcohol and Drug Abuse and Mental Illness: 1985*. DHHS Publication No. (ADM) 90-1694. San Francisco: University of California, Institute for Health and Aging.

Rice DP, Max W, Novotny T, Shultz J, Hodgson T. 1992. *The Cost of Smoking Revisited: Preliminary Estimates*. Paper presented at the American Public Health Association Annual Meeting, November 23, 1992. Washington, DC.

SAMHSA (Substance Abuse and Mental Health Services Administration). 1993. *Improving Treatment for Drug-Exposed Infants: Treatment Improvement Protocol (TIP) Series*. Washington, DC: U.S. Department of Health and Human Services.

SAMHSA (Substance Abuse and Mental Health Services Administration). 1995. *National Household Survey on Drug Abuse: Population Estimates 1994*. Washington, DC: U.S. Department of Health and Human Services.

Schelling TC. 1992. Addictive drugs: The cigarette experience. *Science* 255:431–433.

Tonry M. 1990. Research on drugs and crime. In: Morris N, Tonry M, eds. *Drugs and Crime. Vol. 13*. Chicago: University of Chicago Press.

Volkow ND, Fowler JS, Wang G-J, Hitzemann R, Logan J, Schlyer DJ, Dewey SI, Wolf AD. 1993. Decreased dopamine D2 receptor availability is associated with reduced frontal metabolism in cocaine abusers. *Synapse* 14:169–177.

Wall PD, Melzack R. 1994. *Textbook of Pain*. 3rd ed. Edinburg: Churchill-Livingstone.

WHO (World Health Organization). 1992. *International Statistical Classification of Diseases and Related Health Problems*. Tenth Revision. Geneva: WHO.

2

Behavioral Research

Behavioral research has contributed to our understanding of many of the factors involved in drug abuse, including initiation, maintenance, cessation, and relapse. Prior to the 1960s, the general belief held by professionals and lay people was that drug abuse was caused by an underlying psychopathology that could be studied only in humans. Behavioral researchers, however, took advantage of the knowledge gained about the control of appetitive behaviors and developed an animal model of drug abuse. Although early work on drug abuse and drug-taking behaviors assumed that only those animals[1] already physically dependent on opiates could be induced to take them (Thompson and Schuster, 1964), it soon became clear that when drugs were made available, drug-naive animals took them readily and to excess.

This chapter highlights some of the major accomplishments in behavioral research (including the development of behavioral models) and discusses opportunities for future research. Insights from behavioral research have made major contributions to our understanding of the addictive process, enabling researchers to study the behavior of drug taking separately from its pharmacological sequelae and making it possible to integrate the findings of other research disciplines (e.g., treatment and neurosciences).

---

[1] The terms "animals" and "nonhumans" are used interchangeably throughout this chapter to refer to nonhuman laboratory animals.

BEHAVIORAL MODELS

The major contribution of behavioral research to the study of drug abuse has been the development of the self-administration model and the use of this model to test for abuse liability and to expand our understanding of addiction. This basic model has been augmented by other models based on the principles of learning and conditioning such as drug classification (drug discrimination); the relationship between drug use and variables controlling use (behavioral economics); the nature of transition states in drug abuse (initiation, abstinence, withdrawal); motivational states (e.g., incentive motivation); and the roles of tolerance and physical dependence in drug-seeking behavior.

Drug Self-Administration Model

The drug self-administration model is based on the learning principle that behavior is maintained by its consequences, called reinforcers. Laboratory animals (humans and nonhumans) will work to receive a range of different drugs administered orally, intramuscularly, intravenously, by smoking, or by insufflation. In this model, the laboratory animal performs some action, such as depressing a lever, to trigger the administration of a drug (e.g, through an indwelling catheter or a solution to drink). In general, those drugs (e.g., cocaine, heroin, nicotine, alcohol) that maintain drug taking in nonhumans are also commonly abused by humans, and those that are avoided by humans (e.g., antipsychotics) are also avoided by nonhumans. These results are replicable in virtually every species tested with the model and with different routes of administration. Such findings brought into question the traditional explanations of the etiology of drug abuse, such as psychopathology or various social deprivations.

This model also allows behavioral researchers to control past history and current environmental conditions, thus demonstrating that it is the interaction of the drug's pharmacological effects with past history and current environmental conditions (i.e., setting) that determines whether sampling an abusable drug will proceed to persistent use or abuse (e.g., Barrett and Witkin, 1986). This model points to the importance of a confluence of variables in drug-taking behavior and has broadened the clinician's understanding of the various causal factors that might be involved in drug abuse.

Drug Discrimination

The drug discrimination paradigm is considered a model of the subjective effects of drugs in humans. In this paradigm, research subjects are trained to respond differently to the test drugs (e.g., drug versus placebo or drug versus drug). For example, a research subject might be trained to press the left lever after a dose of amphetamine and the right lever after a dose of placebo. After training, research subjects (nonhuman or human) will respond differentially to drug and placebo, allowing for comparison among drugs and for conclusions about pharmacological and behavioral similarity, depending on the manner in which the trained research subject responds.

Animal Models of Drug Dependence

Drug dependence has also been modeled in laboratory animals. Drug dependence (or addiction), as noted in Chapter 1, is characterized in both the *Diagnostic and Statistical Manual of Mental Disorders* (DSM-IV; APA, 1994) and the International Classification of Diseases (ICD-10, WHO, 1992) as drug-seeking behavior involving compulsive use of high doses of one or more drugs, for no clear medical indication. Dependence is usually accompanied by tolerance and withdrawal; physicians often confuse the presence of a withdrawal syndrome (i.e., physical dependence) with the compulsive drug taking that is a part of the behavioral dependence syndrome. Models have been developed in which animals are maintained on specific drugs of abuse (e.g., opiates) for some period of time, either via self-administered or experimenter-administered drug, and then observed for the effects of abrupt cessation (e.g., Woods and Schuster, 1968). Manipulations using animal models have provided information about the relationship between repeated drug use and toxicity, as well as the likelihood that the drug will be taken in the future.

ACCOMPLISHMENTS

Dopamine Transporter

In addition to being a useful tool for investigating basic biobehavioral mechanisms underlying drug abuse, the drug self-administration model has provided the foundation for research in many other areas of drug abuse. For example, it has been shown that there is a significant positive correlation between the potencies of cocaine (and other stimulants) as dopamine reuptake blockers and their ability to maintain self-administration behavior, although the same is not true for norepinephrine and serotonin (Ritz et al., 1987; Bergman et al., 1989). This finding suggests that the action of cocaine at its binding site, which results in dopamine uptake blockade, mediates the effects that contribute to abuse (Fischman and Johanson, 1996).

Neuroscientists have taken advantage of this model to investigate the brain loci mediating the reinforcing and dependence-producing properties of morphine (Bozarth and Wise, 1984), the dopaminergic contributions to drug reinforcement, and the brain areas activated by specific drugs (Koob and Bloom, 1989; Cerruti et al., 1994; Nestler, 1994). Geneticists have used this technology to evaluate the heritability of drug abuse (e.g., Froelich et al., 1988); similarly, neurochemists have examined specific behavioral correlates in this model (Kalivas and Duffy, 1993; see Chapter 3).

Excitatory Amino Acids

Research on phencyclidine (PCP) provides a good example of the way in which behavioral studies provide a body of data for understanding the neural basis of learning and memory, as well as the development of novel medication strategies. In the early 1970s, the introduction of PCP as a drug of abuse was immediately recognized as different and potentially more devastating than abuse of other hallucinogens. Initial studies evaluated this drug and its analogues in self-administration and drug discrimination paradigms (reviewed in Balster and Willetts, 1996). It became obvious that PCP was a noncompetitive antagonist at the NMDA (*N*-methyl-*D*-aspartate) receptor. PCP became an important research tool for understanding the role of excitatory amino acid neurotransmission initiated by glutamate in the control of a variety of behaviors and in the pathophysiology of neuronal death.

Current work in this area has the potential to lead to novel treatment medication strategies for preventing neurotoxicity following brain trauma. As excitatory amino acid antagonists are developed for therapeutic uses, an important goal will be to avoid the abuse liability (the likelihood that a drug will be abused) and psychological disturbances produced by PCP; the animal models developed by drug abuse researchers are now being relied on in this area of medications development. An exciting research development suggests that excitatory amino acids may play an important role in the development of tolerance to and dependence on drugs of abuse such as the opiates, alcohol, and stimulants (Balster and Willetts, 1996). It is possible that this research will lead to completely novel strategies for the treatment of the addictions.

Development of Therapeutic Drugs Without Abuse Liability

A major concern in the development of new psychotropic medications is to maximize therapeutic efficacy while reducing the risks of abuse and dependence. In the 1920s, substitutes for morphine were sought that lacked abuse liability. That research measured physical dependence and focused on the withdrawal syndrome by collecting behavioral and physiological data on both objective and self-reported measures. Work in that area led to the important discovery that physical dependence and abuse liability were not the same and that abuse liability could not be assessed solely on the basis of chemical structure.

The drug self-administration model continues to provide a bioassay for the evaluation of abuse liability. Animal self-administration studies have been used widely to predict the abuse liability of new drugs (Brady and Lukas, 1984). Self-administration data are frequently a part of the information submitted to the Food and Drug Administration (FDA) by pharmaceutical companies as part of their applications for approval of psychoactive drugs, including those targeted for psychiatric disorders (e.g., anxiety, depression). Those data are used by the FDA (and ultimately the Drug Enforcement Administration) in their scheduling recommendations.[2] Behavioral assays using this model provide critical data for determining the appropriate regulatory status of drugs, since such determinations cannot be made simply on the basis of chemical structure or *in vitro* data. Because the particular schedule in which a drug is placed strongly influences the marketing success of the new compound, the pharmaceutical industry has been a major supporter of behavioral research. In fact, different preparations of the same medications, with the same active chemical constituent, are often regulated and scheduled differently based on their behavioral effects. For example, nicotine gum is unscheduled and sold over the counter; approval is pending for over-the-counter sale of nicotine patches; however, nicotine nasal spray may be placed in Schedule IV or V.

Medications for the Treatment of Drug Abuse

The drug self-administration model has been of major importance in the search for potentially useful pharmacological interventions to treat drug abusers. Early research, for example, demonstrated the efficacy of immunizing rhesus monkeys with an antigen that caused the formation of antibodies that bound morphine when it was injected intravenously (Bonese et al., 1974). Rates of heroin self-administration decreased almost to zero in immunized animals, although the toxicity of the procedure

[2] Under the Controlled Substances Act (Public Law 91-513, October 27, 1970), a drug with a potential for abuse is placed into one of five schedules, depending on the magnitude of the abuse potential, whether the drug has accepted medical uses, and the extent to which abuse of the drug will lead to physical or psychological dependence.

limited its utility in humans. Other researchers, using monoclonal antibody techniques, recently reported the development of an artificial enzyme that inactivates cocaine by cleaving it into two inactive metabolites (Landry et al., 1993). This technique is effective in the test tube, but it must now be demonstrated in nonhumans before it proceeds to human trials; researchers are pursuing this work in conjunction with behavioral researchers experienced in drug self-administration research and medications development (J. Woods, University of Michigan, personal communication, 1995). Further evidence for the promising nature of immunopharmacotherapy is given in a recent report (Carrera et al., 1995) describing suppression of locomotor activity and stereotyped behavior in rats after active immunization with a cocaine immunogen. This response was specific to cocaine and was not seen after amphetamine administration.

Administration of antagonists or immunization against specific drugs, although clearly potentially important tools in our armamentarium against drug use (see discussion on behavioral economics, below), promises no more success than the available opiate antagonist naltrexone[3] for the treatment of heroin addiction. It is very clear that nonhumans, treated with naltrexone, will show extinction in their opiate responding (Koob et al., 1984), and humans, under residential laboratory conditions, also will stop using heroin after treatment with naltrexone (Mello et al., 1981). However, after leaving the structured setting of a residential laboratory individuals relapse to heroin use. Although laboratory studies on naltrexone, with nonhuman and human subjects, demonstrate the utility of the drug self-administration model in the initial assessment of the utility of a new medication, the model does not allow for an evaluation of the contextual (social and environmental) factors that could ultimately affect drug-taking behavior. Thus, there is a need for behavioral models that pattern complex behaviors (e.g., studies that give heroin users the choice of taking naltrexone and explore the range of conditions under which it is taken). Studies focused on compliance are becoming increasingly important because the most efficacious medications are useless if the patient does not take them.

The National Institute on Drug Abuse (NIDA) Medications Development Program relies on drug self-administration and drug discrimination models for its preclinical evaluation of new medications (IOM, 1995; Mello

---

[3]Naltrexone acts to block or reverse the effects of mu opioids, such as heroin. Patients taking naltrexone cannot feel the effects of heroin if they take it; so heroin's positive reinforcing effects are reduced or eliminated (IOM, 1995). Naltrexone has proven most useful in highly motivated, dependent patients who have a great socioeconomic risk or other risk associated with relapse.

and Negus, in press). Animal models of self-administration (versus human models) have several advantages for medications development. For example, drugs that are not approved for use in humans can be evaluated; the effects of new treatment medications on patterns of drug self-administration can be evaluated quantitatively under controlled experimental conditions; social factors such as peer pressure or expectancy do not complicate interpretation of data; and accurate baseline measures of the daily dose and patterns of drug self-administration can be determined before, during, and after administration of the treatment medication. Additionally, the safety of the medication can be evaluated continually. Thus, the use of animal models for those aspects of medications development is parallel in importance to the earlier reliance on animal models of drug self-administration for evaluation of the abuse liability of new drugs. To the extent possible, however, these laboratory models should be employed across species to include humans.

Learning and Conditioning

A major contribution of behavioral research has been an understanding of the ways in which basic principles of learning and conditioning can be used to modify drug-taking behavior. These principles have been precisely defined so that they can be studied and replicated across conditions and species.

For example, research on drug effect expectancies suggests that learned beliefs and attitudes may serve as risk factors for the initiation and use of drugs (Brown, 1993). Further, epidemiological research has pointed to the importance of social modeling and attitudes as having strong impacts on drug use and abuse. Research on learning and conditioning has led to successful treatment models for drug abusers, including relapse prevention, community reinforcement, and focused techniques such as extinction training, relaxation training, contingency management, and job skills training. Two well-studied behavioral interventions are discussed below: contingency management and relapse prevention.

Contingency management research is based on the fact that, although drugs are potent reinforcers, there are non-drug reinforcers that can compete with drug use (see discussion of behavioral economics, below). Manipulation of the environment can shift the focus toward or away from drug reinforcers (e.g., Azrin et al., 1966; Barrett and Witkin, 1986). In the laboratory, monkeys will choose saccharine over phencyclidine if they are required to work substantially harder for the drug (Carroll and Rodefer, 1993). Research with humans has shown that experienced cocaine users will choose money or tokens over cocaine when the appropriate quantity and quality of alternative reinforcers are available (Foltin and Fischman,

1994; Higgins et al., 1994). In addition, direct reinforcement of drug abstinence can be effective in methadone maintenance programs (Iguchi et al., 1988), and drug consumption can be reduced significantly when valued alternatives (commodities and recreational activities) are provided in exchange for clean urine (Higgins et al., 1993).

Relapse prevention research also combines cognitive and behavioral approaches (e.g., Marlatt and Gordon, 1985; Carroll KM et al., 1991). Behavioral analysis of drug abusers has demonstrated that learning and conditioning (both classical and operant) play an important role in the initiation, maintenance, cessation, and relapse to drug use. Early work in rats (Wikler and Pescor, 1967) and in humans (O'Brien et al., 1977) showed that signs of abstinence can become classically conditioned to the specific environmental conditions under which withdrawal has occurred in the past. Thus, even though a previously opiate-dependent person has remained drug free for a prolonged period of time, specific environmental conditions could trigger opiate withdrawal symptoms, which in turn might motivate relapse. This effect has been modeled in the laboratory, where rhesus monkeys, dependent in the past on morphine, showed clear signs of physical dependence and relapse in the presence of stimuli that in the past signaled opiate withdrawal (Goldberg and Schuster, 1967, 1969; Goldberg et al., 1970, 1971). Conditioned opiate withdrawal and craving have also been demonstrated experimentally in humans (O'Brien et al., 1977; Childress et al., 1988). Although Wikler (1973), for example, observed that conditioned withdrawal plays a substantial role in relapse to opiate use, even years after the drug-dependent person has ceased using opiates, the role of conditioned responses in relapse in the nonlaboratory setting is not yet clear.

Drug Administration and Withdrawal

A variety of behavioral studies have been used to characterize and quantitate the potential deleterious effects of drug administration and withdrawal for both illicit and licit drug use and have been useful in guiding policy development. For example, while cigarette smoking has long been associated with increased alertness, sustained performance in situations of fatigue, and increased cognitive performance (Rusted and Warburton, 1992), dependent individuals experience decreases in performance stemming from nicotine withdrawal. These decrements are reversed rapidly by the readministration of tobacco or medically approved forms of nicotine such as nicotine gum or patch (Henningfield, 1994). Characterizing the course and timing of this behavioral degradation has been critical in determining how to manage nicotine-dependent airline pilots. Since performance decrements do not emerge until approximately four hours after the last cigarette, the prohibition of smoking by pilots would not be expected to compromise their performance on flights of two hours or less, and non-disrupted pilot behavior might be sustained by nicotine-delivering medications in the absence of tobacco (Fiore et al., 1994). Those findings point the way to research with other drugs of abuse where similar effects may cause a reluctance to stop use.

RESEARCH OPPORTUNITIES

Motivation

Behavioral research has revealed the complexity of drug use and has shown that the conditions under which drugs are used may be as powerful in motivating drug use as the drug itself. It has been observed that even noxious stimuli in the environment will serve as reinforcers and result in the self-administration of drugs. Thus, the concept of motivation—why people use drugs—is far more complicated than initially believed and may include adjunctive behaviors, non-drug reinforcers, appetitive behaviors, and single priming doses.

Adjunctive Behaviors

Although drug abuse is frequently described as a direct consequence of exposure to a drug with abuse liability, the great majority of people experimenting with such drugs do not become abusers (Anthony et al., 1994). The intrinsic effects produced by certain drugs (i.e., their physiological and subjective effects) can serve as motivating factors for drug abuse, but there is another, less direct, yet powerful way in which drugs can gain control over a person's life. Drug taking can develop as an adjunct to another strongly motivated behavior when that behavior becomes intermittently blocked or cannot be completed. When so blocked, that person may turn to an easy, satisfying alternative—an adjunctive behavior (Falk, 1984, 1993).

In the laboratory, excessive adjunctive behavior (e.g., excessive water drinking, aggression, eating, smoking) is related to the intermittent availability of an important commodity or activity. The conditions or "generator schedules" under which such behaviors become excessive are similar to conditions in natural and social environments that provide what we need, but only in small amounts, and with delay intervals. The adjunctive behavior generated may be noninjurious (e.g., drinking water) or creative (e.g., an intense hobby), but it also can result in aggression or drug taking, depending upon personal history, skills, and currently available alternatives. Drug abuse can arise from conditions already generating behavioral excesses, and this may be one of the reasons that drug abusers often have other behavioral problems.

Adjunctive behavior studies indicate that drug abuse may stem more from environmental-generating conditions, together with a lack, or poor utilization, of other opportunities, than from any intrinsic attractiveness of drugs with abuse liability. Those studies clarify how drugs can become so attractive to some individuals, and the abuse behavior so persistent, in light of the trouble it causes for them. Understanding the conditions that comprise economically or socially restricted schedules of reinforcement and, therefore, can generate and sustain drug abuse behavior has important implications for the design of therapeutic and prevention strategies. Adjunctive behavior research procedures may also serve as models of limited opportunities in the natural ecology.

Alternative Reinforcers

Drug use has an obvious effect on motivation. Individuals who, in the absence of drug use, will go to work, support a family, seek an education, and engage in other aspects of a productive life style, can become totally involved in drug seeking and drug taking, neglecting all other activities they previously found rewarding. Behavioral research with human subjects is now focusing on understanding the determinants of the reinforcing effects of drugs in an environment in which alternative reinforcers are available.

Research on the factors controlling the choice to use drugs is best carried out in the laboratory, where multiple behaviors can be measured and manipulated (see Fischman et al., 1991). Such research has established some of the determinants of choice both between drugs and between drugs and non-drug reinforcers. For example, the frequency of drug choice depends on dose (Johanson, 1975; Nader and Woolverton, 1991), as well as on environmental factors such as the availability of a non-drug option (Carroll ME et al., 1991), simultaneous delivery of an adverse consequence (e.g., electric shock) (Johanson, 1975), or increased response requirement for the drug (Nader and Woolverton, 1991).

Research with humans has shown that the choice between cocaine and alternative reinforcers can be a sensitive assay for the efficacy of new medications (e.g., Foltin and Fischman, 1994). The question then becomes whether a specific medication increases the likelihood that drug abusers will choose non-drug rather than drug options, a question much closer to the natural ecology of a treatment setting. This type of research is highly complex, and methodologies for conducting research, analyzing data, and developing theoretical frameworks must be developed in order to elucidate interactions among the organism, the drug, and the environment.

The behavioral economics approach, described below, is one such possibility, but others must also be considered.

Appetitive Behaviors

Research into other appetitive behaviors may be directly relevant to drug abuse. For example, studies have shown that food deprivation can increase drug intake (Carroll, 1995), but it is not known whether this is true for deprivation of money, social factors, or other commodities. It may well be that research into disorders such as bulimia and anorexia is directly relevant to the study of drug abuse: they have similar topographies, although there are currently no data indicating that their underlying processes are also similar.

Priming Doses

Research with nonhumans has repeatedly shown that a single (priming) dose of a drug can reinstate drug-reinforced responses even after the animal has ceased responding to that drug due to extinction (e.g., de Wit and Stewart, 1981; Slikker et al., 1984). This phenomenon is believed to occur in humans as well, which is why most drug abuse treatment programs stress the need for total abstinence. Recent studies have shown that nonalcoholic human research subjects chose an ethanol-containing beverage over money on days when they were pretreated with an ethanol-containing beverage but not on days when they were pretreated with placebo (de Wit and Chutuape, 1993; Chutuape et al., 1994). These observations support the hypothesis that priming doses of a drug can reinstate drug taking in those who are currently not seeking or taking a drug.

It is possible that priming effects are not specific to drugs but may be a more general phenomenon. For example, food-satiated humans presented with a specific food "prime" will choose to eat more of that food but not of other foods (Cornell et al., 1992). This phenomenon, in the context of incentive motivational theory, suggests that drugs of abuse (specifically heroin and cocaine) produce their motivational effects by acting directly on the central nervous system, and that administration of such drugs has the ability to induce motivation (incentive) for them (Stewart et al., 1984). It has been suggested that after repeated use, the conditioned incentive effect of a drug can mimic its neural activity, which can initiate drug-taking behavior. Research in this area has the potential to provide information about the neural substrates underlying appetitive motivation and offers opportunities for integrated behavioral and neurobiological research into the mechanisms underlying relapse.

Craving

Patients seeking treatment for their drug use report irresistible craving that leads to continued use, despite firm resolutions to remain abstinent. From the perspective of the drug abuser, this motivation to continue use is a major impediment to abstinence. Drug treatment specialists refer to drug craving by their patients as an important determinant of success or failure in treatment. Despite the clear importance of this concept from a descriptive perspective, it is an extremely difficult concept to measure in the laboratory (or the clinic) in a meaningful fashion. Clinicians try to gauge the efficacy of treatment interventions by assessing changes in reports of drug craving by their patients. Studies attempting to correlate reported craving with actual use of cocaine in a laboratory setting have not been successful. Under some conditions, use remained unchanged as reported craving decreased (Fischman et al., 1990); under other conditions, use decreased while craving remained unchanged (Foltin and Fischman, 1994). A similar dissociation has been found in tobacco smokers: nicotine chewing gum decreased tobacco intake, but measures of the desire to smoke were unaffected (Nemeth-Coslett and Henningfield, 1986). Studies of heroin addicts found that craving increased under conditions of precipitated withdrawal, but the choice of self-administering an opiate was unaffected (Schuster et al., 1995).

Conditioned craving has been reported in former opiate addicts (O'Brien, 1975) and in former cocaine addicts (O'Brien et al., 1990) when presented with stimuli associated with prior drug use. This phenomenon has been used to screen medications for potential anticraving activity (Robbins et al., 1992; Berger et al., 1996). Reports of craving in response to drug-related stimuli have been accompanied by significant changes in skin temperature, skin resistance, pulse, and other autonomic measures. Recently, specific limbic system activation has been noted using oxygen-15 PET (positron-emission tomography) measures of regional cerebral blood flood (Childress et al., 1995). Although the relationship of the conditioned craving phenomenon to actual relapse is unclear, it has been possible to demonstrate an effect on drug-taking behavior in nicotine-dependent smokers. Droungas and colleagues (1995) demonstrated that smoking cues provoked craving for cigarettes and a reduced latency to smoke in smokers who were not aware that they were being observed.

In the context of a cocaine treatment intervention, reports of craving during the first week of treatment were only weakly predictive of treatment outcome, and changes in craving over the course of the treatment intervention were uncorrelated with success in abstaining from cocaine use (S.T. Higgins, University of Vermont, personal communication, 1995). Data collected thus far suggest that craving and the increased probability of drug self-administration may both be related to other variables (e.g., withdrawal states, drug-associated environmental cues) but that craving is not causally related to increased drug taking. In fact, one author has suggested that drug use may be mediated by processes different from those mediating craving and that craving may represent the cognitive "battle" going on in the drug abuser related to whether or not to seek and take the drug (Tiffany, 1990). Based on these insights, a new multi-item questionnaire has been developed that might more accurately reflect the multidimensional aspect of what drug users are reporting, thus better predicting treatment-related behavior (Tiffany et al., 1993). At this time, although attempts to understand craving may be important clinically, it seems unwarranted to employ drug craving as a surrogate measure of drug self-administration.

Patients frequently report craving that is associated with increased thoughts about drugs and drug use. Modification or alleviation of those thoughts, while not resulting in abstinence, may well shift their focus away from drug seeking and drug taking toward more acceptable behaviors that are in keeping with the goals of a treatment program. Because of the belief, shared by patients and clinicians, that craving has a major impact on relapse, craving should be studied further. An understanding of the nature of craving, what it is and how it impacts behavior, is an important opportunity for drug abuse research.

Violence and Aggression

Although illicit drugs (particularly cocaine) have been associated with a dramatic upsurge in violence in the United States, it has been difficult to attribute causality to the pharmacological effects of the drugs being used (see Chapter 7). Animal models have shown that acute cocaine administration enhances aggressive responding (Miczek et al., 1994), but the majority of data on humans has been based on epidemiological rather than experimental findings. The ethical issues involved in actually engendering violent or aggressive behavior are formidable, and substantial creativity is required to design ethically acceptable and valid models.

One such laboratory model has demonstrated differential effects related to the drug being tested (Cherek, 1981; Cherek et al., 1991). In this model, each research participant is told that responding on one lever will earn points exchangeable for money, whereas responding on the second lever will subtract points from an unseen research participant in another location. The person making this latter (aggressive) response gains no points by making the response and, in fact, there is no second person. Although the model appears to have face validity, it has not undergone rigorous testing to verify that it models aggressive behavior. Recent efforts to verify the model by studying prisoners found guilty of either violent or nonviolent crimes suggest that the model shows behavioral differences in these two subpopulations (D. Cherek, University of Texas, personal communication, 1995). Continued research is needed to develop models of aggression in animals and humans.

Vulnerability to Drug Use

Animal models of drug self-administration have identified factors that facilitate the addiction process. For example, genetic strain (e.g., George and Goldberg, 1989) and individual differences in activity level (e.g., Piazza et al., 1993) can predict vulnerability to repetitive drug use. Environmental conditions such as lack of alternative reinforcers, restricted access to food (e.g., Carroll, 1995), and drug history (e.g., Horger et al., 1991) can accelerate the onset of drug self-administration. Behavioral studies to delineate those facilitating variables in animals may lead to data-based programs for targeting high-risk human populations, making education and prevention efforts more focused and presumably more effective.

Research in the area of etiology has focused on risk factors, with the underlying assumption that some drug use is pathological. However, one of the messages from animal research using the self-administration model is that drugs easily serve as reinforcers and that conditions do not need to be pathological for drugs to be repeatedly self-administered by all animals. Research in the area of neurobiology is beginning to demonstrate that drug-taking behavior is controlled by brain mechanisms developed through evolution to ensure the reinforcing effects of biologically essential activities of eating, drinking, and copulating. The implication of these research findings is that, were it not for countervailing influences, drug use would be the norm, not an aberration. That inference may be somewhat strong, since there are individual differences in those brain systems that contribute to vulnerability, but it points to a research effort in prevention that takes into account the biological foundations against which these efforts are made.

For example, a variety of environmental risk factors can affect responsivity to drugs, including personality, family, and peer influences. Etiological research has identified issues of interest in these areas, including questions related to risk taking, impulsivity, and deviance (see Chapter 5). Those areas have received attention from behavioral researchers in other contexts, and it should be possible to adapt existing models or to develop new ones with direct relevance to drug abuse and dependence. One etiological hypothesis that might be tested with these models is drug effect expectancy. It has been hypothesized that individuals learn about the effects of drugs directly or from other sources (e.g., media, others), creating a memory network (i.e., an expectancy) that can be activated by drug-related cues. These cognitively developed networks are associated with a drug or drugs and potentially can change as new learning occurs. Use of this construct has important implications for treatment, since it implies that changes in cognition can result in changes in drug abuse behavior. Little research has been carried out in this area, with most of it currently concentrated on alcohol use, and the paradigms for implementing and measuring these changes are not yet well developed. As the role of expectancies in the development and maintenance of drug abuse is delineated more clearly, procedures for preventing or changing drug effect expectancies may well be a useful aspect of a more general cognitive-behavioral approach to drug abuse treatment.

Behavioral Economics

Drug self-administration models have been developed to provide finer-grained analyses of the dynamic interplay among variables. One example is the application of behavioral economics, which focuses on concepts from consumer demand theory. This approach provides a way of understanding the relationship between consumption (i.e., drug use or self-administration) and variables such as price, income, and the characteristics of the goods to be consumed. The utility of this approach stems from its ability to integrate the effects of multiple independent variables (e.g., unit price and the conditions under which the subject chooses reinforcers) into a single term—elasticity of demand[4]—that may be used to better understand the consequences of various treatments.

Drug taking occurs in the context of multiple interacting and competing reinforcers. Some are directly related, in that the consumption of one leads to the consumption of others (e.g., cigarettes and alcohol), whereas some show an inverse relationship (e.g., involvement in some religious activities and drug use). It has been generally assumed that providing individuals, particularly children and adolescents, with alternative sources of reinforcement will decrease the use of drugs. Behavioral economic analysis can use the concept of cross-price elasticity to quantify precisely whether each reinforcer acts as a substitute (a viable alternative) for, serves as a complement (a promoter) to, or is independent (ineffective) of the one against which it is compared. Making sense of the relationships among qualitatively different reinforcers will give us the ability

[4] Defined here as the degree of responsiveness of drug consumption to changes in price (see Chapter 10).

to suggest concrete ways in which drug use can be affected in both animals and humans (Bickel et al., 1993; Carroll, 1993).

The concepts of elasticity and cross-elasticity and the behavioral methods that have been developed to study drug taking from this perspective can also be utilized in the development of medications. The use of behavioral economics could provide information about whether a specific medication, in addition to directly decreasing drug use, also increases sensitivity to other factors of the treatment regimen (e.g., counseling). The opportunity to screen potential new medications by using this conceptual approach, as well as the objective measure of drug self-administration, expands the utility of laboratory analyses and makes them invaluable screening procedures prior to the use of uncontrolled and expensive clinical trials.

CONCLUSION AND RECOMMENDATION

In summary, there are opportunities for continued progress in behavioral approaches to drug abuse research. Behavioral models are useful for developing drug abuse pharmacotherapies; improving treatment engagement and compliance; developing novel procedures for both strengthening weak positive behaviors and attenuating strong drug-related behaviors; addressing questions related to mechanisms of craving and relapse; and promoting better understanding of drug use over the life span of drug users. Increased understanding of various drugs' mechanisms of action can also lead to better understanding of behavior and of vulnerability to drug abuse, which may not be elucidated with familial and drug use histories. The continued development of behavioral models is necessary to improve integration of data and variables being studied. To this end, combining neurobiological and behavioral models should be a primary research goal of the future.

Identification of the mechanisms by which drugs produce behavioral effects is important in the development of new treatment approaches, especially medications development. Behavioral assays, including drug self-administration by animals and humans, as well as subjective effects assessment in humans, are the cornerstone of medications development research because they enable efficient means of screening new chemicals that are highly predictive in their effects on human drug taking. The opportunities for future behavioral research are in the continued development and utilization of those behavioral assays of drug effects.

Although current research into the development of new medications for the treatment of drug abuse is important, drug abuse will likely continue to be treated with a combination of treatment modalities (i.e., behavioral and pharmacological interventions). Research on the modification of drug-taking behavior must continue, with special emphasis on the use of alternative reinforcers. Outcomes should be analyzed with sophisticated approaches that integrate the effects of multiple variables (e.g., behavioral economic analyses). This area of research has only begun to be applied within the clinic, and more sophisticated interventions must be developed based on carefully collected data.

Although a number of animal models have been developed, the use of behavioral models with human participants is a necessary step in expanding the field of drug abuse research. The models being developed should combine a range of behavioral approaches including conditioning, social learning, and cognitive models, integrating them to emulate most effectively the complex behaviors represented by the various aspects of drug seeking and taking. Controlled environment research, behavioral economic analyses, and vulnerability studies are a first step toward addressing some of the complex behaviors associated with drug abuse.

The committee recommends the use of behavioral models (involving both humans and nonhumans) to further our understanding of the various aspects of drug use, abuse, and dependence (such as initiation, relapse, prolonged abstinence, craving, and transitions from drug use to abuse); to develop improved behavioral and pharmacological interventions for the treatment of drug abuse and dependence; and to inform prevention efforts.

Although research in this area is difficult, it is an important investment, and researchers should be encouraged to explore new paradigms to model complex behaviors related to drug abuse. Importantly, the models must be validated if they are to have utility for the field and should combine a range of behavioral approaches including conditioning, social learning, and cognitive models, integrating them to most effectively emulate the complex behaviors represented by the various aspects of drug seeking and taking.

REFERENCES

Anthony JC, Warner LA, Kessler RC. 1994. Comparative epidemiology of dependence on tobacco, alcohol, controlled substances, and inhalants: Basic findings from the National Comorbidity Survey. *Experimental and Clinical Psychopharmacology* 2:244–268.

APA (American Psychiatric Association). 1994. *Diagnostic and Statistical Manual of Mental Disorders.* 4th ed. Washington, DC: APA.

Azrin NH, Hutchinson RR, Hake DF. 1966. Extinction-induced aggression. *Journal of the Experimental Analysis of Behavior* 9:191–204.

Balster RL, Willetts J. 1996. Phencyclidine: A drug of abuse and a tool for neuroscience research. In: Schuster CR, Gust SW, Kuhar MJ, eds. *Pharmacological Aspects of Drug Dependence: Towards an Integrated Neurobehavioral Approach. Handbook of Experimental Pharmacology* 118:233–262.

Barrett JE, Witkin JM. 1986. The role of behavioral and pharmacological history in determining the effects of abused drugs. In: Goldberg SR, Stolerman IP, eds. *Behavioral Analysis of Drug Dependence*. Orlando: Academic Press. Pp. 195–224.

Berger SP, Hall S, Mickalian JD, Reid MS, Crawford CA, Delucchi K, Carr K, Hall S. 1996. Haloperidol antagonism of cue-elicited cocaine craving. *Lancet* 347:504–508.

Bergman J, Madras BK, Johnson SE, Spealman RD. 1989. Effects of cocaine and related drugs in nonhuman primates. Part III. Self-administration by squirrel monkeys. *Journal of Pharmacology and Experimental Therapeutics* 251:150–155.

Bickel WK, Degrandpre RJ, Higgins ST. 1993. Behavioral economics: A novel experimental approach to the study of drug dependence. *Drug and Alcohol Dependence* 33:173–192.

Bonese KR, Wainer BH, Fitch FW, Rothberg RM, Schuster CR. 1974. Changes in heroin self-administration by rhesus monkey after morphine immunization. *Nature* 252:708–710.

Bozarth MA, Wise RA. 1984. Anatomically distinct opiate receptor fields mediate reward and physical dependence. *Science* 224:516–517.

Brady JV, Lukas SE. 1984. *Testing Drugs for Physical Dependence Potential and Abuse Liability. NIDA Research Monograph 52*. Rockville, MD: NIDA.

Brown SA. 1993. Drug effect expectancies and addictive behavior change. *Experimental and Clinical Psychopharmacology* 1:55–67.

Carrera MRA, Ashley JA, Parsons LH, Wirsching P, Koob GF, Janda KD. 1995. Suppression of psychoactive effects of cocaine by active immunization. *Nature* 378:727–730.

Carroll KM, Rounsaville BJ, Keller DS. 1991. Relapse prevention strategies for the treatment of cocaine abuse. *American Journal of Drug and Alcohol Abuse* 17:249–265.

Carroll ME. 1993. *Drugs and Environment*. Netherlands: Open University Press.

Carroll ME. 1995. Interactions between food and addiction. In: Niesink RJM, Kornet ML, eds. *Behavioral Toxicology and Addiction: Food, Drugs and Environment*. Netherlands: Open University Press.

Carroll ME, Rodefer JS. 1993. Income alters choice between drug and an alternative nondrug reinforcer in monkeys. *Experimental and Clinical Psychopharmacology* 1:110–120.

Carroll ME, Carmona GG, May SA. 1991. V. Cocaine self-administration in rats: Effects of non-drug alternative reinforcers on acquisition. *Psychopharmacology* 110:5–12.

Cerruti C, Pilotte NS, Uhl G, Kuhar MJ. 1994. Reduction in dopamine transporter MRNA after cessation of repeated cocaine administration. *Molecular Brain Research* 22:132–138.

Cherek DR. 1981. Effects of smoking different doses of nicotine on human aggressive behavior. *Psychopharmacology* 75:339–345.

Cherek DR, Bennett RH, Grabowski J. 1991. Human aggressive responding during acute tobacco abstinence: Effects of nicotine and placebo gum. *Psychopharmacology* 104:317–322.

Childress AR, McLellan AT, Ehrman R, O'Brien CP. 1988. Classically conditioned responses in opioid and cocaine dependence: A role in relapse? *NIDA Research Monograph* 84:25–43.

Childress AR, Mozley D, Fitzgerald J, Reivich M, Jaggi J, O'Brien CP. 1995. Limbic activation during cue-induced cocaine craving. *Society for Neuroscience Abstracts* 21(3):1956.

Chutuape MA, Mitchell S, de Wit H. 1994. Ethanol preloads increase ethanol preference under concurrent random-ratio schedules in social drinkers. *Experimental and Clinical Psychopharmacology* 2:310–318.

Cornell CE, Rodin J, Weingarten H. 1992. Stimulus-induced eating when satiated. *Physiology and Behavior* 45:695–704.

de Wit H, Chutuape MA. 1993. Increased ethanol choice in social drinkers following ethanol preload. *Behavioural Pharmacology* 4:29–36.

de Wit H, Stewart J. 1981. Drug reinstatement of heroin-reinforced responding in the rat. *Psychopharmacology* 79:29–31.

Droungas A, Ehrman RN, Childress AR, O'Brien CP. 1995. Effect of smoking cues and cigarette availability on craving and smoking behaviors. *Addictive Behaviors* 20:657–673.

Falk JL. 1984. The environmental generation of excessive behavior. In: Mule SJ, ed. *Behavior in Excess: An Examination of the Volitional Disorders*. New York: Free Press. Pp. 313–337.

Falk JL. 1993. Schedule-induced drug self-administration. In: Van Haaren F, ed. *Methods in Behavioral Pharmacology*. Amsterdam: Elsevier. Pp. 301–328.

Fiore M, Shi FY, Heishman SJ, Henningfield JE. 1994. *The Effect of Smoking and Smoking Withdrawal on Flight Performance: A 1994 Update*. Submitted by the Centers for Disease Control to the Federal Aviation Administration.

Fischman MW, Johanson CE. 1996. Cocaine. In: Schuster CR, Gust SW, Kuhar MJ, eds. *Pharmacological Aspects of Drug Dependence: Towards an Integrated Neurobehavioral Approach. Handbook of Experimental Pharmacology* 118:159–195.

Fischman MW, Foltin RW, Nestadt G, Pearlson GD. 1990. Effects of desipramine maintenance on cocaine self-administration by humans. *Journal of Pharmacology and Experimental Therapeutics* 253:760–770.

Fischman MW, Kelly TH, Foltin RW. 1991. Residential laboratory research: A multidimensional evaluation of the effects of drugs on behavior. *NIDA Research Monograph* 100:113–128.

Foltin RW, Fischman MW. 1994. Effects of buprenorphine on the self administration of cocaine by humans. *Behavioural Pharmacology* 5:79–89.

Froelich JC, Harts J, Lumen L, Li T-K. 1988. Differences in response to the aversive properties of ethanol in rats selectively bred for oral ethanol preference. *Pharmacology, Biochemistry and Behavior* 31:215–222.

George FR, Goldberg SR. 1989. Genetic approaches to the analysis of addiction processes. *Trends in Pharmacological Sciences* 10:78–83.

Goldberg SR, Schuster CR. 1967. Conditioned suppression by a stimulus associated with nalorphine in morphine-dependent monkeys. *Journal of the Experimental Analysis of Behavior* 10:235–242.

Goldberg SR, Schuster CR. 1969. Nalorphine: Increased sensitivity of monkeys formerly dependent on morphine. *Science* 166:1548–1549.

Goldberg SR, Woods JH, Schuster CR. 1970. Conditioned nalorphine-induced abstinence changes: Persistence in post morphine-dependent monkeys. *Journal of the Experimental Analysis of Behavior* 14:33–46.

Goldberg SR, Woods JH, Schuster CR. 1971. Nalorphine-induced changes in morphine self-administration in rhesus monkeys. *Journal of Pharmacology and Experimental Therapeutics* 176:464–471.

Henningfield JE. 1994. Comments on West's editorial, "Beneficial effects of nicotine: fact or fiction?" *Addiction* 89:135–146.

Higgins ST, Budney AJ, Bickel WK, Hughes JR, Foerg F, Badger G. 1993. Achieving cocaine abstinence with a behavioral approach. *American Journal of Psychiatry* 150:763–769.

Higgins ST, Bickel WK, Hughes JR. 1994. Influence of an alternative reinforcer on human cocaine self-administration. *Life Science* 55:179–187.

Horger BA, Wellman PJ, Morien A, Davies BT, Schenk S. 1991. Caffeine exposure sensitizes rats to the reinforcing effects of cocaine. *Neuro Report* 2:53–56.

Iguchi MY, Stitzer ML, Bigelow GE, Liebson IA. 1988. Contingency management in methadone maintenance: Effects of reinforcing and aversive consequences on illicit polydrug use. *Drug and Alcohol Dependence* 22:1–7.

IOM (Institute of Medicine). 1995. *The Development of Medications for the Treatment of Opiate and Cocaine Addictions*. Washington, DC: National Academy Press.

Johanson CE. 1975. Pharmacological and environmental variables affecting drug preference in monkeys. *Pharmacology Reviews* 27:343–355.

Kalivas PW, Duffy P. 1993. Time course of extracellular dopamine and behavioral sensitization to cocaine. I. Dopamine axon terminals. *Journal of Neuroscience* 13:266–275.

Koob GF, Bloom FE. 1989. Nucleus accumbens as a substrate for the aversive stimulus effects of opiate withdrawal. *Psychopharmacology* 98:530–534.

Koob GF, Pettit HO, Ettenberg A, Bloom FE. 1984. Effects of opiate antagonists and their quaternary derivatives on heroin self-administration in the rat. *Journal of Pharmacology and Experimental Therapeutics* 229:481–486.

Landry DW, Zhao K, Yang GX-Q, Glickman M, Georgiadis TM. 1993. Antibody-catalyzed degradation of cocaine. *Science* 259:1899–1901.

Marlatt GA, Gordon JR. 1985. *Relapse Prevention: Maintenance Strategies in the Treatment of Addictive Behaviors*. New York: Guilford Press.

Mello NK, Negus SS. In press. Preclinical evaluation of pharmacotherapies for treatment of cocaine and opiate abuse using drug self-administration procedures. *Neuropsychopharmacology*.

Mello NK, Mendelson JH, Kuehnle JC, Sellers MS. 1981. Operant analysis of human heroin self-administration and the effects of naltrexone. *Journal of Pharmacology and Experimental Therapeutics* 216:45–53.

Miczek KA, DeBold JF, Haney M, Tidey J, Vivian J, Weerts E. 1994. Alcohol, drugs of abuse, aggression and violence. In: Reis AJ, Miczek KA, Roth JA, eds. *Understanding and Preventing Violence: Biobehavioral Perspectives on Violence, Vol. 2*. Washington, DC: National Academy Press. Pp. 245–514.

Nader MA, Woolverton WL. 1991. Effects of increasing the magnitude of an alternative reinforcer on drug choice in a discrete-trials choice procedure. *Psychopharmacology* 105:169–174.

Nemeth-Coslett R, Henningfield HE. 1986. Effects of nicotine chewing gum on cigarette smoking and subjective and physiologic effects. *Clinical Pharmacology and Therapeutics* 39:625–630.

Nestler EJ. 1994. Molecular neurobiology of drug addiction. *Neuropsychopharmacology* 11:77–87.

O'Brien CP. 1975. Experimental analysis of conditioning factors in human narcotic addiction. *Pharmacological Reviews* 27:535–543.

O'Brien CP, Testa T, O'Brien TJ, Brady JP, Wells B. 1977. Conditioned narcotic withdrawal in humans. *Science* 195:1000–1002.

O'Brien CP, Childress AR, McLellan AT, Ehrman R. 1990. Integrating systemic cue exposure with standard treatment in recovering drug dependent patients. *Addictive Behaviors* 15:355–365.

Piazza PV, Deroche V, Deminiere JM, Maccari S, Le Moal M, Simon H. 1993. Corticosterone in the range of stress-induced levels possesses reinforcing properties: Implications for sensation-seeking behaviors. *Proceedings of the National Academy of Sciences (USA)* 90:11738–11743.

Ritz MC, Lamb RJ, Goldberg SR, Kuhar MJ. 1987. Cocaine receptors on dopamine transporters are related to self-administration of cocaine. *Science* 237:1219–1223.

Robbins S, Ehrman R, Childress AR, O'Brien CP. 1992. Using cue reactivity to screen medications for cocaine abuse: Amantadine hydrochloride. *Addictive Behaviors* 17:491–499.

Rusted JM, Warburton DM. 1992. Facilitation of memory by post-trial administration of nicotine: Evidence for an attentional explanation. *Psychopharmacology (Berl)* 108(4):452–455.

Schuster CR, Greenwald MK, Johanson CE, Heishman S. 1995. Measurement of drug craving during naltrexone-precipitated withdrawal in methadone-maintained volunteers. *Experimental and Clinical Psychopharmacology* 3:424–431.

Slikker W, Brocco MJ, Killam KF. 1984. Reinstatement of responding maintained by cocaine or thiamylal. *Journal of Pharmacology and Experimental Therapeutics* 228:43–52.

Stewart J, de Wit H, Eikelboom R. 1984. Role of unconditioned and conditioned drug effects in the self-administration of opiates and stimulants. *Psychological Review* 91:251–268.

Thompson T, Schuster CR. 1964. Morphine self-administration, food-reinforced and avoidance behaviors in rhesus monkeys. *Psychopharmacology* 5:87–94.

Tiffany ST. 1990. A cognitive model of drug urges and drug-use behavior: Role of automatic and nonautomatic processes. *Psychological Review* 97:147–168.

Tiffany ST, Singleton E, Haertzen CA, Henningfield JE. 1993. The development of a cocaine craving questionnaire. *Drug and Alcohol Dependence* 34:19–28.

WHO (World Health Organization). 1992. *International Statistical Classification of Diseases and Related Health Problems.* Tenth Revision. Geneva: WHO.

Wikler A. 1973. Dynamics of drug dependence: Implications of a conditioning theory for research and treatment. *Archives of General Psychiatry* 28:611–616.

Wikler A, Pescor F. 1967. Classical conditioning of the morphine abstinence phenomenon. Reinforcement of opioid drinking behavior and relapse in morphine addicted rats. *Psychopharmacologia* 10:255–284.

Woods JH, Schuster CR. 1968. Reinforcement properties of morphine, cocaine, and SPA as a function of unit dose. *International Journal of the Addictions* 3:231–236.

3

Neuroscience

Over the past 20 years, drug abuse research has contributed to impressive gains in the neurosciences and in our understanding of brain function. Neuroscience research as it relates to drug abuse has advanced knowledge about neurotransmitters and neural pathways, and has yielded information about brain mechanisms both under normal conditions and when affected by drugs of abuse. That knowledge has already been translated into improved clinical care and has had significant impacts on other scientific disciplines.

The goal of neuroscience research in the area of drug dependence is to determine the actions of abusable drugs on the brain that result in dependence and to determine the neural substrates that make one individual inherently vulnerable to such actions and others relatively resistant. That knowledge can have an impact on the ways in which drug abuse and dependence are managed clinically and on the way they are viewed by our society. Neuroscience research can add to the knowledge base in the science of addiction and provide information for the development of more effective medications to treat drug dependence. New pharmacotherapies will significantly improve the effectiveness of psychosocial interventions. It must be emphasized that it is impossible to predict all of the benefits of ongoing fundamental neuroscience research in the drug abuse field. Many of the advances that will be discussed throughout this chapter were unanticipated, yet clearly improved public health in many ways.

The interface between basic neurobiology and the applied neuroscience of drug abuse research has been a rich and fruitful part of the approach termed integrative neuroscience. Drug abuse research has contributed to many discoveries in neuroendocrinology and the neurobiology of stress including the discovery of opioid peptides and stress neurotransmitters, the neurochemical control of stress hormone, and reproductive hormone release. In addition, drug abuse research impacts on disciplines as diverse as molecular biology, the neurobiology of emotional behavior, and the neurobiology of cognitive function in the effort to understand the complex phenomena associated with a course of drug dependence.

The following chapter contains a technical overview illustrating the complexity of the neurotransmission processes involved in the neurobiology of drug dependence, a description of the many advances in understanding the neurobiological basis for drug dependence, a summary of gaps and needs, and finally recommendations for future research. The technical overview provides the vocabulary and basic concepts necessary to understand how drugs can interact at many different functional levels including the molecular, cellular, and systems levels. The section on accomplishments details the significant advances in understanding the neurobiology of drug reinforcement and the beginnings of our understanding of the processes of neuroadaptation to these systems associated with dependence. In addition, the chapter describes progress in human imaging research and the recent developments in understanding brain mechanisms of pain and analgesia. Gaps and needs are identified that focus on the chronic consequences of drug exposure in brain systems implicated in the motivational effects of drug dependence at the molecular, cellular, and system levels of analysis. Finally, the chapter identifies numerous areas for research opportunities that will aid in our understanding of the neurobiology of drug dependence and help integrate this basic research with the applied problems of vulnerability, treatment, and prevention of drug abuse. These areas include molecular neurobiology, genetics research, animal models of dependence, brain imaging, co-occurring psychiatric disorders, HIV models, neurotoxicity of drug dependence, immunology, analgesia and pain, and relapse and prolonged abstinence.

NEUROTRANSMISSION AND ITS EFFECTS

The human brain is composed of an enormous number of neurons, with estimates ranging from 10 billion to 10 trillion (reviewed by Kandel et al., 1991; Hyman and Nestler, 1993). These neurons are organized in such a way that they communicate with one another in a highly intricate and specific manner. This process of communication is referred to as synaptic transmission.

In a simplified scheme, neurons consist of a cell body or soma; multiple dendrites that arise from the cell body to receive incoming signals; and usually a single axon that also arises from the cell body. Axons can be very long and give rise to outgoing signals through their branched ends (terminals). A single neuron can possess thousands of axon terminals and thereby form connections (called synapses) with up to thousands of other neurons. The brain utilizes a chemical process of neurotransmission to transfer information across synapses. Briefly, an electrochemical impulse produced by changes in concentrations of ions across the axon membrane travels down the axon of one neuron, invades the axon's nerve terminals, and triggers the release of a chemical substance, called a neurotransmitter, from the terminals. The neurotransmitter diffuses across the synaptic cleft (the space between the two neurons) and binds to specific receptor proteins located on the surface of the cell, or plasma membrane, of the next neuron. The binding of a neurotransmitter to its receptor activates the receptor and causes a change in the flow of ions across the cell membrane, which can either lead to or inhibit the generation of electrical impulses in that next neuron. The neurotransmitter stimulus is then "turned off" either by enzymatic degradation in the synaptic cleft or by protein-mediated reuptake of neurotransmitter into the nerve terminal. Neurons receive incoming signals from hundreds or thousands of nerve terminals. Whether a neuron fires an impulse is determined by the summation of those numerous inputs.

Neuronal membranes contain classes of proteins, termed ion pumps, that maintain unequal concentrations of ions (e.g., Na^+, K^+, Ca^{2+}, Cl^-) between the outside and inside of the cell. The most important pump is termed the Na^+–K^+ ATPase (adenosine triphosphatase). Neurons are polarized, meaning that the inside of the cell is negatively charged with respect to the outside. Neurons also possess other proteins in their plasma membrane, termed ion channels, that allow passage of specific ions across the cell membrane. Neurotransmitters regulate the electrical properties of neurons by activating or inhibiting the activity of specific types of ion channels.

Neurotransmitters and Their Receptors

The majority of neurotransmission in the brain is performed by amino acid neurotransmitters, which are contained in two-thirds of all synapses in the brain. Glutamate is the major excitatory neurotransmitter in the brain because its receptor channel permits Na^+ (and in some cases Ca^{2+}) to flow into the cell; the major inhibitory neurotransmitter in the brain is gamma-aminobutyric acid (GABA) (GABA's receptor channel carries Cl^- into the cell).

Most other neurotransmitters in the brain bind to receptor proteins that do not contain ion channels within their structures. Rather, these receptors produce their physiological effects by interacting with a special class of proteins, called G proteins, which are composed of three variable molecules, called alpha, beta, and gamma subunits. When a neurotransmitter binds to a G protein-coupled receptor, the G protein dissociates into a free alpha and free beta-gamma subunit, which then interacts with many other cellular proteins to produce a variety of physiological effects. For example, specific types of ion channels can be induced to increase or decrease their activity by the action of G protein subunits.

Second Messengers and Protein Phosphorylation

The G protein-coupled receptors also influence many other neural processes through complex pathways of intracellular messengers. The first steps in these pathways are "second messengers" (the neurotransmitter is considered the first messenger, and the G protein a coupling factor). Prominent second messengers in the brain are cAMP (cyclic adenosine monophosphate), cGMP (cyclic guanosine monophosphate), Ca^{2+}, nitric oxide, and metabolites of arachidonic acid (e.g., prostaglandins) and phosphatidylinositol. The G protein-coupled receptors control the levels of these second messengers by regulating the activity of enzymes that catalyze the synthesis and degradation of second messengers, with different effects produced depending on the G protein involved.[1] For example, neurotransmitters that increase cAMP levels act through Gs, which binds to and stimulates adenylyl cyclase, the enzyme that catalyzes the synthesis of cAMP. Other neurotransmitters decrease cAMP levels by acting through Gi, which binds to and inhibits adenylyl cyclase. Still other neurotransmitters do not affect cAMP, but instead increase the generation of phosphatidylinositol-derived second messengers.

The next step in these intracellular pathways is the regulation, by second messengers, of protein phosphorylation, the process by which phosphate groups are added to or removed from specific amino acid residues by protein kinases and protein phosphatases, respectively. Phosphate groups, because of their large size and negative charge, affect the conformation and charge of proteins, which in turn affect their physiological function. For example, phosphorylation of ion channels and pumps affects their ability to open or close or to allow ions to pass through them. Phosphorylation of receptors affects their ability to bind to their

---

[1]There are three subtypes of G proteins (guanine nucleotide-binding membrane proteins). Gs is stimulatory in that it stimulates adenylyl cyclase, and Gi is inhibitory in that it inhibits adenylyl cyclase. Gq is the third subtype but the "q" has no implicit meaning.

neurotransmitters or interact with their G proteins. Phosphorylation of enzymes affects their catalytic activity (e.g., phosphorylation of adenylyl cyclase can increase its capacity to synthesize cAMP).

The brain contains many types of protein kinases and protein phosphatases that exhibit differential regulation. For example, cAMP activates cAMP-dependent protein kinases, Ca^{2+} activates Ca^{2+}-dependent protein kinases, etc. Each type of protein kinase then phosphorylates a specific array of target proteins and thereby produces many additional effects of the original neurotransmitter–G protein–second messenger stimulus.

Due to the multiple effects of phosphorylation on a number of important intracellular processes, a neurotransmitter stimulus can influence virtually every chemical process that occurs within its target neurons. Some effects, such as alterations in electrical activity, are very rapid (within seconds) and short-lived. Other effects, such as alterations in gene expression, can develop more slowly (over minutes or hours) and last for a long time. These more long-lasting effects of a neurotransmitter stimulus alter the manner in which the target neuron responds to subsequent stimuli—both the original neurotransmitter and others—and presumably represent the basis of neural adaptation and change, called plasticity. Together, these types of responses of widely differing time courses allow neurons to exert very complex control over other neurons operating within neural circuits.

Neurotrophic Factor Signaling Pathways

Second-messenger–regulated protein phosphorylation is just one component of a neuron's complex intracellular regulatory mechanisms. Neurons contain many protein kinases and protein phosphatases in addition to those regulated by second messengers, and these enzymes also contribute to the diverse effects that a neurotransmitter stimulus exerts on its target neurons. For example, neurotrophic factors were first studied for their important role in neural development and differentiation. However, it is now known that neurotrophic factors also play an important role in the regulation of the fully differentiated adult brain. One important family of neurotrophic factors, called neurotrophins, binds to a class of receptor that contains a special type of protein kinase within its structure, a protein tyrosine kinase, which phosphorylates proteins specifically on tyrosine residues. Binding of neurotrophin to its protein tyrosine kinase receptor activates the kinase activity and leads to the phosphorylation of specific cellular proteins and, eventually, to a cascade of protein kinase activity. Thus, neurotrophic factor-related signaling pathways are another example of the complexity of a neuron's intracellular regulatory machinery, and serve to highlight the complex types of effects that a neurotransmitter stimulus produces in its target neurons which ultimately contributes to the short- and long-term effects of neurotransmitters on the brain.

Understanding Drug Dependence in the Context of Neurotransmission

All drugs of abuse interact initially with receptor or reuptake proteins, summarized in Table 3.1 (Nestler et al., 1995). For example, opiates activate opioid receptors, and cocaine inhibits reuptake proteins for the monoamine neurotransmitters (which include dopamine, norepinephrine, and serotonin). These initial effects lead to alterations in the levels of specific neurotransmitters, or to different activation states of specific neurotransmitter receptors, in the brain. Opiate activation of opioid receptors, for example, leads to recruitment of inhibitory and related G proteins. This, in turn, leads to activation of K^+ channels and inhibition of Ca^{2+} channels. Both are inhibitory actions, because more K^+ flows out of the cell and less Ca^{2+} flows into the cell. Thus, the electrical properties of the target neurons are affected relatively rapidly by opiates. Recruitment of the inhibitory G protein also inhibits adenylyl cyclase, and reductions in cellular Ca^{2+} levels decrease Ca^{2+}-dependent protein phosphorylation cascades, altering the activity of still additional ion channels. These effects, along with changes in many other neural processes within target neurons, contribute further to the acute effects of opiates. The sum of such

TABLE 3.1 Acute Effects of Abused Drugs on Neurotransmitters

Drug	Action
Opiates	Agonist at opioid receptors
Cocaine	Inhibits monoamine reuptake transporters
Amphetamine	Stimulates monoamine release
Alcohol	Facilitates $GABA_A$ receptor function and inhibits *N*-methyl-*D*-aspartate (NMDA) glutamate receptor function[a]
Nicotine	Agonist at nicotinic acetylcholine receptors
Cannabinoids	Agonist at cannabinoid receptors[b]
Hallucinogens	Partial agonist at $5\text{-}HT_2$[c] serotonin receptors
Phencyclidine (PCP)	Antagonist at NMDA glutamate receptors

[a]The mechanism by which alcohol produces these effects has not been established but would not appear to involve direct alcohol binding to the receptors as is the case for the other drugs listed in this table.

[b]Although a specific receptor for cannabinoids has been identified in the brain, the endogenous ligand for this receptor has not yet been identified with certainty.

[c]5-Hydroxytryptamine-2.

changes presumably triggers the longer-term effects of the drugs that eventually lead to abuse, dependence, tolerance, and withdrawal.

ACCOMPLISHMENTS

Significant advances in understanding the neurobiological basis of drug dependence in the past 25 years are now beginning to provide a strong scientific basis for drug abuse treatment, prevention, and etiology. Drug dependence has long been associated with some perturbation of the brain reward systems. At the systems level, specific neural circuits within the midbrain–forebrain connection of the medial forebrain bundle have been identified that mediate the acute reinforcing effects of drugs (Figure 3.1) (Koob, 1992a). These neural circuits are composed of specific chemical neurotransmitters and include the midbrain dopamine systems, the endogenous opioid peptide systems, and other neurotransmitters such as serotonin, GABA, and glutamate. These systems appear to be modified during the development of dependence and appear to remain sensitive to future perturbations. Cellular studies have identified specific changes in the function of different components of that midbrain–forebrain system and are beginning to provide a framework for the adaptive changes within neurons that are associated with withdrawal and sensitization (Nestler, 1992). Molecular studies not only have identified the specific neurotransmitter receptors and receptor subtypes important for mediating those reinforcement actions, but also have begun to provide a molecular basis for the long-term plasticity associated with relapse and vulnerability (Nestler, 1994). The remainder of this section highlights some of the neurobiological advances resulting from research on individual differences; neural substrates of reinforcement, withdrawal, tolerance, and relapse; pharmacotherapy; and brain imaging.

Individual Differences

It is widely presumed that individuals differ in their predilection for drug dependence (see Chapter 5). This has been demonstrated in epidemiological studies of alcoholism, but it remains largely unproven for other addictive disorders. There is, however, growing evidence of individual differences in responsiveness to drugs of abuse in laboratory animals.

Genetic Factors

Genetically inbred strains of mice and rats exhibit clearly different behavioral responses to one or another drug of abuse (Li and Lumeng, 1984; Pickens and Svikis, 1988; George and Goldberg, 1989; Guitart et al.,

1993; Kosten et al., 1994). Such strain differences have been demonstrated with respect to numerous behavioral measures, including locomotor activity and sensitization, physical dependence, drug self-administration, conditioned place preference, and brain stimulation reward (Li et al., 1986; Crabbe et al., 1994). These observations suggest that there are likely genetic determinants of diverse aspects of drug action, including drug reinforcement. Researchers have also observed that genetically inbred strains of mice and rats differ not only in acute responses to drugs of abuse but also in responses to repeated drug exposure (e.g., George and Goldberg, 1989; Nestler, 1992; Guitart et al., 1993; Kosten et al., 1994), indicating that pharmacodynamic differences may reside in part at the level of gene expression. This research has implications for the treatment of drug abuse discussed later in the chapter.

Environmental Factors

In animal models, environmental factors also contribute to an individual's responses to drugs of abuse. First, exposure to a drug of abuse itself influences an animal's subsequent responses to the drug, including the reinforcing effects of a drug (Piazza et al., 1989; Horger et al., 1992). Second, other types of environmental factors have been shown to influence an animal's responses to drugs of abuse. One prominent example is stress, which can enhance the reinforcing and locomotor activating effects of several drugs of abuse, including cocaine and other stimulants, opiates, and alcohol (Volpicelli et al., 1986; Piazza et al., 1989; Vezina and Stewart, 1990; Cunningham and Kelley, 1992; Hamamura and Fibiger, 1993; Koob and Cador, 1993; Sorg and Kalivas, 1993; Goeders and Guerin, 1994; Shaham and Stewart, 1994). The effects of stress may be mediated, at least in part, via stress systems such as the hypothalamic–pituitary–adrenal axis, which is known to be activated by stress, and extrahypothalmic stress systems because mediators of those systems, including corticotropin-releasing factor (CRF) and glucocorticoids, alter drug reinforcement and drug-induced locomotor activity (Cole et al., 1990; Piazza et al., 1991). These findings have relevance in the clinical setting for the treatment of drug dependence since continued exposure to environmental factors increases an individual's risk for drug abuse and dependence (see Chapter 2). More work is needed, however, in the area of environmental factors on drug dependence and their neurobiological impact.

Genetic-Environmental Interactions

One way to understand these observations is that genes determine an individual animal's potential responses to drugs of abuse, whereas environmental factors shape that genetic potential. That is, environmental exposures (e.g., a drug or stress) alter the brain in different ways depending on the genetic template of the brain. Particularly powerful environmental exposures (e.g., high levels of a drug of abuse) may lead to the same types of changes in the brain despite genetic differences (Nestler, 1992). Together, genetic and environmental factors combine to set an individual's responses to drugs of abuse. Identification of the specific genetic and environmental factors that influence the actions of drugs of abuse in animal models can provide insight into the types of genetic factors that contribute to an individual vulnerability for drug dependence in humans (Hilbert et al., 1991).

Neural Substrates of Drug Abuse

Neural Substrates of Reinforcement

A multineurotransmitter system called the medial forebrain bundle, which courses from the ventral midbrain to the basal forebrain, has long been associated with reinforcement and reward (Olds and Milner, 1954; Olds, 1962; Stein, 1968; Wise, 1989). Electrical stimulation through electrodes implanted along this bundle is considered to be pleasurable or rewarding because animals will perform certain tasks repeatedly (e.g., pressing a bar) to trigger the stimulation (self-stimulation). Thresholds for that intracranial self-stimulation are lowered by drugs of abuse, suggesting that they "sensitize" the brain reward system. Recent advances exploring the neurobiological basis for the positive reinforcing effects of drugs of abuse have focused on specific neurochemical systems that make up the medial forebrain bundle reward system.

Psychomotor stimulants, such as cocaine and amphetamine, appear to depend on an increase in the synaptic release of dopamine in the mesolimbic dopamine system (Koob, 1992b). This system has its cell bodies of origin in the ventral tegmental area and projects to the nucleus accumbens, olfactory tubercle, frontal cortex, and amygdala. Cocaine is thought to act mainly to block reuptake of dopamine by binding to a specific protein, the dopamine transporter protein, involved in reuptake; amphetamines both enhance dopamine release and block its reuptake. Three of the five cloned dopamine receptor subtypes have been implicated in the reinforcing actions of cocaine (Woolverton, 1986; Koob, 1992b; Caine and Koob, 1993).

Opiate drugs bind to opioid receptors to produce their reinforcing effects.[2] The mu receptor appears to be most important for the reinforc-

[2]Three known receptor subtypes have been cloned: mu, delta, and kappa.

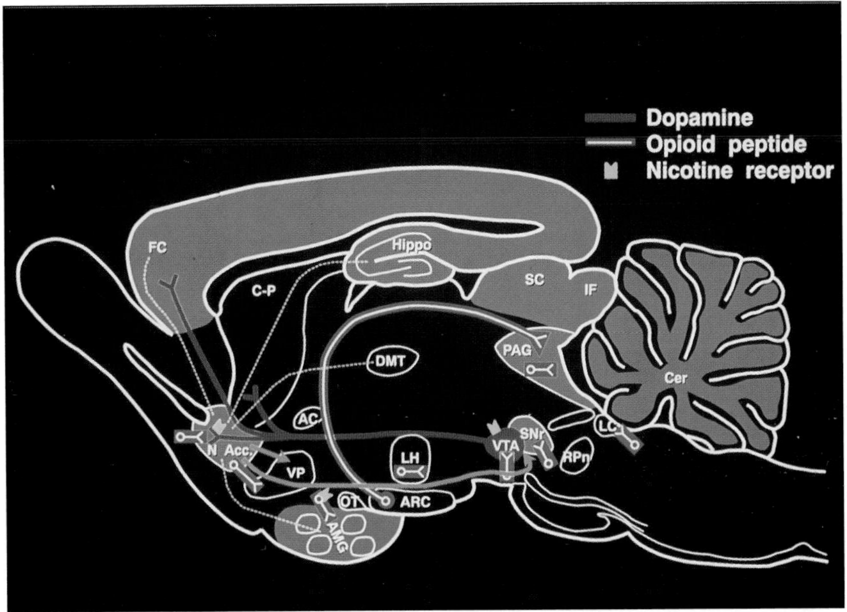

FIGURE 3.1 Sagittal rat brain section illustrating a drug (cocaine, amphetamine, opiate, and alcohol) neural reward circuit that includes a limbic-extrapyramidal motor interface. Yellow dotted lines indicate limbic afferents to the nucleus accumbens (N Acc.), and orange represents efferents from the nucleus accumbens thought to be involved in psychomotor stimulant reward. Red indicates projection of the mesocorticolimbic dopamine system thought to be a critical substrate for psychomotor stimulant reward. This system originates in the A10 cell group of the ventral tegmental area (VTA) and projects to the N. Acc., olfactory tubercle, and ventral striatal domains of the caudate-putamen (C-P). Green indicates opioid peptide-containing neurons, systems that may be involved in opiate and ethanol reward. These opioid peptide systems include the local enkephalin circuits (short segments) and the hypothalamic midbrain beta-endorphin circuit (long segment). Blue indicates the approximate distribution of GABA-A receptor complexes, some of which may mediate sedative/hypnotic (ethanol) reward, determined by both tritiated flumazenil binding and expression of the alpha, beta, and gamma subunits of the GABA-A receptor. Yellow refers to nicotinic receptors hypothesized to be localized on dopamine and opioid peptide systems. AC, anterior commissure; AMG, amygdala; Cer, cerebullum; DMT, dorsomedial thalamus; FC, frontal cortex; Hippo, hippocampus; LC, locus coeruleus; LH, lateral hypothalamus; OT, olfactory tract; PAG, periaqueductal gray; SNr, substantia nigra pars reticulata; VP, ventral pallidum. Modified with permission of Elsevier Science LTD., from Koob, 1992a.

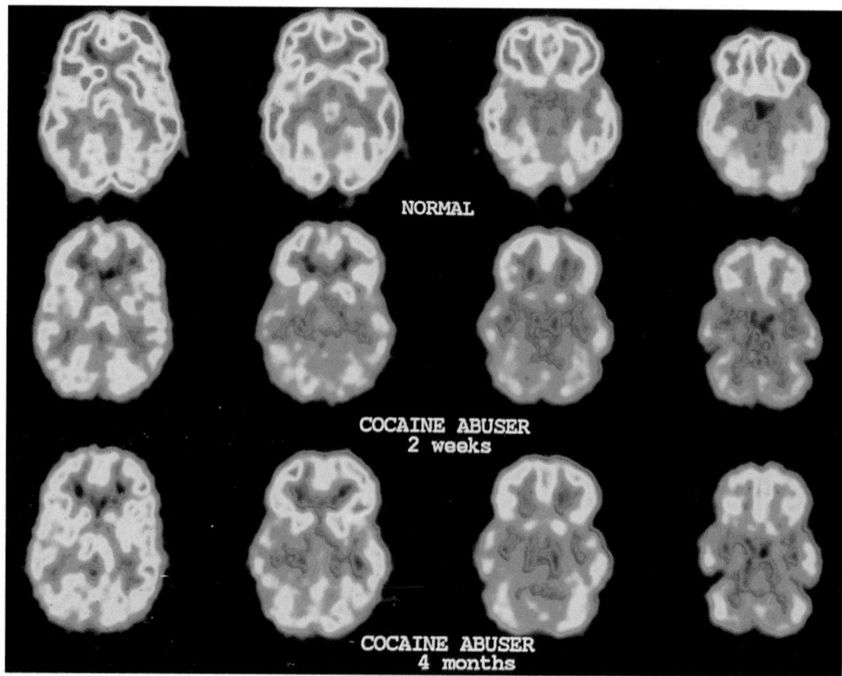

FIGURE 3.2 Metabolic images obtained with FDG in a normal control and in a cocaine abuser tested 3 months after cocaine discontinuation. Notice the reductions in metabolism in frontal brain regions when compared with the control. Reprinted with permission from N. Volkow, Brookhaven National Laboratory.

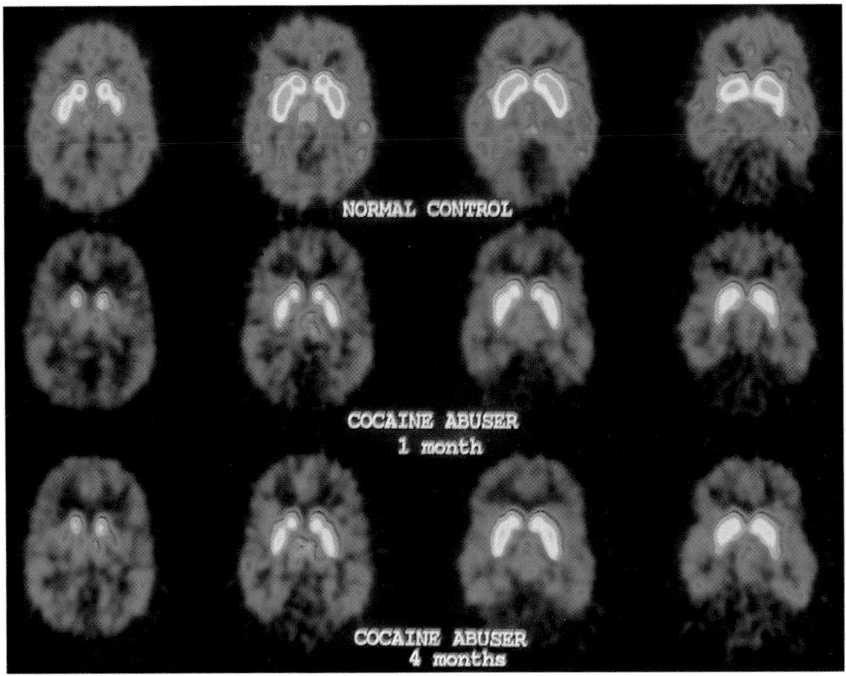

FIGURE 3.3 [18F]N-methylspiroperidol images in a normal control and in a cocaine abuser tested 1 month and 4 months after last cocaine use. The images correspond to the four sequential planes where the basal ganglia are located. Notice the lower uptake of the tracer in the cocaine abuser when compared with the normal control. Notice the persistence of the decreased uptake even after 4 months of cocaine discontinuation (Reprinted by permission of John Wiley & Sons, Inc. from Volkow et al., 1993).

ing effects of heroin and morphine, and the most important brain sites for the acute reinforcing actions of those drugs appear to be in the ventral tegmental area and the nucleus accumbens. Opiates stimulate the release of dopamine in the terminal areas of the mesolimbic dopamine system, and there also appears to be a dopamine-independent action in the region of the nucleus accumbens on neuronal systems that receive a dopaminergic input (Koob, 1992a).

Ethanol and other sedative hypnotics clearly have multiple sites of action for their acute reinforcing effects, which depend on facilitation of GABAergic neurotransmission, stimulation of dopamine release at low doses, activation of endogenous opioid peptide systems, and antagonism of serotonergic and glutamatergic neurotransmission. The exact sites for these actions are under study but appear again to involve the mesolimbic dopamine system and its connections in the basal forebrain, particularly in limbic areas such as the amygdala.

Nicotine is a direct agonist at brain nicotinic acetylcholine receptors, which are widely distributed throughout the brain. Nicotine self-administration is blocked by dopamine antagonists and opioid peptide antagonists, and both a nicotinic acetylcholine antagonist and an opiate antagonist have been shown to precipitate nicotine withdrawal in rodents (Malin et al., 1993, 1994). Nicotine is thus thought to activate both the mesolimbic dopamine system and opioid peptide systems in the same neural circuitry associated with other drugs of abuse (Corrigall et al., 1992).

The neurobiological substrates for the acute reinforcing actions of psychedelic drugs are less well understood. Indeed, rodents and nonhuman primates will not self-administer psychedelic drugs. Lysergic acid diethylamide (LSD) clearly involves a serotonergic action, possibly as a postsynaptic agonist. However, the brain sites and specific subtypes involved are still under study. Little is known about the neurobiology of the acute reinforcing actions of marijuana, but the cloning of the tetrahydrocannabinol (THC) receptor and the discovery of endogenous THC compounds in the brain offer exciting new approaches to this question, discussed below (Matsuda et al., 1990; Devane et al., 1992).

Neural Substrates for Drug Tolerance

The neural substrates for drug tolerance overlap significantly with those associated with dependence because tolerance and dependence may be components of the same neuroadaptive process. Tolerance also involves associative processes (processes of learning where previously neutral stimuli come to acquire significance through pairing with biologically significant events), however, and the role of associative processes has been most explored in the context of opiate drugs and sedative-hypnotics such as alcohol (Young and Goudie, 1995). Both operant (behavioral tolerance) and classical (context-dependent tolerance) conditioning have been shown to play a role in drug tolerance, and mechanisms for these associative processes may involve several neurotransmitters independent of their role in dependence. Norepinephrine and serotonin have long been known to be involved in the development of tolerance to ethanol and barbiturates (Tabakoff and Hoffman, 1992). More recently, administration of glutamate antagonists has been shown to block the development of tolerance, again consistent with an associative component of tolerance (Trujillo and Akil, 1991).

Mechanisms of tolerance at the molecular level often overlap with those of dependence (Nestler et al., 1993).[3] For example, up-regulation of the cAMP pathway could be a mechanism of tolerance; the changes would be expected to oppose the acute actions of opiates of inhibiting adenylyl cyclase. In addition, tolerance seems to involve the functional uncoupling of opioid receptors from their G proteins. The mechanisms underlying this uncoupling remain unknown but could involve drug-induced changes in the phosphorylation state of the receptors or G proteins that reduce their affinity for each other. Another possible mechanism of tolerance involves drug-induced changes in the ion channels that mediate the acute effects of drugs. For example, alterations in the phosphorylation state, amount, or even type of channel conceivably could contribute to drug tolerance (Nestler, 1992).

Neural Substrates of Withdrawal

Withdrawal from chronic use of drugs of abuse is characterized by a dependence syndrome that is made up of two elements. The objectively observable physical signs of alcohol withdrawal are tremor and autonomic hyperactivity; abdominal discomfort and pain are associated with opiate withdrawal. The self-reported "psychological" signs of drug withdrawal, which may be considered more motivational, are usually different components of a negative emotional state including dysphoria, depression, anxiety, and malaise (Koob et al., 1993) and are difficult to measure directly in animals. Behavioral history is a primary determinant of whether withdrawal and the negative affective state associated with it produce drug-seeking behavior. For individuals with a history of self-medication of opiates and alcohol, physical dependence is an important

[3]Tolerance and dependence can be separated operationally at the molecular level in vitro, but at the systems level they are usually related when the same dependent variable is measured for both constructs.

factor in motivating individuals to seek out and self-administer opiates and alcohol. The phenomenon of physical dependence, however, does not produce drug-seeking behavior in the majority of individuals made physically dependent in the course of treatment with an opiate for a medical condition. The neural substrates for the physical signs of withdrawal are, in fact, not well understood. There is evidence that the changes in body temperature associated with opiate withdrawal may be due to interactions in the hypothalamus. The neural substrates for many of the other physical signs are distributed widely throughout the brain. Much evidence implicates the nucleus locus coeruleus (a nucleus containing exclusively norepinephrine neurons located in the brain stem region called the pons) in the activational properties and stresslike effects of opiate withdrawal (Aghajanian, 1978; Taylor et al., 1988; Maldonado et al., 1992). Little evidence exists for the neural substrates of ethanol withdrawal, but some neuropharmacological mechanisms have been identified including a decrease in GABAergic function, an increase in glutamatergic function (Grant et al., 1990; Tabakoff and Hoffman, 1992; Koob et al., 1994b), and related changes in calcium channel function (Littleton et al., 1992).

Additional research has begun to focus on the neural substrates and neuropharmacological mechanisms of the negative affective states associated with drug withdrawal—effects that probably produce much of the negative reinforcement associated with drug dependence. The same neural systems implicated in the positive reinforcing effects of drugs of abuse have been shown to be involved in those motivational effects. Evidence suggests that reward thresholds are increased (decrease in reward) following chronic administration of all major drugs of abuse, including opiates, psychostimulants, alcohol, nicotine, and THC. These effects reflect changes in the activity of the same mesolimbic system (midbrain–forebrain system) implicated in the positive reinforcing effects of drugs and can last up to 72 hours (Schaefer and Michael, 1986; Markou and Koob, 1991; Koob et al., 1993, 1994b; Schulteis et al., 1994, 1995).

The neurobiology of the change in reward function associated with drug dependence is a very active area of current research. Decreases in the function of neurochemical systems associated with the same neurotransmitters implicated in the acute reinforcing effects of drugs have been observed during withdrawal following chronic administration of cocaine, opiates, and ethanol. One example is where dopamine function in the nucleus accumbens appears to be decreased during cocaine, opiate, and ethanol withdrawal as measured by in vivo microdialysis (Weiss et al., 1992). Also, there is evidence of decreased opioid peptide receptor function in the nucleus accumbens during opiate withdrawal (Nestler, 1992). Serotonin function also appears to be decreased during acute withdrawal from psychostimulants and ethanol in the nucleus accumbens

(Parsons et al., 1995). As noted above, both GABAergic and glutamatergic systems have been implicated in ethanol withdrawal and may be of motivational significance for the changes occurring in the mesolimbic system and its connections. All of those transmitter systems have been implicated in the acute reinforcing effects of those drugs of abuse. However, evidence also exists for the recruitment of other neurotransmitter systems associated with stress-like responses during drug dependence. One example is the increased functional activity of the opioid peptide dynorphin in the nucleus accumbens following chronic cocaine administration, and this may contribute to the negative affective state of withdrawal (Hurd et al., 1992; Spanagel et al., 1992). Also, corticotropin releasing factor function appears to be activated during acute withdrawal to cocaine, alcohol, and opiates, and thus may mediate aspects of stress associated with abstinence (Koob et al., 1994a). More prolonged post-acute withdrawal changes have been observed in the mesolimbic dopamine system that may subserve the phenomenon of sensitization. Animals previously exposed to stress or psychostimulant drugs show enhanced responsiveness to the activating and rewarding effects of psychostimulants after the acute withdrawal period. This behavioral sensitization is paralleled by increased dopamine activity in the mesolimbic dopamine system (Robinson and Berridge, 1993).

Significant insight is now available concerning the molecular and cellular mechanisms of drug dependence. A model of such mechanisms is the locus coeruleus, the major noradrenergic nucleus in the brain, which plays an important role in physical dependence on opiates (Aghajanian, 1978; Taylor et al., 1988; Rasmussen et al., 1990; Koob et al., 1992; Maldonado and Koob, 1993). Activation of the locus coeruleus has been shown to mediate many of the signs and symptoms of physical opiate withdrawal in rodents and nonhuman primates. In fact, it was the identification of opiate action in the locus coeruleus that led to the introduction of clonidine, an alpha-2-adrenergic agonist, as the first nonopiate treatment that decreases the autonomically mediated signs of opiate withdrawal (Aghajanian, 1978; Gold et al., 1978).

We now know that the activation of the locus coeruleus during withdrawal is due to a combination of intrinsic (arising within the specific brain region) and extrinsic (arising from another brain region) factors. The intrinsic mechanisms involve up-regulation of the cAMP pathway (Sharma et al., 1975; Nestler, 1992; Nestler et al., 1993). Acutely, opiates inhibit the cAMP pathway in the locus coeruleus by inhibiting adenylyl cyclase, a molecular site of action for opiate neuroadaptation described above (Collier, 1980). In contrast, chronic exposure to opiates increases the amount of adenylyl cyclase and cAMP-dependent protein kinase expressed in the neurons. This up-regulated cAMP pathway has been shown to contribute to the increase in the electrical excitability of locus coeruleus neurons associated with withdrawal. A major unanswered question is the precise mechanism (e.g., at the level of transcription, translation, or protein modification) by which chronic opiate exposure leads to up-regulation of the cAMP pathway (Nestler, 1992).

The extrinsic mechanisms of withdrawal activation of the locus coeruleus involve increased activation of the major glutamatergic input to the locus coeruleus, which arises from a brain stem area called the paragigantocellularis (Rasmussen and Aghajanian, 1989; Akaoka and Aston-Jones, 1991). A major unanswered question is what drives this increase in glutamatergic tone. Presumably, chronic opiate exposure leads to changes in the glutamatergic neurons of the paragigantocellularis themselves or in neurons that drive those neurons in some neural circuit (Nestler, 1992).

Much less is known about the molecular and cellular mechanisms of changes in the negative affective state associated with drug dependence, although there is some evidence to suggest that similar mechanisms may be involved. Several drugs of abuse up-regulate the cAMP pathway in the nucleus accumbens after chronic administration (Nestler et al., 1993; Nestler, 1994; Self and Nestler, 1995). This up-regulation could mediate some of the documented electrophysiological changes in the nucleus accumbens associated with chronic drug exposure, such as enhanced responsiveness of D-1 dopamine receptors after chronic cocaine treatment (Henry and White, 1991). Moreover, studies involving direct administration of activators or inhibitors of the cAMP pathway into the nucleus accumbens are consistent with the interpretation that up-regulation of the cAMP pathway in this brain region may contribute to the negative affective state during drug withdrawal (Self and Nestler, 1995). The development of improved animal models will enable further study of negative affective states associated with drug withdrawal.

Neural Substrates of Relapse

Neurobiological mechanisms associated with relapse have been hampered by limited development of animal models. The term relapse is often used to describe a return to drug use despite an individual's attempt to remain abstinent. Thus, incorporation of some motivation to remain abstinent in animal models is necessary. The few studies that exist, using neuropharmacological probes to reinstate self-administration in animals trained and then extinguished on intravenous drug self-administration, have shown that drugs that activate the mesolimbic dopamine system rapidly reinstate intravenous self-administration (de Wit and Stewart, 1981; Stewart and de Wit, 1987). Further progress in understanding relapse will require better animal models.

Pharmacotherapy

Antagonists

The hypothesis that antagonizing the positive reinforcing actions of drugs of abuse would prevent relapse and effectively treat drug dependence has received significant preclinical attention. Basic neuropharmacology has shown that all the behavioral effects of opiate drugs, including their positive reinforcing actions, can be reversed by the opiate antagonist naloxone (Di Chiara and North, 1992; Koob, 1992a). The opiate receptor subtype involved in heroin and morphine reinforcement appears to be largely the mu receptor. For cocaine, no specific competitive antagonist has been identified, but antagonism of dopamine receptors in the mesolimbic system appears to block competitively the reinforcing effects of cocaine (Woolverton and Johnson, 1992). Three of the five dopamine receptor subtypes have been implicated in these reinforcing effects, particularly the D-1 and D-3 receptors.

For benzodiazepines, a selective competitive antagonist has been characterized, but not studied in the context of benzodiazepine reinforcement, and it has little effect on ethanol reinforcement (Samson and Harris, 1992). Ethanol reinforcement can be blunted by antagonists and agonists to a number of neurotransmitter systems (Samson and Harris, 1992; Koob et al., 1994b), but none to date has proven wholly specific to or competitive with ethanol. Ethanol reinforcement can be decreased by GABA antagonists, dopamine antagonists, serotonin agonists, and opioid antagonists. Opiate antagonist effects appear to involve both mu and delta receptors, which has led to the introduction of naltrexone, the first new pharmacotherapeutic treatment for alcoholism in 40 years. Recent identification of a competitive THC antagonist will most certainly lead to its testing in reinforcement models. However, the clinical value of such an approach clearly still needs to be established, given the very limited success of opiate antagonists in treating opiate dependence.

Work on the development of antagonists for animal models of relapse (e.g., animal models for the conditioned positive and conditioned negative reinforcement associated with dependence) has only just begun (Koob, 1995). Limited studies suggest that dopamine antagonists can block the reinstatement induced by other drugs of abuse in the intravenous self-administration reinstatement model. For the negative reinforcement associated with drug withdrawal, there is evidence that clonidine can block conditioned withdrawal from opiates (Kosten, 1994) and chlordiazepoxide can block conditioned withdrawal from ethanol (Baldo et al., 1995). Much more work is needed in this area, particularly in developing better models and identifying mechanisms at the systems, cellular, and molecular levels of analysis.

Agonists

An alternative approach to the treatment of drug dependence is the use of pharmacotherapies to alleviate the signs and symptoms of abstinence and, thus, alleviate at least part of the motivational state driving the dependence. One model for this approach that has met with significant clinical success is methadone detoxification and methadone maintenance. Early animal studies identified methadone as an orally active, long-acting opioid agonist that could block and prevent opiate withdrawal (Bigelow and Preston, 1995). An even longer-acting opiate agonist *levo*-alpha-acetylmethadol (LAAM) has long been under clinical investigation and is now approved by the Food and Drug Administration (FDA) for the treatment of opiate dependence (Bigelow and Preston, 1995). Nonopioid drugs, developed preclinically which also block some of the signs and symptoms of opiate withdrawal, include alpha-2-noradrenergic agonists such as clonidine. Little success has been reported, however, in preclinical attempts to block the withdrawal associated with cocaine in either animals or humans, largely because the withdrawal models have been limited (Markou and Koob, 1991); thus, development of a better model of withdrawal is also critical for progress in this area. There is some evidence that dopamine agonists can attenuate cocaine withdrawal, but the dopamine receptor subtype involved is unknown. Given the limited success of bromocriptine in the clinic, D-1 agonists, partial agonists, or even less selective dopamine agonists should be explored. Recent evidence suggests that D-1 agonists are more effective than D-2 agonists in blunting the reinstatement of cocaine self-administration in animals subjected to extinction (Self et al., 1996). Ethanol withdrawal can be effectively blocked by benzodiazepines, and they continue to be the treatment of choice for detoxification (O'Brien et al., 1995). Nicotine withdrawal can be effectively eliminated by chronic, slow-release forms of nicotine delivery, an approach that forms the basis for the nicotine patch, nicotine gum, and nicotine spray in humans (Russell, 1991; Fiore et al., 1992).

Brain Imaging

Until recently, the contribution of regional brain function and neurotransmitter systems to the causes and consequences of drug abuse and other brain diseases could be addressed only indirectly through measurement of blood and cerebrospinal fluid neurotransmitter metabolites, drug challenges, and gross neurophysiological measures such as the electroencephalogram (EEG). In the past decade, however, technological advances in the field of functional brain imaging have presented an opportunity to bridge the gap between basic neuroscience and clinical research. Positron-emission tomography (PET), single-photon emission computed tomography (SPECT), and more recently, functional magnetic resonance imaging (fMRI) are being used in studies of the mechanisms of action of abusable drugs and of the metabolic and neurochemical changes in the brain associated with dependence.

PET and SPECT employ instruments that measure the spatial distribution and movement of radioisotopes in tissues of living subjects (Mullani and Volkow, 1992; Rogers and Ackermann, 1992). Functional magnetic resonance imaging is one of the most recent and exciting advances in brain imaging, and with PET, blood flow scans can be used to infer the activity of focal brain regions by measuring changes in blood flow by several techniques (Kaufman et al., 1996).

The fMRI procedure offers the advanced spatial resolution of MRI combined with great temporal resolution, since repeated images taken over seconds or minutes reveal discrete brain regions serially and specifically affected (e.g., during the performance of cognitive tasks or exposure to a psychotropic drug). Also, because it does not involve the use of a radioisotope, fMRI can be repeated readily. The repitition allows for measurement of changes in brain activity in response to a task or drug and how such changes may differ between normal individuals and those with neuropsychiatric disorders. Additionally, fMRI equipment is more widely available than PET or SPECT cameras. However, interpreting the evidence may not be straightforward, and a major limitation of fMRI is uncertainty as to what its signal actually reflects with respect to brain function.

There is no doubt that studies of the neurochemical state of the brains of neuropsychiatric patients made possible by PET and SPECT imaging will one day provide novel and essential information on neuropsychiatric disorders. Additional brain imaging methodologies, notably magnetic resonance spectroscopy (MRS), also promise to provide anatomical and neurochemical information that has until very recently been completely inaccessible in neuropsychiatric patients. Some of the accomplishments of these advances follow.

The availability of the short-lived positron emitter carbon-11 has made it possible to label drugs of abuse, so that PET can then be used to measure their pharmacokinetics in the human brain. The labeled drug and whole-body PET also can be used to determine the target organs for the drug and its labeled metabolites and, thus, to provide information on potential toxic effects as well as tissue half-lives. They also allow the evaluation of the relation between the kinetics of an abused drug in the brain and the temporal relation to its behavioral effects.

Different labeled tracers can be used to assess the effects of drugs on brain function and neurochemistry, including metabolism and cerebral blood flow (CBF), neurotransmitter activity, transporter or receptor occupancy, and enzyme activity. The most widely utilized approach has been to assess the effects of acute drug administration on brain glucose metabolism and on CBF. This allows analysis of the brain regions that are most sensitive to the effects of the drug, and because the studies are done in awake human subjects, it allows analysis of the relationship between functional changes and behavioral changes in addicted and nonaddicted subjects. This strategy has been used to investigate the effects on brain glucose metabolism and/or CBF for most of the drugs of abuse.

The measurement of brain glucose metabolism with ^{18}FDG (^{18}fluoro-D-glucose) provides an index of brain activity that is not confounded by CBF changes and hence is useful in the assessment of changes in brain function that may occur during withdrawal. For example, studies in cocaine abusers done at different times after cocaine discontinuation have shown that regional glucose metabolism changes as a function of the withdrawal phase at which the studies are performed. Cocaine abusers, and polydrug abusers, tested within one week of their last cocaine use showed significantly higher metabolic activity in frontal brain regions and in basal ganglia than normal controls (Volkow et al., 1991). In contrast, cocaine abusers tested one to four months after cocaine discontinuation showed marked reduction in frontal metabolism (Figure 3.2) (Volkow et al., 1993).

Specific receptor radioligands are useful in assessing the extent to which a particular neurotransmitter system is affected in addicted subjects. For example, in cocaine dependence (where a dysfunction in brain dopamine activity has been postulated to underlie dependence), imaging studies have documented decrements in dopamine D-2 receptor ligand binding during early and protracted cocaine withdrawal (Figure 3.3) (Volkow et al., 1993), as well as decrements in dopamine metabolism (Baxter et al., 1988). Multiple tracer studies that measure glucose metabolism and/or CBF in conjunction with specific dopamine tracers (i.e., receptors and/or transporters) permit researchers to assess the functional significance of changes in these dopamine elements. Such studies have been done to investigate the relation between brain glucose metabolism and dopamine D-2 receptors in cocaine abusers. A significant correlation was reported between dopamine D-2 receptors and glucose metabolism in orbitofrontal cortex, cingulate gyrus, and superior frontal cortex (Volkow et al., 1993). Lower values of dopamine D-2 receptor concentration were associated with lower metabolism in these brain regions.

Pain and Analgesia

Relieving Pain

Some drugs that have high abuse liability, most notably the opioid analgesics, have essential medical uses. Since its founding, NIDA has been the major supporter of research into brain mechanisms of pain and analgesia, analgesic tolerance, and analgesic pharmacology. The resulting discoveries have led to an understanding of the brain circuits that are required to generate pain and pain relief, have revolutionized the treatment of postoperative and cancer pain (Foley and Inturrisi, 1986), and have led to improved treatments for many chronic pain conditions. The major accomplishments of drug abuse research that have a significant impact on managing and relieving pain are described below.

Clinical Pharmacology of Opioids

The investigation of the potency, metabolism, analgesic effects, and side effects of opioid drugs has been a major research target of the drug abuse field since its inception. National Institute on Drug Abuse (NIDA)-supported research has revealed the range of plasma opioid concentrations required for effective pain relief. Based on this research, clinicians have developed new methods of drug administration that maintain optimal levels of analgesic, including sustained-release tablets, transdermal patches, continuous drug infusions, and patient-controlled analgesic pumps. Those methods have now made it possible to keep more than 90% of cancer patients relatively comfortable for their entire course, and to eliminate most of the pain following major surgical procedures (Carr et al., 1992; Jacox et al., 1994).

Research into the Neural Circuitry Underlying Pain and Analgesia

NIDA-supported studies of the mechanism of opioid analgesia have also led to the discovery of endogenous pain-relieving circuits in the brain and spinal cord. Opioids activate analgesic areas in the brainstem, causing descending axons to release pain-inhibiting neurotransmitters in the spinal cord, blocking the entry of pain signals into the central nervous system. The finding that those inhibitory circuits use the neurotransmitters norepinephrine, serotonin, and enkephalins has led to the development of new treatments for acute and chronic pain (Wall and Melzack, 1994), including spinal administration of opioids for surgical and cancer pain (Yaksh and Malmberg, 1994) and the tricyclic antidepressants for pain caused by nerve injury (Max et al., 1992).

Molecular Biology of Pain and Analgesia

Drug abuse research has begun to elucidate the changes in gene regulation caused by acute and chronic pain and its treatment by opioids and other analgesics in animals (Hunt et al., 1987; Draisci et al., 1991). Those results provide direct applications to pain research and treatment. The amount of expression of immediate-early genes such as c-*fos* correlates well with the amount of tissue injury and pain behavior, offering another type of measure of pain, especially applicable to experiments in which it may be difficult to monitor behavior (Abbadie and Besson, 1994). The availability of cloned receptors from neural components mediating pain and analgesia, as well as the elucidation of second and third messenger systems provides new targets for the design of analgesic agents. In addition, the knowledge of the effects of opioids, *N*-methyl-*D*-aspartate (NMDA) antagonists, and other commonly abused drugs on genes involved in acute and chronic pain (Gogas et al., 1991) may offer insights into their effects in drug dependence and withdrawal, which like pain can have extremely aversive states.

GAPS AND NEEDS

A wealth of information has been gained concerning the actions of drugs of abuse on the brain. However, the field of drug abuse research has not, until relatively recently, taken full advantage of the revolutionary advances in molecular and cell biology and basic neuroscience that have occurred over the past two decades. New developments in molecular and cell biology open new possibilities for more basic understanding of drug abuse.

Basic Research at the Molecular Level

There are several gaps in current knowledge of drug dependence at the molecular level. One area includes genes that contribute to individual responsiveness to drugs of abuse. This includes genes encoding proteins that affect an individual's acute and chronic responses to drug exposure. A major deficiency in the field has been the choice of genes targeted for study. Most studies have focused on genes that control levels of neurotransmitters or receptors; in contrast, relatively little attention has been given to the host of genes involved in controlling intra- and intercellular signaling. Identification of genes that confer vulnerability for drug dependence would be expected to lead to the development of novel pharmacotherapies for addictive disorders.

Similarly, although progress is being made in identifying adaptations that occur in specific brain regions in response to long-term exposure to drugs of abuse, more work is needed in this area. Identifying these adaptations will provide a more complete understanding of the ways in which drugs alter neuronal function and lead to the many long-term effects of drugs on the brain. In addition to elaborating the pathophysiology of drug dependence, a more complete knowledge of drug-induced adaptations in the brain will facilitate medication development efforts. In identifying these adaptations, an expansion of our knowledge of proteins, and of cellular and molecular processes of drug actions is needed.

Finally, only recently has there been any hint of the mechanisms by which chronic drug exposure induces adaptations in specific target proteins. The major challenge in the future will be to study many types of transcription factors and other nuclear proteins for their potential regulation by drugs of abuse, and then to relate changes in a specific transcription factor to changes in specific target proteins. In addition, increased attention should be given to posttranscriptional mechanisms, because we know that levels of a particular gene product can be influenced at the level of RNA splicing and transport to the cytoplasm, stability of the mRNA, rate of translation of the mRNA, and stability of the encoded protein. Each of these mechanisms represents a potential target for drug action.

Drug abuse research should use the potent new methods of molecular and cellular biology and the neurosciences to pay particular attention to the host of genes that control intra- and intercellular signaling following exposure to drugs of abuse, including effects on second-, third-, and fourth-messenger cascades; changes in levels of transcription factors and posttranscriptional processing; and further adaptations in target proteins.

Basic Research at the Cellular Level

Although a significant amount is known about the acute actions of opiates in certain neuronal cell types, there is a relative paucity of similar information available with respect to other drugs of abuse. For example, we still know very little about the ionic basis of the currents elicited by most dopamine receptors in the brain. A major focus of future research, then, is to utilize the most sophisticated electrophysiological methodologies available, such as patch clamping, to delineate the ionic basis of acute drug actions on the brain and the postreceptor signaling pathways through which the drugs produce these effects.

There is an even greater need to study the chronic consequences of drug exposure on the activity of target neuronal populations. Most is known about the effects of chronic stimulant exposure on activity of the mesolimbic dopamine system and its post-synaptic targets, implicated in the motivational aspects of cocaine and other drug addictions (see above). This work has had an important impact on evolving molecular and systems analyses of drug dependence, and continued efforts are needed. Moreover, very little is known about the long-term effects of other drugs of abuse. For example, whereas considerable information is available concerning chronic opiate action on certain neuronal cell types, virtually no information is available concerning the long-term effects of opiates on neurons in the mesolimbic dopamine system and its connections. Even less is known about the consequences of chronic cannabinoid, nicotine, and psychotomimetic exposure. This type of information is critical to understand molecular phenomena within a functional context and to understand interactions among neurons at the systems level. Translation of molecular events to cellular interactions is essential to link drugs, which are molecular entities, to behavior.

Sophisticated electrophysiological methodologies should be used to delineate the ionic basis of acute and chronic effects of drugs on a variety of neuronal populations, including the linkage between changes in effects at ion channels and postreceptor signaling pathways. Studies of molecular and cellular mechanisms in brain tissue of animals with chronic drug dependence, prolonged abstinence, and relapse are of particular interest. In addition, cellular physiology, neuronal cell loss, and more subtle forms of neural injury and glial adaptations should be studied.

Basic Research at the Systems Level

A great deal has been learned in the past decade about the structure of the striatum and nucleus accumbens, the latter in particular being an important neural substrate of the acute reinforcing effects of drugs of abuse and of the motivational aspects of drug dependence. This work has delineated different subsets of neurons within these structures and has begun the arduous process of defining each subtype based on its chemical constituents (e.g., the types of proteins such as dopamine receptors and neuropeptides it expresses) and on its afferent and efferent connections. Given the important role of the nucleus accumbens in drug-related behaviors, continued efforts in this area are needed, and these efforts must be integrated more effectively with ongoing research at the molecular and cellular levels as outlined above. For example, the chemical constituents of selected subtypes of nucleus accumbens neurons represent potential targets for medication development and human genetic analyses.

In addition, the field needs to go beyond the mesolimbic dopamine system to identify other neural substrates that contribute to the complex behavioral effects of drugs of abuse. As animal models are developed that more accurately measure these aspects of dependence, the relevant brain regions can then be identified, and these regions can be targeted for molecular and cellular analyses to understand the underlying mechanisms involved. Understanding the role of these brain structures in drug dependence will provide key information linking the well-studied mesolimbic system to other limbic structures implicated in emotions and motivated behavior and will provide a rich substrate for understanding etiology, vulnerability, and relapse.

RESEARCH OPPORTUNITIES

Genetics Research

A major goal of future research is to identify genes that contribute to individual vulnerability to drug addiction. The identification of drug addiction vulnerability genes, like the identification of any disease vulnerability gene, will require careful and thorough policy analysis and implementation. Although most research in this area has involved genetic studies in people, the focus has been on candidate genes for which there is little preclinical evidence for a role in vulnerability to dependence. For example, much of the effort in the field has focused on alleles of monoamine receptors or transporters as candidate genes. Yet, there is little if any evidence in animals or people that individual differences in the functioning of those proteins contribute to individual differences in drug responsiveness.

A promising strategy, however, which has not been employed sufficiently to date, is the use of animal models for genetic studies. This strategy is analogous to that used with success in other medical specialties. Mapping of the mouse genome, and more recently the rat genome, is proceeding at a rapid pace. By use of a variety of experimental strategies such as quantitative trait locus analysis (Belknap et al., 1993), it is now feasible to begin the process of identifying genetic loci associated with specific behavioral phenotypes related to drug dependence. It is likely that genes identified through this process will include those that encode for proteins not currently thought of as being involved in drug dependence. Identification of drug dependence vulnerability genes in animals may reveal the types of genes involved in people. Even if the same homologous genes are not involved in people, genes that encode proteins along the same biochemical pathways would be additional candidate genes for investigation. This approach would involve the targeting of far more sophisticated candidate genes for analysis, rather than a continuation of the current approach. Thus, studies of inbred rodent strains could be used to identify genes leading to different preferences for initiating or chronically maintaining self-administration of commonly abused drugs.

Such genes could then become targets for molecular and cellular genetic studies.

Transgenics and Knockouts

The advent of engineering genetic mutations in mice has been an area of explosive research interest in recent years (Capecchi, 1994; Takahashi et al., 1994). Transgenic mice refer to those in which a new, exogenous gene is expressed in the animal. Knock-out mice refer to those in which the expression of an endogenous gene has been abolished in the animal. There are also combinations of those approaches, for example, an animal in which a normal gene is removed by knock-out technology and replaced by a mutant gene with transgenic technology. It is easy to see how these genetic approaches will revolutionize the study of the normal physiological function of a given gene and its encoded protein, as well as the role of mutations in the gene in leading to various disease states (Aguzzi et al., 1994).

Research with homozygous mice, in which the gene encoding the DAT (dopamine transporter) has been disrupted, establish the central importance of the transporter as the key element controlling synaptic dopamine levels. Additionally, this research demonstrates the role of the transporter as an obligatory target for the behavioral and biochemical action of amphetamine and cocaine. The DAT knock-out mice provide a tool for the study and development of drugs used in management of dopaminergic dysfunction. These mice may also aid in determining the role of dopaminergic neurotransmission in complex behavioral paradigms such as reward, addiction, and tolerance of drugs of abuse (Giros et al., 1996).

However, the use of those genetic techniques in the neurosciences, while possessing great promise, is hindered by serious limitations. The genetic mutation is present from very early stages of development, and can lead to several layers of adaptive processes to compensate for the mutation. This is particularly problematic for the brain, where these compensations may involve altered development of synaptic connections between various neuronal cell types and even aberrant development of entire brain regions. This makes it difficult to study the physiological function of a protein (targeted by the original mutation) in the adult state. One important area for future research is to validate behavioral models of drug dependence in mice as opposed to rats. Another important need is to identify mouse strains that are useful for the generation of gene knockouts, but in which behavior has been characterized and can be reliably studied.

With these caveats, research on transgenic and knock-out animals is underway at an increasing rate. Once genetic mutant mice are generated, the next step is to identify phenotypic abnormalities. The field of drug abuse has been and will continue to be one important component of this research, because animal models of drug dependence are among the most accurate and straightforward to interpret with respect to clinical and physiological phenomena.

Signal Transduction Pathways

Progress is being made in identifying adaptations in signal transduction proteins that occur in specific brain regions following chronic exposure to drugs of abuse. One major challenge for future research is to identify and investigate a broader range of molecular and cellular targets of drugs of abuse than those currently under scrutiny. A second major challenge is to relate specific molecular and cellular adaptations to specific behavioral features of dependence, particularly drug reinforcement and motivational aspects of dependence. This will first require the development of rodent animal models that more accurately reflect the phenomenon of drug craving, which is a core clinical feature of addictive disorders. These animal models can then be used to study the functional relevance of adaptations in the cellular physiology of specific neuronal cell types; adaptations in specific signaling and structural proteins within these neurons; and ultimately, specific transcriptional, translational, and posttranslational mechanisms of the adaptive changes. The information gained may provide clues for the development of more effective medications and may aid in genetics research.

Animal Models

As described above, one of the major gaps in the neurobiology of drug dependence research is the integration of clinical phenomena with basic research. One area that needs attention is the further validation of current animal models (see Chapter 2) and, perhaps more importantly, the anchoring of the basic neurobiology in such models. Much of the current research focuses on the acute or semiacute administration of drugs, no validation of functional dependence (behavioral or physiological measures combined with biochemistry or molecular biology) is provided. Thus, large amounts of data are gathered on the effects of drug use, but how this is related to drug abuse and dependence is unclear.

Although models of drug self-administration and drug discrimination have provided an excellent basis for behavioral research (Chapter 2), models that can reliably reproduce the more complex behaviors of dependence, relapse, withdrawal, and craving are needed. The development of animal models is a high priority, because it will enable characterization of these phenomena at the molecular, cellular, and systems levels.

Additionally, primate models have the promise of advancing knowledge in the neurobiology of drug abuse research. Primates can be trained readily in more sophisticated choice tasks that eliminate the need for controlling the rate of response, motivational, and motor confounds. The use of primate models could provide neural substrates more closely linked to the human brain from a comparative physiological perspective. Primates provide much more highly developed limbic and associative cortices for studying the neurobiology of cognitive effects of drugs of abuse and the interaction of cognition and drug development (e.g., craving and relapse). Therefore, the development of nonhuman primate models is desirable because the cortical anatomy and behavioral repertoire of primates more closely resembles those of humans.

Brain Imaging

The new imaging techniques discussed above can be used to assess the distribution of drugs of abuse in the human brain and to study neural mechanisms directly in the addicted individual. Because imaging studies are done in awake human subjects, it is possible to investigate the relation between behavior and regional brain effects, as well as between drug pharmacokinetics in the brain and the temporal course of pharmacological effects. Although the studies described above reveal the power of imaging, the field has not yet taken advantage of all of its potential.

Technologies of particular promise include fMRI because of is exceptional sensitivity and MRS because of its ability to estimate directly the concentration of many chemical components of brain tissue. Magnetic resonance also offers the ability to image brain vasculature (magnetic resonance angiography, MRA) and fluid motion (diffusion-weighted imaging, DWI). Since most drugs of abuse are vasoactive and some of the clinical sequelae associated with drug abuse may be associated with brain perfusion abnormalities, both MRA and DWI might also play important roles in understanding the mechanisms and consequences of drug abuse (Kaufman et al., 1996). Such studies may, for example, allow the initiation of investigations into the mechanism(s) by which certain drugs facilitate the emergence of aggressive behaviors.

Imaging may also prove to be valuable in the evaluation of therapeutic agents for drug dependence, for example, labeling them with positron emitters to assess their pharmacokinetics and bioavailability and to characterize their binding in the human brain. Similarly, imaging could be used to assess drug combinations and their potential toxicity, the mechanisms by which environmental factors (including behavioral therapy) might affect drug abuse, or the mechanisms by which genetic factors predispose to drug abuse.

Ultimately, brain imaging and neurobiological studies have a singular purpose—to better understand drug dependence and other neuropsychiatric disorders so that more effective treatments can be developed. In this scheme, studies in molecular and cellular neurobiology identify candidate neuropathic processes relevant to neuropsychiatric disorders. Such information is validated by the tools of behavioral neuroscience in animal models of the disorders. These studies in animals then direct human genetic studies aimed at identifying specific genes that contribute to the disorders in people. Identification of proteins relevant to the disorders directs brain imaging studies to examine the status of the proteins and related systems in patients' brains. Such knowledge then defines further clinical studies of the course and treatment of specific illnesses. Of course, insight evolving from the clinical work, including brain imaging, feeds back and informs ongoing preclinical studies of the underlying mechanisms involved.

Co-Occurring Psychiatric Disorders

The major psychiatric disorders associated with drug dependence are depression and personality disorders (see Chapter 5). Epidemiological data indicate that the rates of affective disorders among drug abusers are substantially higher than the expected rates of co-occurring disorders based in the general population (see Chapters 4 and 5). For example, lifetime rates of major depressive disorders range up to 50 percent in drug dependent patients compared with only 7 percent in a community sample (Rounsaville et al., 1982, 1987, 1991), and some form of drug abuse has been identified in more than 83 percent of individuals with personality disorders (Regier et al., 1990). Psychotic disorders, such as schizophrenia, represent only about 3 percent of drug abusers, but up to 50 percent of psychotic patients have addictive disorders.

The underlying neurobiology may differ for each of those disorders and for each drug of abuse. A number of neurochemical hypotheses are based largely on pharmacological interactions with these disorders or the symptoms of these disorders. For example, people with schizophrenia taking dopamine antagonists may use cocaine to relieve the antagonist-induced dysphoria, presumably because cocaine makes dopamine available to stimulate other dopamine receptors (e.g., D-1) that can also lead to euphoria. Another speculation about schizophrenia involves excitatory amino acids and PCP (phencyclidine) leading to psychotic illnesses (Javitt and Zukin, 1991). For depression, the underlying neurobiology is less clear because both serotonergic and adrenergic medications are helpful. Dopaminergic medications have little antidepressant efficacy, however, although dopamine seems so critical for hedonic tone or at least euphoria. Direct evidence for neurobiological connections between drug dependence and psychiatric disorders remains to be elucidated and may be studied with newly developed tools (e.g., functional brain imaging).

HIV Models

The utility of an animal model rests in its ability to permit the study of a disease process under controlled conditions. Animal models that recapitulate the pathogenic and functional outcomes seen with HIV infection in humans can then be used to examine the influence of drugs of abuse on HIV disease progression. Direct neurotoxic effects of drugs, in addition to their effects on immunocompetence, may contribute to an enhancement of neurological sequelae of AIDS (called neuroAIDS disease) or accelerate its onset. These studies also will help determine the nature of viral neuropathogenesis to specific brain systems relevant to drug reward. That may have significant clinical outcomes related to risk reduction in terms of altered behavioral and pharmacological sensitivity to drugs of abuse in infected individuals. Thus, behavioral analysis in animal models of viral neuropathogenesis provides a unique opportunity to study the interaction between drugs of abuse and the immune system and should go far in identifying critical viral- and host-derived factors associated with increased susceptibility to the pathobiological effects of drugs of abuse and consequent synergistic neurotoxicity. Continued development of animal models of the effects of HIV infection on the brain would be useful for studying the links between AIDS and drug abuse—e.g., effects of drugs on disease progression, and the effect of HIV on brain reward systems and behaviors relevant to risk.

Neurotoxicity of Drug Dependence

There were early reports that chronic exposure to drugs of abuse led to neuronal death. Most reports proved to be spurious, however this is still a controversial area. One example of drug-induced neurotoxicity remains well established, namely the ability of certain amphetamine derivatives to kill central monoaminergic neurons. Methamphetamine and to a lesser extent amphetamine are toxic to midbrain dopamine neurons (Seiden et al., 1975), and methylenedioxymethamphetamine (MDMA, also known as Ecstasy) is toxic to midbrain serotonin neurons (Ricaurte et al., 1988).

More recently, subtler forms of neural injury have been detected in the brain under a variety of conditions. Chronic stress, perhaps mediated by glucocorticoids, causes pruning of dendritic spines in certain hippocampal neurons (Sapolsky, 1992). Recent work raises the possibility that neural adaptation, perhaps forms of learning, may be associated with changes in the numbers of dendrites and dendritic spines (Woolley and McEwen, 1995; Yuste and Denk, 1995). Recent evidence suggests that such subtle forms of neural injury may be induced in midbrain dopamine neurons by chronic exposure to drugs of abuse (Sklair-Tavron et al., 1995). Further work is needed to better characterize these adaptations in animal models of drug dependence and eventually to extend these studies to people by using evolving brain imaging procedures. Thus, cell loss and more subtle forms of neural injury should be studied in animal models of drug dependence.

Neurobiology of Relapse After Prolonged Abstinence

There is evidence in the clinical literature for physiological changes in people with a history of drug abuse that persist for years following the last drug exposure (Jaffe, 1990). These changes have been referred to as "prolonged abstinence" or "protracted abstinence syndrome." Individuals who have been abstinent for years can return to a place associated with past drug exposure and quickly relapse to drug abuse (O'Brien, 1976). Individuals who took years to develop a hard-core dependence can, even after years of abstinence, descend back to that hard-core addicted state far more rapidly than before. There are relatively few preclinical studies of such types of phenomena; however, one example reports that sensitization to the locomotor activating effects of stimulants can persist for several months in rats (Robinson and Berridge, 1993). Given the clinical importance of prolonged abstinence, more preclinical research on this phenomenon is needed.

One difficulty is that it is not at all clear that the same brain regions that mediate acute drug reinforcement and, perhaps, some motivational aspects of drug dependence are involved in prolonged abstinence. Such persisting adaptations may be more likely to reside in cortical, hippocampal, and amygdaloid regions as opposed to the mesolimbic dopamine system. Again the first step in this process must be the development of animal models of prolonged abstinence.

However, we may not yet have the neurobiological resolution necessary to reveal the kinds of adaptations responsible for such long-lived phenomena as prolonged abstinence. Prolonged abstinence can be considered a form of long-term memory, and very little progress indeed has been made in establishing the neurobiological basis of long-term memory in general. Long-term memory may involve changes in the numbers or sizes of dendritic spines of certain hippocampal and cortical neurons, or changes in the numbers and even types of synaptic terminals that innervate those neurons. Although the work is very tedious, it is possible to investigate such types of adaptation once behavioral models are developed and the relevant brain regions are identified.

A Role for Immunology in Drug Treatment

Another approach to drug abuse treatment is the development of antidrug vaccination, by which an immune response is induced in the organism that would effectively remove the drug from circulation and thus block its actions in the brain. Early work showed that immunizations can be used to blunt the reinforcing effects of morphine or heroin (Bonese et al., 1974; Killian et al., 1978). Recent evidence in cocaine abuse research suggests that synthetic analogues of cocaine can be used to produce active immunization in animals against the parent compound sufficient to block its stimulant effects (Carrera et al., 1995). Unknown at this time is how long such treatments will last and how they would affect other aspects of models of dependence. Other immunotherapies now being pursued include the development of passive immunizations (e.g., monoclonal antibodies or even catalytic antibodies could be injected into a subject to prevent a drug's action) (Landry et al., 1993). Again, the efficacy, duration of action, and impact of monoclonal or catalytic antibodies on drug dependence models remain to be explored.

Research in Analgesia and Pain

Finally, research in analgesia and pain has both informed neuroscience research on drug abuse and benefited from advances in drug abuse research. Four areas in analgesia and pain research have been highlighted for future research.

Molecular Substrates of Analgesia and Tolerance

New molecular research techniques are allowing investigators to identify some of the genes and intracellular messenger systems that are activated or suppressed by pain and analgesics (Hunt et al., 1987; Draisci et al., 1991; Gogas et al., 1991; Abbadie and Besson, 1994). These new techniques will allow a new level of analysis of the action of the body's many endogenous pain-modulating systems mediated by endorphins, enkephalins, serotonin, norepinephrine, GABA, acetylcholine, and other transmitters (Fields and Liebeskind, 1994). This in turn could lead to novel treatments for pain and make possible the prevention of tolerance to and dependence on opioids. For example, evidence from animal models suggests that excitatory amino acid neurotransmission plays a role in tolerance to analgesia, which can be reversed or prevented by coadministration with NMDA antagonists (Elliott et al., 1994). Clinical trials of NMDA antagonist–opioid combinations in humans are just beginning.

Development of Analgesics Acting at Opioid Receptors Other than the Mu Receptor

In animals, agonists at delta, kappa, and epsilon receptors provide analgesia. In humans, such drugs might have fewer side effects or abuse liability than conventional analgesics (which act predominantly at the mu receptor). Animal studies suggest that opioids acting at different receptors may produce analgesic synergism if combined (Miaskowski et al., 1992). Research to clone receptor subtypes, develop specific drugs, and investigate their basic and clinical pharmacology will promote that goal.

Functional Brain Imaging Studies of Pain and Opioid Analgesia

Although our knowledge of pain physiology has emerged largely from studies in small animals, pain and opioid analgesia are complex human phenomena. PET and MRI are beginning to provide unique maps of the involvement of higher human brain centers in pain (Casey et al., 1994; Coghill et al., 1994; Iadarola et al., 1995). These techniques could potentially identify the areas in the brain mediating opioid analgesia and the pain-related effects on emotion, movement, and the endocrine and immune systems. Imaging methods may also be invaluable for predicting the actions of novel analgesic compounds.

Treatment of Chronic Nonmalignant Pain by Opioids

There is a consensus that acute pain and chronic cancer pain should be treated with opioids (Carr et al., 1992; Jacox et al., 1994). However, there is great controversy about the benefits and risks of long-term opioid treatment of various types of nonmalignant pain conditions such as neuropathic pain, low back pain, myofascial pain, and arthritic pain (Wall and Melzack, 1994). There are almost no data on the responsiveness of each type of pain to opioids, the rate of development of analgesic tolerance and physical dependence, and the risk of true abuse and dependence. There is a particular need for data about the risks and outcome of opioid treatment of former addicts with pain, as well as patients with pain related to human immunodeficiency virus (HIV) infection.

CONCLUSION AND RECOMMENDATION

Significant progress has been made in understanding the neural substrates of drug dependence, and yet—due to the complexity of the brain and the difficulties inherent in studying the pathogenesis of any brain disease—there is still much more work to be done. Although physical withdrawal from drugs can now be managed well, all currently available treatments for the behavioral aspects of dependence remain inadequately effective for most people. By utilizing increasingly sophisticated research techniques and methods, future neurobiological studies at all levels of inquiry—molecular, cellular, and systems—will provide essential information for developing drug abuse treatment and prevention measures.

The committee recommends continued support for fundamental investigations in neuroscience on the molecular, cellular, and systems levels. Research should be supported in the following areas: developing better animal models of the motivational aspects of drug dependence (with particular emphasis on protracted abstinence and propensity to relapse); genetics research; brain imaging; the neurobiology of co-occurring psychiatric disorders and drug abuse; animal models of the effects of HIV infection on the brain; the neurotoxicity of drug dependence; immunological approaches to drug abuse treatment; and pain and analgesia.

REFERENCES

Abbadie C, Besson J-M. 1994. Chronic treatment with aspirin or acetaminophen reduces both the development of polyarthritis and fos-like immunoreactivity in rat lumbar spinal cord. *Pain* 57:45–54.

Aghajanian GK. 1978. Tolerance of locus coeruleus neurons to morphine and suppression of withdrawal response by clonidine. *Nature* 276:186–188.

Aguzzi A, Brandner S, Sure U, Ruedi D, Isenmann S. 1994. Transgenic and knock-out mice: Models of neurological disease. *Brain Pathology* 4:3–20.

Akaoka A, Aston-Jones G. 1991. Opiate withdrawal-induced hyperactivity of locus coeruleus neurons is substantially mediated by augmented excitatory amino acid input. *Journal of Neuroscience* 11:3830–3839.

Baldo BA, Heyser CJ, Griffin P, Schulteis G, Stinus L, Koob GF. 1995. Effects of chlordiazepoxide and acamprosate on the conditioned place aversion induced by ethanol withdrawal. *Neuroscience Abstracts* 21:1701.

Baxter LR, Schwartz JM, Phelps ME, Mazziotta JC, Barrio J, Rawson RA, Engel J, Guze BH, Selin C, Sumida R. 1988. Localization of neurochemical effects of cocaine and other stimulants in the human brain. *Journal of Clinical Psychiatry* 49:23–26.

Belknap JK, Metten P, Helms ML, O'Toole LA, Angeli-Gade S, Crabbe JC, Phillips TJ. 1993. Quantitative trait lock (QTL) applications to substances of abuse: Physical dependence studies with nitrous oxide and ethanol in BXD mice. *Behavior Genetics* 23:213–222.

Bigelow GE, Preston KL. 1995. Opioids. In: Bloom FE, Kupfer DJ, eds. *Psychopharmacology: The Fourth Generation of Progress*. New York: Raven Press. Pp. 1731–1744.

Bonese KF, Wainer BH, Fitch FW, Rothberg RM, Schuster CR. 1974. Changes in heroin self-administration by a rhesus monkey after morphine immunization. *Nature* 252:708–710.

Caine SB, Koob GF. 1993. Modulation of cocaine self-administration in the rat through D-3 dopamine receptors. *Science* 260:1814–1816.

Capecchi MR. 1994. Targeted gene replacement. *Scientific American* 270(3):52–59.

Carr DB, Jacox AK, Chapman CR, et al. 1992. *Acute Pain Management: Operative or Medical Procedures and Trauma: Clinical Practice Guideline*. AHCPR Publication No. 92-0032. Rockville, MD: U.S. Public Health Service, Agency for Health Care Policy and Research.

Carrera MRA, Ashley JA, Parsons LH, Wirsching P, Koob GF, Janda KD. 1995. Active immunization suppresses psychoactive effects of cocaine. *Nature* 378:727–730.

Casey KL, Minoshima S, Berger KL, Koeppe RA, Morrow TJ, Frey KA. 1994. Positron emission tomographic analysis of cerebral structures activated specifically by repetitive noxious heat stimuli. *Journal of Neurophysiology* 71:802–807.

Coghill RC, Talbot JD, Evans AC, Meyer E, Gjedde A, Bushnell MC, Duncan GH. 1994. Distributed processing of pain and vibration by the human brain. *Journal of Neuroscience* 14:4095–4108.

Cole BJ, Cador M, Stinus L, Rivier C, Rivier J, Vale W, Le Moal M, Koob GF. 1990. Critical role of the hypothalamic pituitary adrenal axis in amphetamine-induced sensitization of behavior. *Life Science* 47:1715–1720.

Collier HOJ. 1980. Cellular site of opiate dependence. *Nature* 283:625–629.

Corrigall WA, Franklin KBJ, Coen KM, Clarke PBS. 1992. The mesolimbic dopamine system is implicated in the reinforcing effects of nicotine. *Psychopharmacology (Berl)* 107:285–289.

Crabbe JC, Belknap JK, Buck KJ. 1994. Genetic animal models of alcohol and drug abuse. *Science* 264:1715–1723.

Cunningham ST, Kelley AE. 1992. Evidence for opiate-dopamine cross-sensitization in nucleus accumbens: Studies of conditioned reward. *Brain Research Bulletin* 29:675–680.

Devane WA, Hanus L, Breuer A, Pertwee RG, Stevenson LA, Griffin G, Gibson D, Mandelbaum A, Etinger A, Mechoulam R. 1992. Isolation and structure of a brain constituent that binds to the cannabinoid receptor. *Science* 258:1946–1949.

de Wit H, Stewart J. 1981. Reinstatement of cocaine-reinforced responding in the rat. *Psychopharmacology* 75:134–143.

Di Chiara G, North RA. 1992. Neurobiology of opiate abuse. *Trends in Pharmacological Sciences* 13:185–193.

Draisci G, Kajander KC, Dubner R, Bennett GJ, Iadarola MJ. 1991. Up-regulation of opioid gene expression in spinal cord evoked by experimental nerve injuries and inflammation. *Brain Research* 560:186–192.

Elliott K, Hynansky A, Inturrisi CE. 1994. Dextromethorphan attenuates and reverses analgesic tolerance to morphine. *Pain* 59:361–368.

Fields HL, Liebeskind JC, eds. 1994. *Pharmacological Approaches to the Treatment of Chronic Pain: New Concepts and Critical Issues*. Seattle: IASP Press.

Fiore MC, Jorenby DE, Baker TB, Kenford SL. 1992. Tobacco dependence and the nicotine patch. Clinical guidelines for effective use. *Journal of the American Medical Association* 268(19):2687–2694.

Foley KM, Inturrisi CE, eds. 1986. *Opioid Analgesics in the Management of Clinical Pain. Advances in Pain Research and Therapy, Vol. 8*. New York: Raven Press.

George FR, Goldberg SR. 1989. Genetic approaches to the analysis of addiction processes. *Trends in Pharmacological Sciences* 10:78–83.

Giros B, Jaber M, Jones SR, Wightman RM, Caron MG. 1996. Hyperlocomotion and indifference to cocaine and amphetamine in mice lacking the dopamine transporter. *Nature* 379:606–612.

Goeders NE, Guerin GF. 1994. Non-contingent electric footshock facilitates the acquisition of intravenous cocaine self-administration in rats. *Psychopharmacology* 114:63–70.

Gogas KR, Presley RW, Levine JD, Basbaum AI. 1991. The antinociceptive action of supraspinal opioids results from an increase in descending inhibitory control: Correlation of nociceptive behavior and c-fos expression. *Neuroscience* 42:617–628.

Gold MS, Redmond DE, Kleber HD. 1978. Clonidine in opiate withdrawal. *Lancet* 11:599–602.

Grant KA, Valverius P, Hudspith M, Tabakoff B. 1990. Ethanol withdrawal seizures and the NMDA receptor complex. *European Journal of Pharmacology* 176:289–296.

Guitart X, Kogan JH, Berhow M, Terwilliger RZ, Aghajanian GK, Nestler EJ. 1993. Lewis and Fischer rat strains show differences in biochemical, electrophysiological, and behavioral parameters: Studies in the nucleus accumbens and locus coeruleus of drug naive and morphine-treated animals. *Brain Research* 611:7–17.

Hamamura T, Fibiger HC. 1993. Enhanced stress-induced dopamine release in the prefrontal cortex of amphetamine-sensitized rats. *European Journal of Pharmacology* 237:65–71.

Henry DJ, White FJ. 1991. Repeated cocaine administration causes persistent enhancement of D1 dopamine receptor sensitivity within the rat nucleus accumbens. *Journal of Pharmacology and Experimental Therapeutics* 258:882–890.

Hilbert P, Lindpaintner K, Beckmann JS, Serikawa T, Soubrier F, Dubay C, Cartwright P, De Gouyon B, Julier C, Takahashi S, et al. 1991. Chromosomal mapping of two genetic loci associated with blood-pressure regulation in hereditary hypertensive rats. *Nature* 353:521–529.

Horger BA, Giles MK, Schenk S. 1992. Preexposure to amphetamine and nicotine predisposes rats to self-administer a low dose of cocaine. *Psychopharmacology* 107:271–276.

Hunt SP, Pini A, Evan G. 1987. Induction of c-fos-like protein in spinal cord neurons following sensory stimulation. *Nature* 328:632–634.

Hurd YL, Brown EE, Finlay JM, Fibiger HC, Gerfem CR. 1992. Cocaine self-administration differentially alters mRNA expression of striatal peptides. *Molecular Brain Research* 13:165–170.

Hyman SE, Nestler EJ. 1993. *The Molecular Foundations of Psychiatry*. Washington, DC: American Psychiatric Press.

Iadarola MJ, Max MB, Berman KF, Byassmith MG, Coghill RC, Gracely RH, Bennett GJ. 1995. Unilateral decrease in thalamic activity observed with positron emission tomography in patients with chronic neuropathic pain. *Pain* 63:55–64.

Jacox A, Carr DB, Payne R, et al. 1994. *Management of Cancer Pain. Clinical Practice Guideline.* AHCPR Publication No. 94-0592. Rockville, MD: U.S. Public Health Service, Agency for Health Care Policy and Research.

Jaffe JH. 1990. Drug addiction and drug abuse. In: Gilman AG, Rall TW, Nies AS, Taylor P, eds. *The Pharmacological Basis of Therapeutics*. 8th ed. New York: Pergamon Press. Pp. 522–573.

Javitt DC, Zukin SR. 1991. Recent advances in the phencyclidine model of schizophrenia. *American Journal of Psychiatry* 148:1301–1308.

Kandel ER, Schwartz JH, Jessell TM. 1991. *Principles of Neural Science*. 3rd ed. New York: Elsevier.

Kaufman MF, Levin JM, Christensen JD, Renshaw PF. 1996. Magnetic resonance studies of substance abuse. *Seminars in Clinical Neuropsychiatry* 1:1–16.

Killian A, Bonese K, Rothberg RM, Wainer BH, Schuster CR. 1978. Effects of a passive immunization against morphine on heroin self-administration. *Pharmacology, Biochemistry and Behavior* 9:347–352.

Koob GF. 1992a. Drugs of abuse: Anatomy, pharmacology, and function of reward pathways. *Trends in Pharmacological Sciences* 13:177–184.

Koob GF. 1992b. Dopamine, addiction and reward. *Seminars in the Neurosciences* 4:139–148.

Koob GF. 1995. Animal models of drug addiction. In: Bloom FE, Kupfer DJ, eds. *Psychopharmacology: Fourth Generation of Progress*. New York: Raven Press. Pp. 759–772.

Koob GF, Cador M. 1993. Psychomotor stimulant sensitization: The corticotropin-releasing factor-steroid connection. *Behavioural Pharmacology* 4:351–354.

Koob GF, Maldonado R, Stinus L. 1992. Neural substrates of opiate withdrawal. *Trends in Neurosciences* 15:186–191.

Koob GF, Markou A, Weiss F, Schulteis G. 1993. Opponent process and drug dependence: Neurobiological mechanisms. *Seminars in the Neurosciences* 5:351–358.

Koob GF, Heinrichs SC, Menzaghi F, Pich EM, Britton KT. 1994a. Corticotrophin-releasing factor, stress and behavior. *Seminars in the Neurosciences* 7:221–229.

Koob GF, Rassnick S, Heinrichs S, Weiss F. 1994b. Alcohol, the reward system and dependence. In: Jansson B, Jörnvall H, Rydberg U, Terenius L, Vallee BL, eds. *Toward a Molecular Basis of Alcohol Use and Abuse*. Proceedings of Nobel Symposium on Alcohol. Basel: Birhauser Verlag. Pp. 103–114.

Kosten TA. 1994. Clonidine attenuates conditioned aversion produced by naloxone-precipitated opiate withdrawal. *European Journal of Pharmacology* 254:59–63.

Kosten TA, Miserendino MJD, Chi S, Nestler EJ. 1994. Fischer and Lewis rats strains show differential cocaine effects in conditioned place preference and behavioral sensitization but not in locomotor activity or conditioned taste aversion. *Journal of Pharmacology and Experimental Therapeutics* 269:137–144.

Landry DW, Zhao K, Yang GX, Glickman M, Georgiadis TM. 1993. Antibody-catalyzed degradation of cocaine. *Science* 259:1899–1901.

Li TK, Lumeng L. 1984. Alcohol preference and voluntary alcohol intakes of inbred rat strains and the NIH heterogeneous stock of rats. *Alcoholism: Clinical and Experimental Research* 8:485–486.

Li TK, Lumeng L, McBride WJ, Waller MB, Murphy JM. 1986. Studies on an animal model of alcoholism. In: Braude C, Chao HM, eds. *Genetic and Biological Markers in Drug Abuse and Alcoholism*. Washington, DC: National Institute on Drug Abuse. Pp. 41–49.

Littleton J, Little H, Laverty R. 1992. Role of neuronal calcium channels in ethanol dependence: From cell cultures to the intact animal. *Annals of the New York Academy of Sciences* 654:324–334.

Maldonado R, Koob GF. 1993. Destruction of the locus coeruleus decreases physical signs of opiate withdrawal. *Brain Research* 605:128–138.

Maldonado R, Stinus L, Gold LH, Koob GF. 1992. Role of different brain structures in the expression of the physical morphine withdrawal syndrome. *Journal of Pharmacology and Experimental Therapeutics* 261:669–677.

Malin DH, Lake JR, Carter VA, Cunningham JS, Wilson OB. 1993. Naloxone precipitates abstinence syndrome in the rat. *Psychopharmacology* 112:339–342.

Malin DH, Lake JR, Carter VA, Cunningham JS, Hebert KM, Conrad DL, Wilson OB. 1994. The nicotine antagonist mecamylamine precipitates nicotine abstinence syndrome in the rat. *Psychopharmacology* 115:180–184.

Markou A, Koob GF. 1991. Post-cocaine anhedonia. An animal model of cocaine withdrawal. *Neuropharmacology* 4:17–26.

Matsuda L, Lolait SJ, Brownstein MJ, Young AC, Bonner TI. 1990. Structure of a cannabinoid receptor and functional expression of the cloned cDNA. *Nature* 346:561–564.

Max MB, Lynch SA, Muir J, Shoaf SE, Smoller B, Dubner R. 1992. Effects of desirpamine, amitriptyline, and fluoxetine on pain in diabetic neuropathy. *New England Journal of Medicine* 326:1250–1256.

Miaskowski C, Sutters KA, Taiwo YO, Levine JD. 1992. Antinociceptive and motor effects of delta/mu and kappa/mu combinations of intrathecal opioid agonists. *Pain* 49:137–144.

Mullani NA, Volkow ND. 1992. Positron emission tomography instrumentation: A review and update. *American Journal of Physiological Imaging* 7:121–135.

Nestler EJ. 1992. Molecular mechanisms of drug addiction. *Journal of Neuroscience* 12:2439–2450.

Nestler EJ. 1994. Molecular neurobiology of drug addiction. *Neuropsychopharmacology* 11:77–87.

Nestler EJ, Hope BT, Widnell KL. 1993. Drug addiction: A model for the molecular basis of neural plasticity. *Neuron* 11:995–1006.

Nestler EJ, Fitzgerald LW, Self DW. 1995. Neurobiology of substance abuse. *APA Annual Review of Psychiatry* 14:51–81.

O'Brien CP. 1976. Experimental analysis of conditioning factors in human narcotic addiction. *Pharmacological Reviews* 27:533–543.

O'Brien CP, Eckardt MJ, Linnoila VMI. 1995. Pharmacotherapy of alcoholism. In: Bloom FE, Kupfer DJ, eds. *Psychopharmacology: Fourth Generation of Progress.* New York: Raven Press. Pp. 1745–1755.

Olds J. 1962. Hypothalamic substrates of reward. *Physiological Reviews* 42:554–560.

Olds J, Milner P. 1954. Positive reinforcement produced by electrical stimulation of septal area and other regions of rat brain. *Journal of Comparative and Physiological Psychology* 47:419–427.

Parsons LH, Koob GF, Weiss F. 1995. Serotonin dysfunction in the nucleus accumbens of rats during withdrawal after unlimited access to intravenous cocaine. *Journal of Pharmacology and Experimental Therapeutics* 274:1182–1191.

Piazza PV, Deminiere JM, Le Moal M, Simon H. 1989. Factors that predict individual vulnerability to amphetamine self-administration. *Science* 245:1511–1513.

Piazza PV, Maccari S, Deminiere JM, Le Moal M, Mormede P, Simon H. 1991. Corticosterone levels determine individual vulnerability to amphetamine self-administration. *Proceedings of the National Academy of Sciences (USA)* 88:2088–2092.

Pickens RW, Svikis DS. 1988. Genetic vulnerability to drug abuse. *NIDA Research Monograph* 89:1–8.

Rasmussen K, Aghajanian GK. 1989. Withdrawal-induced activation of locus coeruleus neurons in opiate-dependent rats: Attenuation by lesions of the nucleus paragigantocellularis. *Brain Research* 505:346–350.

Rasmussen K, Beitner-Johnson D, Krystal JH, Aghajanian GK, Nestler EJ. 1990. Opiate withdrawal and the rat locus coeruleus: Behavioral, electrophysiological, and biochemical correlates. *Journal of Neuroscience* 10:2308–2317.

Regier DA, Farmer ME, Rae DS, Locke BZ, Keith SJ, Judd LL, Goodwin FK. 1990. Comorbidity of mental disorders with alcohol and other drug abuse. *Journal of the American Medical Association* 264:2511–2518.

Ricaurte GA, Forno LS, Wilson MA, De Lanney LE, Molliver ME, Langston JW. 1988. (±)3,4-Methylenedioxymethamphetamine (MDMA) selectively damages central serotonergic neurons in non-human primates. *Journal of the American Medical Association* 260:51–55.

Robinson TE, Berridge KC. 1993. The neural basis of drug craving: An incentive-sensitization theory of addiction. *Brain Research Reviews* 18:247–291.

Rogers LW, Ackermann RJ. 1992. SPECT instrumentation. *American Journal of Physiological Imaging* 7:105–120.

Rounsaville BJ, Weissman MM, Kleber HD, Wilber CH. 1982. Heterogeneity of psychiatric diagnosis in treated opiate addicts. *Archives of General Psychiatry* 39:161–166.

Rounsaville BJ, Dolinsky ZS, Babor TF, Meyer R. 1987. Psychopathology as a predictor of treatment outcome in alcoholics. *Archives of General Psychiatry* 44:505–513.

Rounsaville BJ, Anton SF, Carroll K, Budde D, Prusoff BA, Gawin F. 1991. Psychiatric diagnoses of treatment-seeking cocaine abusers. *Archives of General Psychiatry* 48:43–51.

Russell MA. 1991. The future of nicotine replacement. *British Journal of Addiction* 86(5):653–658.

Samson HH, Harris RA. 1992. Neurobiology of alcohol abuse. *Trends in Pharmacological Science* 13:206–211.

Sapolsky RM. 1992. *Stress, the Aging Brain and the Mechanisms of Neuron Death*. Cambridge, MA: MIT Press.

Schaefer GJ, Michael RP. 1986. Changes in response rates and reinforcement thresholds for intracranial self-stimulation during morphine withdrawal. *Pharmacology, Biochemistry and Behavior* 25(6):1263–1269.

Schulteis G, Markou A, Gold LH, Stinus L, Koob GF. 1994. Relative sensitivity to naloxone of multiple indices of opiate withdrawal: A quantitative dose-response analysis. *Journal of Pharmacology and Experimental Therapeutics* 271:1391–1398.

Schulteis G, Markou A, Cole M, Koob GF. 1995. Decreased brain reward produced by ethanol withdrawal. *Proceedings of the National Academy of Sciences (USA)* 92:5880–5884.

Seiden LS, Fischman MW, Schuster CR. 1975. Long-term methamphetamine induced changes in brain catecholamines in tolerant rhesus monkeys. *Drugs and Alcohol Dependence* 1:215–219.

Self DW, Nestler EJ. 1995. Molecular mechanisms of drug reinforcement and craving. *Annual Review of Neuroscience* 18:463–495.

Self DW, Barnhart WJ, Lehman DA, Nestler EJ. 1996. Opposite modulation of cocaine-seeking behavior by D1- and D2-like dopamine receptor agonists. *Science* 271:1586–1589.

Shaham Y, Stewart J. 1994. Exposure to mild stress enhances the reinforcing efficacy of intravenous heroin self-administration. *Psychopharmacology* 114:523–527.

Sharma SK, Klee WA, Nirenberg M. 1975. Dual regulation of adenylate cyclase accounts for narcotic dependence and tolerance. *Proceedings of the National Academy of Sciences (USA)* 72:3092–3096.

Sklair-Tavron L, Shi WX, Bunney BS, Nestler EJ. 1995. Morphological evidence of changes induced in the ventral tegmental area (VTA) by chronic morphine treatment. *Society of Neuroscience Abstracts* 21:1059.

Sorg BA, Kalivas PW. 1993. Behavioral sensitization to stress and psychostimulants: Role of dopamine and excitatory amino acids in the mesocorticolimbic system. *Seminars in the Neurosciences* 5:343–350.

Spanagel R, Herz A, Shippenberg TS. 1992. Opposing tonically active endogenous opioid systems modulate the mesolimbic dopaminergic pathway. *Proceedings of the National Academy of Sciences (USA)* 89:2046–2050.

Stein L. 1968. Chemistry of reward and punishment. In: Efron D, ed. *Psychopharmacology, A Review of Progress (1957–1967)*. Public Health Service Publication No. 1836. Washington, DC: U.S. Government Printing Office. Pp. 105–123.

Stewart J, de Wit H. 1987. Reinstatement of drug-taking behavior as a method of assessing incentive motivational properties of drugs. In: Bozarth MA, ed. *Assessing the Reinforcing Properties of Abused Drugs*. New York: Springer-Verlag. Pp. 211–227.

Tabakoff B, Hoffman PL. 1992. Alcohol: Neurobiology. In: Lownstein JH, Ruiz P, Millman RB, eds. *Substance Abuse: A Comprehensive Textbook*. Baltimore: Williams & Wilkins. Pp. 152–185.

Takahashi JS, Pinto LH, Vitaterna MH. 1994. Forward and reverse genetic approaches to behavior in the mouse. *Science* 264:1724–1733.

Taylor JR, Elsworth JD, Garcia EJ, Grant SJ, Roth RN, Redmond DE Jr. 1988. Clonidine infusions into the locus coeruleus attenuate behavioral and neurochemical changes associated with naloxone-precipitated withdrawal. *Psychopharmacology* 96:121–131.

Trujillo K, Akil H. 1991. Inhibition of morphine tolerance and dependence by the NMDA receptor antagonist MK-801. *Science* 251:85–87.

Vezina P, Stewart J. 1990. Amphetamine administered to the ventral tegmental area but not to the nucleus accumbens sensitizes rats to systemic morphine: Lack of conditioned effects. *Brain Research* 516:99–106.

Volkow ND, Fowler JS, Wolf AP, Hitzemann R, Dewey S, Bendriem B, Alpert R, Hoff A. 1991. Changes in brain glucose metabolism in cocaine dependence and withdrawal. *American Journal of Psychology* 148:621–626.

Volkow ND, Fowler JS, Wang G-J, Hitzemann R, Logan J, Schlyer D, Dewey S, Wolf AP. 1993. Decreased dopamine D2 receptor availability is associated with reduced frontal metabolism in cocaine abusers. *Synapse* 14:169–177.

Volpicelli R, Davis MA, Olgin JE. 1986. Naltrexone blocks the post-shock increase of ethanol consumption. *Life Science* 38:841–847.

Wall PD, Melzack R. 1994. *Textbook of Pain*. 3rd ed. Edinburgh: Churchill-Livingstone.

Weiss F, Markou A, Lorang MT, Koob GF. 1992. Basal extraceullular dopamine levels in the nucleus accumbens are decreased during cocaine withdrawal after unlimited-access self-administration. *Brain Research* 493:314–318.

Wise RA. 1989. The brain and reward. In: Liebman JM, Cooper SJ, eds. *The Neuropharmacological Basis of Reward*. Oxford: Clarendon Press. Pp. 377–424.

Woolley CS, McEwen BS. 1995. Estradiol regulates hippocampal dendritic spine density via an N-methyl-D-aspartate receptor-dependent mechanism. *Journal of Neuroscience* 14:7680–7687.

Woolverton WL. 1986. Effects of a D1 and D2 dopamine antagonist on the self-administration of cocaine and piribedil by rhesus monkeys. *Pharmacology, Biochemistry and Behavior* 24:531–535.

Woolverton WL, Johnson KM. 1992. Neurobiology of cocaine abuse. *Trends in Pharmacological Sciences* 13:193–205.

Yaksh TL, Malmberg AB. 1994. Central pharmacology of nociceptive transmission. In: Wall PD, Melzack R, eds. *Textbook of Pain*. 3rd ed. Edinburgh: Churchill-Livingstone. Pp. 165–200.

Young AM, Goudie AJ. 1995. Adaptive processes regulating tolerance to behavioral effects of drugs. In: Bloom FE, Kupfer DJ, eds. *Psychopharmacology: Fourth Generation of Progress*. New York: Raven Press. Pp. 733–742.

Yuste R, Denk W. 1995. Dendritic spines are basic functional units of neuronal integration. *Nature* 375:682–684.

4

Epidemiology

Although originally concerned solely with communicable diseases, epidemiology has broadened its scope with time to encompass the study of the incidence, prevalence, causes, and consequences of a range of health problems and health behaviors (Rogers, 1965; NIDA, 1994a).[1] The application of epidemiology to the study of drug use and abuse is relatively recent. During the outbreak of heroin abuse in the late 1960s, the term "epidemic" began to be used (Kozel and Adams, 1986). After the National Institute on Drug Abuse (NIDA) was established in 1974, epidemiology became one of its earliest priorities, and one of the first publications in NIDA's Research Monograph Series was *Epidemiology of Drug Abuse: Current Issues* (NIDA, 1976). Epidemiological research continues to be one of the most active research programs at NIDA.

Traditionally, two classic triads of concepts serve as an organizational framework for epidemiology: the "epidemiologic triangle" of agent, host, and environment for analytic epidemiology and the specification of the rates of disease by person, place, and time for descriptive epidemiology (Lillienfeld and Stolley, 1994). In the application of the epidemiologic triangle, one would consider the drug as the agent of exposure, the host as the individual taking the drug, and the environment as the setting of

[1]Incidence is the number of new cases of a condition (such as heroin use) in a defined population within a specified period of time. Prevalence is the number of instances of a given condition (such as heroin use) in a defined population at a specified time (Last, 1983).

exposure. Early research applied a narrow traditional epidemiological framework to the study of heroin use (de Alarcon, 1969; Hughes and Crawford, 1972); however, recent studies employ a broader concept of epidemiology in which both descriptive and analytic epidemiological studies are used to address the problems of drug use and abuse in society.

Epidemiological research provides information essential for defining the scope of the problem by identifying populations at risk. Epidemiological data on trends in illicit drug use and abuse over time help to measure the effectiveness of the national drug control program. Epidemiological research provides insights into the etiology of drug initiation and use (Chapter 5). Additionally, epidemiological research provides information on the nature and extent of the multiple consequences of drug abuse (Chapter 7). Data on drug availability and demographics allow prevention and treatment programs to target the needs of those populations identified as at risk for increased alcohol and illicit drug use.

This chapter describes the variety of data systems currently in place that address different aspects of the drug use problem in the United States and discusses accomplishments and future directions in epidemiological research.

DEFINITIONS

One way in which the epidemiology of drug abuse differs from more traditional epidemiological studies of infectious diseases is that drug abuse is not universally accepted as a medical condition. As indicated in Chapter 1, there are differences of opinion about applying the medical model to drug abuse. Researchers and clinicians commonly distinguish three levels of drug behavior: use, abuse, and dependence (see Chapter 1 and Appendix C). The stages of abuse and dependence are most clearly amenable to a diagnostic perspective, whereas the use stage is more readily characterized by its frequency, quantity, and duration. Therefore, use is generally the stage most easily and accurately measured outside clinical practice as described by epidemiological research. A complication in research, however, is that different drugs have different patterns of use, and the transition from use to abuse to dependence may be very different for different drugs (e.g., heroin as compared to marijuana).

ACCOMPLISHMENTS

Clearly, one of the major accomplishments in epidemiology has been to establish a variety of data systems that measure different aspects of drug use and abuse. Two major data systems provide broad-based statistics on trends in drug use in the general population:[2] the National Household Survey on Drug Abuse (NHSDA) and the Monitoring the Future study (MTF). Additionally, a number of surveys and other data collection efforts describe use and abuse in specific populations (Table 4.1). Other major accomplishments of epidemiological research include the development of valid measures and survey methodologies and the collection and analysis of data on co-occurring psychiatric disorders, natural history, and etiology of drug abuse.

General Population Surveys

National Household Survey on Drug Abuse

NHSDA has been conducted periodically since 1971 and is currently an annual survey.[3] It provides national-level estimates of the prevalence of use of illicit drugs, alcohol, and tobacco among members of the household population of the United States (surveys before 1991 excluded Alaska and Hawaii). The survey is estimated to represent 98 percent of the total population age 12 and over; completion rates of the survey in recent years vary between 74 and 84 percent. The subpopulations excluded are homeless persons; persons living in correctional facilities, nursing homes, and treatment centers; and active military personnel (SAMHSA, 1995c).

The NHSDA series was designed to measure the prevalence and correlates of alcohol, tobacco, and illicit drug use in the United States; sufficient continuity has been evident in the core questions of NHSDA to be able to chart trends in drug use since 1972. In each survey, similar questions have been asked about the use of illicit drugs, alcohol, and tobacco in the respondent's lifetime, in the past year, and in the past month. Illicit drug use is defined as use of illegal drugs and nonmedical use of prescription-type psychotherapeutic drugs.

An important aspect of the epidemiology of drug use is the variation among persons (based on gender, age, and other demographic factors), place (region, population density), and time. Table 4.2 shows the prevalence of illicit drug use in the past month among the household popula-

---

[2]It is important to note that the total number of users results from the rates of use in different age groups in the population and from the demographic structure of the population. The actual number of users may increase while the average or overall rate of use are declining.

[3]The survey has been conducted annually since 1990. The National Commission on Marihuana and Drug Abuse sponsored the 1971 and 1972 surveys, NIDA sponsored the NHSDA from 1974 to 1990, and the Substance Abuse and Mental Health Services Administration has been the responsible agency since 1992.

TABLE 4.1 Major Epidemiologic Data Systems

Data System	Target Population	Current Sponsor	Status
Estimates of Use in Various Populations			
National Household Survey on Drug Abuse	General population, 12 years old and older	SAMHSA	Began in 1971; conducted annually
Monitoring the Future Study	Secondary school students, college students, young adults	NIDA	Began in 1975; conducted annually
DC*MADS	Population of District of Columbia Metropolitan Statistical Area, 12 years old and older	NIDA	Conducted in 1991
National Pregnancy and Health Survey	Pregnant women	NIDA	Conducted in 1992–1993
Survey of Health Related Behaviors Among Military Personnel	Active-duty military personnel	DOD	Conducted in 1980, 1982, 1985, 1988, 1992, and 1995
Drug Use Forecasting Program	Arrestees in 23 metropolitan areas	NIJ	Began in 1987; conducted quarterly
Community Epidemiology Work Group	Metropolitan areas	NIDA	Began in 1976; meets semi-annually
Estimates of Diagnoses of Abuse and Dependence			
National Comorbidity Survey	General population, 15–54 years old	NIMH, NIDA, W.T. Grant Foundation	Conducted in 1990–1992
Estimates of Consequences of Use			
Drug Abuse Warning Network	Hospital emergency room visits; deaths	SAMHSA	Began in 1973; data reported semiannually

NOTE: DC*MADS = Washington, D.C., Metropolitan Area Study; DOD = Department of Defense; NIDA = National Institute on Drug Abuse; NIJ = National Institute of Justice; NIMH = National Institute of Mental Health; SAMHSA = Substance Abuse and Mental Health Services Administration.

TABLE 4.2 Percentages Reporting Past Month Use of Any Illicit Drug by Age Group and Demographic Characteristics, 1994-B[a]

Demographic Characteristic	Age Group (years)				
	12–17	18–25	26–34	≥35	Total
Total	8.2	13.3	8.5	3.2	6.0
Race/Ethnicity					
White	8.5	14.6	9.0	3.1	6.0
Black	8.3	12.8	10.2	4.4	7.3
Hispanic	8.1	9.1	5.7	2.9	5.4
Other	2.7	*b*	3.2	*b*	3.1
Sex					
Male	8.5	17.1	11.6	4.3	7.9
Female	7.8	9.6	5.6	2.2	4.3
Population density[c]	7.6	14.0	9.1	3.0	6.1
Large metro	10.4	13.5	8.3	3.9	6.6
Small metro					
Nonmetro	5.7	11.8	7.5	2.4	4.8
Region					
Northeast	6.8	10.8	7.8	2.7	5.1
North Central	9.2	13.8	8.7	2.8	5.8
South	7.7	14.2	8.5	3.5	6.3
West	8.8	13.6	9.0	3.5	6.6
Adult education[d]					
<High school	N/A	15.8	13.3	2.2	5.8
High school graduate	N/A	12.8	9.3	3.2	5.9
Some college	N/A	14.0	7.7	3.5	6.4
College graduate	N/A	9.3	5.8	5.9	4.7
Current employment[d]					
Full-time	N/A	12.4	8.6	4.6	6.7
Part-time	N/A	12.8	7.5	3.8	6.7
Unemployed	N/A	19.9	16.4	8.9	13.9
Other[e]	N/A	13.3	5.8	0.8	2.7

NOTES: "Any illicit drug" is defined as nonmedical use of marijuana or hashish, cocaine (including crack), inhalants, hallucinogens (including LSD [lysergic acid diethlyanide] and PCP [phencyclidine]), heroin or psychotherapeutics at least once. The majority of illicit drug use is marijuana use. N/A = not applicable.

[a]Estimates for 1994-B are derived from the NHSDA new-version questionnaire.
[b]Low precision; no estimate reported.
[c]Population density is based on 1990 metropolitan statistical areas (MSA) classifications and their 1990 census of population counts.
[d]Data on adult education and current employment are not shown for persons aged 12–17. Estimates for both adult education and current employment are for persons aged ≥18.
[e]Retired, disabled, homemaker, student, or "other."

SOURCE: SAMHSA (1995c).

tion in 1994 by age and other demographic characteristics (SAMHSA, 1995c).[4] There are relatively large variations in the prevalence of illicit drug use by age group and by gender. The 18–25 age group is distinctly higher than other age groups, with the group 35 and older being lowest. Males are almost twice as likely as females to have used an illicit drug in the past month. Among other characteristics there are relatively small variations, with the exception that unemployed persons tend to have higher rates of drug use. There is relatively little variation in use rates by population density, indicating that illicit drug use has permeated the society and is not confined to certain areas.

One of the more interesting findings from this study and other population-based epidemiological studies is that African Americans under 25 tend to report rates of drug use that are similar to or lower than those of other racial or ethnic groups. This finding is not consistent with the impressions that many Americans have about rates of drug use, although a number of investigations have supported these findings (Bachman et al., 1991; Anthony et al., 1994; Wallace and Bachman, 1994). However, this may not be generally true for African Americans over 25, who tend to have higher rates of some illicit drug use than other racial or ethnic groups (Table 4.2).

Trends in the percentage of positive responses provide an indication of changes in the prevalence of use. As shown in Figure 4.1 for four age groups, the percentage of those who used any illicit drug in the previous month declined steadily from 1979 to 1991 in all age groups except the over-35 group, which consistently reported very low rates of illicit drug use in the past 30 days. In 1979, approximately 14 percent of the total household population reported having used one or more illicit drugs in the past month, compared with 6 percent in 1994 (SAMHSA, 1995c). The decreases were particularly dramatic among those aged 18 to 25, the age group that has historically had the highest rates of use. The decreases were more rapid in the earlier part of this period and have since leveled off, particularly in the two younger age groups. The most recent survey, conducted in 1994, however, shows a significant increase among the youngest respondents (ages 12–17) (SAMHSA, 1995c).

Monitoring the Future Study

The MTF is a series of surveys funded by NIDA that examines the use of alcohol, tobacco, and illicit drugs among young people from grade 8 through age 32. The core of the study, which began in 1975, consists of

[4]The majority of illicit drug use is marijuana use.

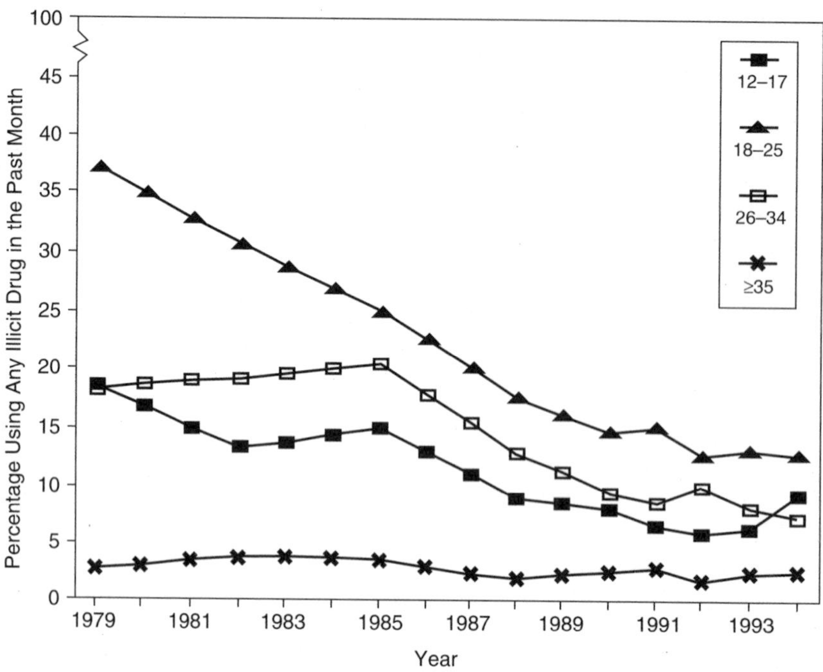

FIGURE 4.1 Trends in Monthly Prevalence of Use of Any Illicit Drug by Age. SOURCE: SAMHSA (1995c).

annual surveys of nationally representative samples of eighth-, tenth-, and twelfth-grade students;[5] in-school questionnaires are administered by professional interviewers to more than 45,000 students in approximately 420 public and private schools each year (Johnston et al., 1995). Since the MTF study targets students in grades 8, 10, and 12, those who have dropped out of school are not eligible. It is estimated that dropouts represent 15–20 percent of the twelfth-grade cohort; dropout rates are much lower for eighth and tenth grades (Johnston et al., 1995). In addition, absentee students are not included; absentee rates average 10 percent for eighth graders, 13 percent for tenth graders, and 16 percent for twelfth graders. School participation rates have ranged from 58 percent to 80 percent, varying by year and grade level.

This series documented a dramatic decrease in marijuana use throughout the decade of the 1980s and a general decline in the use of

[5]Beginning in 1991, students in grades 8 and 10 were added to the survey.

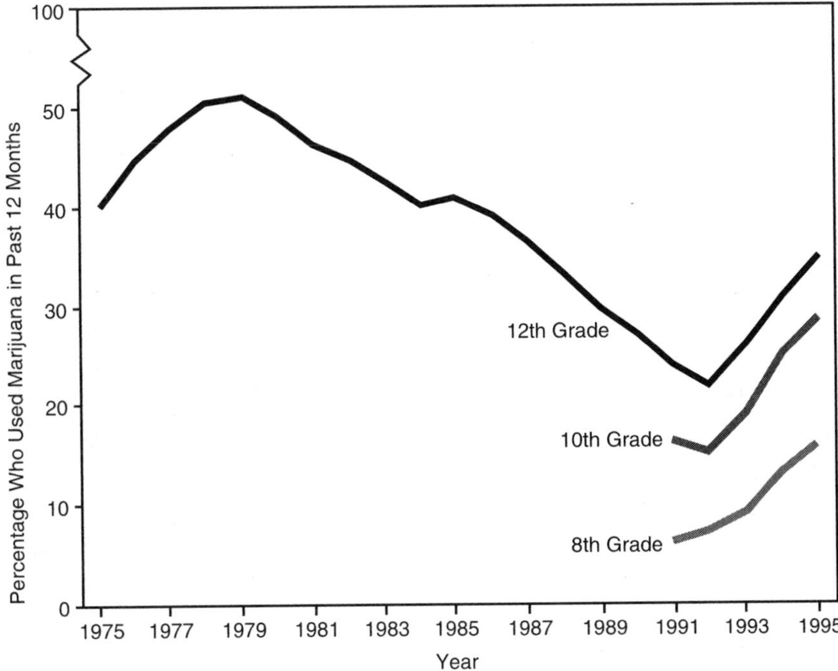

FIGURE 4.2 Trends in annual prevalence of marijuana use (1975–1995) by grade level (Monitoring the Future study, 1995). SOURCE: Johnston et al. (1995).

other illicit drugs. More recent surveys have produced evidence of an important reversal in this trend in the 1990s, particularly among the younger students, for use of several illicit drugs, with marijuana being most notable (Johnston et al., 1995). Figure 4.2 shows the trend lines for annual use of marijuana in the three student samples; all three grades show recent increases in marijuana use (Johnston et al., 1995). MTF also provides a national sample of college students and a national sample of young adult high school graduates. Those groups also showed dramatic decreases in marijuana use throughout the 1980s, although their rates have remained just about level or increased slightly in the early 1990s.

National Comorbidity Survey

NHSDA and MTF provide reasonably accurate epidemiological data on the use of alcohol, tobacco, and illicit drugs among the general population and the trends in those measures. However, they do not include measures of the numbers in the general population whose drug use has progressed to a psychiatric diagnosis of abuse or dependence. The National Comorbidity Survey (NCS) used a psychiatric diagnostic perspective to obtain population-based estimated rates of diagnoses of abuse and dependence.[6] NCS was sponsored primarily by the National Institute of Mental Health (NIMH), with supplemental support from NIDA and the W.T. Grant Foundation. NCS, conducted from 1990 to 1992, was a collaborative epidemiological investigation of the prevalence, causes, and consequences of psychiatric morbidity and comorbidity in the United States.

Results from this survey of more than 8,000 Americans age 15–54 show that a significant 7.5 percent had developed dependence on illicit drugs or inhalants; 4.2 percent were dependent on cannabis and 2.7 percent were dependent on cocaine (Anthony et al., 1994). One in four (24.1 percent) members of the study population had been or were dependent on tobacco; one in seven (14.1 percent) had a diagnosis of dependence on alcohol. Men were more likely than women to be diagnosed as dependent on illicit drugs. One in eleven men (9.2 percent) reached a (lifetime[7]) diagnosis of dependence on illicit drugs, compared with 5.9 percent of women.

Surveys of Specific Populations

Washington, D.C., Metropolitan Area Drug Study

The 1991 Washington, D.C., Metropolitan Area Drug Study (DC*MADS), funded by NIDA, examined the nature and extent of drug use among all types of persons residing in a single metropolitan area, with a special focus on groups that are underrepresented or unrepresented in NHSDA (NIDA, 1994b). These special samples included homeless people, transients, and institutionalized individuals. The objectives of DC*MADS were to estimate the prevalence, correlates, and consequences of drug use among the diverse populations residing in the metropolitan area and to develop a research model for similar data collection in other major metropolitan areas (NIDA, 1994b).

Additionally, DC*MADS data on homeless and institutionalized populations were analyzed to determine the impact of those results on estimates of the number of injection drug users derived from studies such

---

[6]There have been other important and significant efforts to determine the epidemiology of drug abuse and dependence; the most notable is the Epidemiology Catchment Area studies (Eaton and Kessler, 1985), but these were not nationally representative.

[7]The term "lifetime" is used to indicate a disorder occurring at any time during the life span to date and does not indicate a chronic, lifelong condition.

as NHSDA. DC*MADS data on homeless and institutionalized could be added to NHSDA estimates to determine the degree to which the household survey missed injection drug users. The conclusion was that incorporating DC*MADS data would have increased the NHSDA estimated prevalence of past year needle use from 0.2 to 0.3 percent, a small absolute difference (NIDA, 1994b). The number of needle users[8] among the household population was estimated at 5,987; after including homeless, transient, and institutionalized populations, the number was 8,740. The difference is too small to change prevalence estimates noticeably but is a significant difference (an increase of approximately 3,000 needle users) in the population estimates often used by providers for estimating the number of people in need of treatment. As with any survey of drug use, there will be some unknown portion of needle users who either deny use or refuse to participate, resulting in some degree of error when estimating injection drug use.

Drug Use Forecasting Program

The Drug Use Forecasting Program (DUF), launched in 1987 by the National Institute of Justice (NIJ), collects self-report and urinalysis testing information from selected samples of arrestees brought to booking facilities in 23 cities around the country (NIJ, 1994). DUF data identify the illicit drugs that are being used and how usage changes over time among arrestees. The target audiences for these data are state and local policymakers, court administrators, law enforcement officials, and drug treatment program staff. DUF data are collected for two weeks each quarter by trained individuals who interview booked arrestees and obtain voluntary, anonymous urine specimens (NIJ, 1994). Approximately 225 males are sampled quarterly in booking facilities. At some sites, female arrestees, juvenile arrestees, and detainees are also sampled. Typically, more than 90 percent of the arrestees approached agree to be interviewed, and approximately 80 percent of these provide urine specimens (NIJ, 1994). Selection of male adult offenders ensures a wide distribution across charges, with an emphasis on felony charges; female adults and all juvenile arrestees are included, regardless of charge.

The DUF program's major strength is its use of urinalysis to validate the self-reports of recent drug use. This is particularly important given the program's population of arrestees who often underreport their recent drug use. Because this is not a random sample and procedures may vary

---

[8] Needle use is defined as injection of cocaine, hallucinogens, heroin, or psychotherapeutics for nonmedical reasons at least once in the previous 12 months.

between sites, DUF data are not very useful for tracking prevalence or trends, but they are extremely useful regarding the use of drugs by arrestees. In 1993, the percentage of male booked arrestees testing positive for at least one drug ranged from 54 to 81 percent; there was a similar range for female booked arrestees, from 42 to 83 percent (NIJ, 1994).[9] In 21 of the 23 data collection sites, more than half of male and female booked adult arrestees tested positive for a drug at the time of arrest.

Department of Defense Survey of Health Related Behaviors Among Military Personnel

The Survey of Health Related Behaviors Among Military Personnel was conducted in 1980, 1982, 1985, 1988, 1992, and 1995. The eligible population for the survey consists of all active-duty military personnel except recruits, service academy students, persons absent without official leave (AWOL), and those personnel who had a permanent change of station at the time of the survey (Bray et al., 1995). In 1995 the sample consisted of 16,193 personnel selected to represent military personnel in all pay grades of the active-duty U.S. military throughout the world. Military personnel complete self-administered questionnaires, which include questions on the frequency of use of alcohol, tobacco, or illicit drugs in the past 30 days and within the past 12 months. There are also questions on the negative consequences of drug use and questions on a number of other health behaviors.

Trends from this survey show significant reductions in alcohol, tobacco, and illicit drug use since 1980. Use of any illicit drugs declined from 27.6 percent in 1980 to 3.0 percent in 1995. Cigarette smoking in the past 30 days prior to the survey declined from 51.0 percent in 1980 to 31.9 percent in 1995, and heavy drinking declined from 20.8 percent in 1980 to 17.1 percent in 1995 (Bray et al., 1995). Marijuana remained the most commonly used illicit drug: 1.7 percent of military personnel reported marijuana use in the past month and 4.6 percent in the past year.

A comparison of results of this survey with the general civilian population NHSDA shows consistently lower rates of illicit drug use among military personnel when demographic variations[10] are taken into account (Bray et al., 1995). Reasons for these differences include the military's

---

[9]Urine specimens are sent to a central laboratory and analyzed for ten drugs: cocaine, opiates, marijuana, PCP (phencyclidine), methadone, benzodiazepines, methaqualone, propoxyphene, barbiturates, and amphetamines.

[10]The military population is predominantly young males, a population with higher rates of illicit drug use.

strong emphasis on zero tolerance for illicit drug use and the use of random urinalysis testing among military personnel.

National Pregnancy and Health Survey

The first nationally representative survey of alcohol, tobacco, and illicit drug use among pregnant women was conducted in 1992 and sponsored by NIDA. This survey gathered self-report data from a national sample of 2,613 women who delivered babies in 52 urban and rural hospitals during 1992. The results indicate that more than 5 percent of the 4 million women who gave birth in the United States in 1992 used illicit drugs while they were pregnant (NIDA, 1996). This survey is discussed in more detail in Chapter 7.

Community-Level Assessments

Since the mid-1970s, semiannual community-level assessments of illicit drug use have been provided through the Community Epidemiology Work Group (CEWG)—a NIDA-sponsored surveillance network composed of researchers from major metropolitan areas in the United States. CEWG is not itself a data collection system; it synthesizes epidemiological and ethnographic research information from a variety of sources (including public health agencies, medical and treatment facilities, criminal justice and correctional offices, and law enforcement agencies) and provides current descriptive and analytic information on the nature and scope of drug abuse, emerging trends, consequences of illicit drug use and abuse, and characteristics of vulnerable populations. By focusing on specific communities, the CEWG is able to monitor illicit drug use trends and to document regionally specific illicit drug use patterns.

Recent CEWG proceedings include discussion of at least two trends that may significantly influence the epidemiology of drug abuse, particularly the prevalence of injection drug users. The first is AIDS-related mortality, which has already begun to deplete the number of individuals included within this population (NRC, 1995). The second, and potentially countervailing, trend is a resurgence in the prevalence of heroin use, which has been associated with an increasing number of initiates who are using the drug intranasally (NIDA, 1995).

Another community-level report *Pulse Check* is issued by the Office of National Drug Control Policy (ONDCP). This quarterly report is based on observations by ethnographers, law enforcement officials, and treatment providers throughout the United States on the use and distribution of illicit drugs (ONDCP, 1995).

Drug Abuse Warning Network

From a public health standpoint, it is particularly pertinent to know the mortality and morbidity statistics associated with drug abuse (Crowley, 1988). One mechanism for assembling and analyzing this data is the Drug Abuse Warning Network (DAWN), conducted annually by the Substance Abuse and Mental Health Services Administration (SAMHSA) to collect information on drug-related emergency department visits and medical examiner reports (SAMHSA, 1995a,b).[11] The data collected provide information on the estimated number of episodes in which a visit to a hospital emergency room[12] was related directly to the use of an illegal drug or the nonmedical use of a legal drug, or in which a death was drug related or a drug was mentioned in connection with death. Difficulties in data collection, including changes in sample composition, nonresponse from data collectors, changes in data collectors, and coding errors, place limitations on interpreting DAWN data.

Other Epidemiological Data Systems

A number of other data systems are relevant to the epidemiology of alcohol, tobacco, and illicit drug use and abuse and provide a variety of additional perspectives. The National Longitudinal Survey of Youth, sponsored by the U.S. Department of Labor, annually collects occupational information and asks about the relationship of alcohol use to occupational activities. The 1991 National Health Interview Survey of Drug and Alcohol Use and the Third National Health and Nutrition Examination Survey (NHANES III), sponsored by the National Center for Health Statistics, provide information on the correlation of alcohol, cigarette, and illicit drug use and abuse with other health conditions. The Youth Risk Behavior Surveillance System was developed by the Centers for Disease Control and Prevention. It includes national school-based surveys of high school students and has been conducted biennially since 1991. The National AIDS Demonstration Research Project and the National Cooperative Agreement for AIDS Community Based Outreach Intervention

---

[11] Although DAWN has existed since the early 1970s, prior to 1988 the sample was not representative of eligible hospitals (i.e., nonfederal, short-stay general hospitals that have a 24-hour emergency department). Statistical adjustments have been made to allow for some comparisons to be made from 1978 through 1987.

[12] It is important to note that emergency room data are collected on the number of visits to the emergency room but not collected on the extent to which the visits represent repeated contacts with the same patients. Additionally, each drug abuse episode or visit may have multiple drug mentions.

Research Program (sponsored by NIDA) use a targeted sample approach to study injection drug users who are not in treatment.

There are also a variety of attempts to assess the supply of illicit drugs and the success of efforts to reduce the supply. The data of greatest interest from a public health perspective are those that generate informed estimates of the overall amount of illicit drugs consumed and the amount spent by consumers of illicit drugs. Those data collection efforts include the Drug Enforcement Administration (DEA) System to Retrieve Information from Drug Evidence (STRIDE), which compiles data on illicit drugs purchased, seized, or acquired in DEA investigations and includes information on drug purity, street price, and location of confiscation.

RESEARCH OPPORTUNITIES

Refinement of Data Systems

As discussed above, the current epidemiological data collection surveys have made significant contributions to drug abuse research. However, opportunities exist for continued refinement of the data systems to provide more detailed information and analyses of the nature and extent of drug abuse and dependence. This information is critical to determine the extent of need for treatment and to provide information on trends over time in drug abuse and dependence.

As noted above, NHSDA and MTF provide reasonably accurate epidemiological data on alcohol, tobacco, and illicit drug use among the general population, but they are limited in assessing the extent of abuse or dependence. Although both surveys ask questions about frequent use and the resulting consequences of use, neither one allows for diagnosis of DSM (*Diagnostic and Statistical Manual of Mental Disorders*; APA, 1994) disorders; moreover, neither one achieves full coverage of individuals who are drug abusers or drug dependent.

Given the variations in drug use patterns (e.g., binges by cocaine users), it is important to collect additional data on the frequency of use within the span of a day or a week. Increasing the focus of data collection on drug use frequency, consequences of drug use, and other items designed to measure DSM criteria for drug abuse and dependence (e.g., withdrawal and relapse) will provide much needed information on the extent of drug abuse and dependence.

Co-Occurring Psychiatric Disorders

A major accomplishment of epidemiological research has been the collection and analysis of data on the co-occurrence of drug abuse with other illnesses, particularly psychiatric disorders. The Epidemiologic Catchment Area Program sponsored by NIMH documented the high co-occurrence of alcohol and illicit drug use disorders and other psychiatric disorders (Regier et al., 1990). The NCS (see above) provides the first nationally representative estimates on the co-occurrence of drug abuse and psychiatric disorders. The principal finding is that there is a significant overlap in diagnoses. Roughly half of those age 15–54 who had a lifetime addictive disorder (as defined by DSM-III-R) also had a lifetime psychiatric disorder. Similarly, about half of those with a lifetime psychiatric disorder also had a lifetime addictive disorder. The great majority (84 percent) of those with lifetime co-occurrence reported that their first psychiatric disorder occurred prior to their first addictive disorder (Kessler et al., 1996). Further, the NCS found that all the psychiatric disorders (identified) are consistently more strongly associated with dependence as opposed to abuse. Compared to other affective disorders and anxiety disorders, mania is more strongly associated with dependence on alcohol or illicit drugs. Conduct disorders and adult antisocial behavior were more strongly associated with both abuse and dependence than the anxiety disorders or any of the affective disorders other than mania (Kessler et al., 1996). Those extremely high rates of co-occurrence obviously have great implication for treatment, prevention, and understanding the nature of addictive disorders (Chapters 5 and 8).

Although the NCS studied comorbidities with psychiatric disorders, addictive disorders also co-occur with other health and physical disorders. For example, tuberculosis, hepatitis, sexually transmitted diseases, and AIDS are all more prevalent among alcoholics or illicit drug abusers than nonabusers. Other conditions such as homelessness and victimization may also be co-occurring, but await further epidemiological study.

As with any epidemiological study, the fact of co-occurrence does not indicate a causal connection. There are a variety of possible causal relationships. An important task for future research is to provide analysis of the possible reasons for co-occurring disorders in an effort to improve treatment and prevention strategies.

Natural History of Drug Use

Epidemiological research also has contributed to knowledge of the natural history, or life course, of drug use and abuse in the general population, including delineation of stages of involvement with different drugs and degrees of involvement with different types of drugs. Such natural histories require longitudinal studies of individuals over time to discern changes with age; however, there are relatively few studies that span a broad age range. Moreover, it is preferable to utilize a cohort sequential design to isolate classes of probable causes and the time period during which they operate in an individual's life. This research methodology allows for differentiation among age-, history-, or cohort-related factors.

There has been one recent report from a single cohort delineating the natural history of drug use from adolescence to the midthirties in a general population sample (Chen and Kandel, 1995). That study was based on a cohort of adolescents (born from 1954 to 1956) in grades 10 and 11 in New York State public schools. An important finding was that there was little initiation into illicit drug use after age 29, the age by which most use had ceased. Among heavier users, the proportions of heavy use declined for alcohol and marijuana, but not for cigarettes. Because this is a study of a single cohort (and therefore confounds historical effects with age effects), it will be important to confirm the findings with data from other ongoing and future studies.

Currently more is known about the initiation of drug use than about the transition from use to abuse and dependence. Although investigation of the transition between the stages from use to dependence is primarily in the purview of etiological research (see Chapter 5), large-scale epidemiological studies can provide a fertile ground for generating hypotheses, as well as for testing them. The NCS has found differences in the sociodemographic correlates of first use and dependence among users and in the persistence of abuse and dependence (Warner et al., 1995). The cohort effects seen in the NCS emphasize the need to incorporate designs that allow for differentiation of age, cohort, and historical factors. The natural history of drug use, especially focusing on abuse and dependence, is an area for continued research. If the variables associated with the transition from drug use to abuse and dependence can be identified (and are amenable to manipulation), prevention programs and strategies may be developed that target those variables.

Causal Relationships and Societal Norms

Epidemiological research has provided an important source of information regarding the etiology of drug use and the social attitudes and norms pertaining to use. Data from the MTF study have been used to demonstrate a close link between certain attitudes or beliefs about drugs and use. At the aggregate level there is a very close association between perceived harm and use, and an extensive series of analyses of data at the individual level supported a causal interpretation of the belief–behavior link (Bachman et al., 1988, 1990). There appears to be clear evidence that, as the perceived risk of harm associated with marijuana use increased, the prevalence of marijuana use decreased. It is important to note that the recent upturn in use in 1993 was accompanied, and even preceded, by a downturn in perceived risk.

The MTF study also measures perceived availability of alcohol, cigarettes, or illicit drugs, but analyses of that data did not show changes in perceived availability that could account for the changes in use. Without such data and analyses, the declines in marijuana and cocaine use might have been attributed to putative successes in reducing availability. Thus, the epidemiological data provide a means to generate hypotheses and also to refute hypotheses.

Epidemiological data can also be used to address more fundamental issues having to do with "norms" related to illicit drug use.[13] Epidemiological research can be very useful in assessing what the norms are for particular drug-related behaviors and how those norms vary by person, place, and time. Most researchers in the field would emphasize the role of social factors, including broad social-cultural norms, in influencing initiation and experimental use of alcohol, tobacco, or illicit drugs, while intra-individual factors (biological and psychological) would be emphasized in influencing the transition to abuse or dependence (Glantz and Pickens, 1992). Epidemiological research in this field continues to go beyond descriptive documentation of occurrences of a condition according to persons, place, and time by contributing causal analyses of the occurrences.

Ethnographic Research

The patterns, prevalence, and consequences of alcohol, tobacco, and illicit drug use and abuse within youth populations are not fully understood. As mentioned above, young African Americans have significantly lower levels of cigarette and illicit drug use than most of their peers. The 1993 MTF study found that 4.9 percent of African American high school seniors reported daily cigarette use, compared with 22.9 percent of white students (Johnston et al., 1995). The reasons for those differences are not yet understood, and it would be useful to elucidate the reasons for low use among African Americans to determine if that information could be transferred across cultural lines. Further, ethnographic research could provide important data on local-level illicit drug use that could be used to identify potential trends; study the natural history and progression of alcohol, tobacco, and illicit drug use; and provide greater detail than more quantitative surveys.

Studying the problem of illicit drug use and abuse in a variety of

---

[13]The term "norm" is used to refer to both the prescriptive sense (i.e., guidelines for behavior considered to be acceptable) and the statistical sense (i.e., behavior that is approved or practiced by a majority).

cultures would be useful from a number of perspectives. Comparing prevalences of illicit drug use and abuse across cultures may provide information on the universality or generalizability of risk and protective factors. It may also be easier to study the role of specific factors, such as drug availability, by comparing countries such as Colombia (where cocaine is more readily available) with Asian countries (where heroin is more widely available). Additionally, cultural differences offer the opportunity to learn more about the nature and consequences of specific histories (e.g., by comparing U.S. drug abusers, many of whom are multiple drug abusers, with cultures such as China, where it is easier to find individuals who are heavy users of only one illicit drug).

Measurement and Analysis

Research Design and Data Analysis

Research designs and analytical procedures developed for epidemiological research on drug use have further advanced the field of epidemiology in general. Epidemiological data are often collected under conditions of less than complete control (e.g., missing data, attrition, errors of measurement, including deliberately inaccurate reporting), which contribute to analytic problems. However, various research designs and data analysis methods have been implemented to improve the confidence in epidemiological reporting. For example, a structural equation computer program was developed (Bentler and Wu, 1993) from theoretical statistics, algorithmic experiments, and applied data analysis; multilevel analysis, missing data analysis, and meta-analysis have been developed or improved (Collins et al., 1994).

Improved analytical techniques and increasingly sophisticated models will provide more focused and accurate data. Traditional epidemiological survival analysis methods could elucidate aspects of timing of onset of abuse, time to cessation, and time to relapse (Singer and Willett, 1994). Latent growth curve modeling (Duncan and Duncan, 1995), latent class analysis (Uebersax, 1994), and latent transition analysis (Collins et al., 1994) are currently areas of promise for refinement in data analysis. Strategies and software for dealing with missing data are developing at a rapid pace (Graham et al., 1994). A particularly active area is the extension of structural equation methods to accommodate multilevel models; models that do not require traditional assumptions of additivity or linearity; and models that do not require variables that are normally distributed, continuous, and independently measured (e.g., Muthén, 1993). Thus, by using the same level of data collection, it will now be possible to perform increasingly sophisticated analyses that provide additional information regarding alcohol, tobacco, and illicit drug use and abuse problems.

Furthermore, it is critical that future research coordinate both quantitative (e.g., probability-based surveys) and qualitative (trained-observer or ethnographic) approaches in an effort to maximize both their unique contributions and their synergistic potential (see section above). Optimizing the use of both approaches will provide a fuller picture of the nature and extent of alcohol, tobacco, and illicit drug use, abuse, and dependence.

Self-Reports and Biological Indicators

Self-report methods have been shown to be generally reliable and valid when gathered under proper conditions. Such conditions include clear and understandable interview procedures and questionnaires, confidence by the respondent that responses will be kept confidential, and some degree of willingness by the respondent to provide accurate information. However, under some conditions, self-reports are likely to be far less valid. For example, research has shown that higher rates of illicit drug use are found with the use of self-administered questionnaires instead of direct reporting to the interviewer (Turner et al., 1992) and with the use of in-school questionnaires as compared to in-home interviews of adolescents (Rootman and Smart, 1985). Other examples include questioning arrestees or pregnant women about recent drug use. Thus, biological indicators are useful tools to support the validity of self-reports. It would be useful to know the degree to which standard survey techniques underrepresent actual use.

Currently, there are a number of efforts to improve the reliability and validity of self-reported data. The use of computers in collecting data is being explored, including the development of computer-assisted self-administered instruments (CASI) that may produce improved reports of alcohol, tobacco, or illicit drug use. Audio-CASI would incorporate an audio component and would allow minimally literate respondents to hear the questions and respond directly to the computer (e.g., verbally, via keypad or touch-screen); this technique would also facilitate the use of multiple languages. Such procedures need to be researched carefully so that there is an assessment of benefits (improved reliability and validity), costs, and impacts on privacy and confidentiality. Another line of self-report research is the use of principles of cognitive psychology to inform survey methodology (Turner et al., 1992). Those principles include recognition that memory is essentially a reconstructive process, awareness that respondents employ different strategies for reconstructing needed information, and adoption of techniques such as "bounding" to improve memory reconstruction. Substantial changes were made in the 1994 NHSDA as a result of applying those principles.

Biological indicators are useful tools to support the validity of self-reports. Urinalysis testing can now detect with a very high degree of accuracy if illicit drugs have been used recently. Institution of random testing of urine samples is likely responsible, in part, for the dramatic decline in use of illicit drugs in the U.S. Armed Forces, indicating that drug testing can be useful both for epidemiological surveillance and for deterrence (Bray et al., 1992). Saliva, sweat patches, and expired breath can also be used to detect a range of licit and illicit drugs.

Although biological indicators are generally considered to be more valid than self-reports, they are more complicated and more expensive to implement. Additionally, for drugs that are rapidly metabolized, they may detect use only within a limited time frame. To increase the validity of reports of alcohol, tobacco, and illicit drug use, continued investigation of biological markers will be important. Saliva and hair samples are more easily obtained in field studies than urine or blood samples. Drug testing by hair analysis is a particularly active area of research; NIDA and NIJ have recently published the results of a series of collaborative efforts on hair testing financed under an interagency agreement (Cone et al., 1995).

CONCLUSION AND RECOMMENDATION

Significant progress has been made in collecting and analyzing data on the extent, incidence, prevalence, and trends of alcohol, tobacco, and illicit drug use. Major data systems are in place that allow incipient changes in use to be detected and provide information for policymakers to prioritize prevention and treatment efforts. However, although use has been studied extensively, it has been more difficult to determine the nature and extent of abuse or dependence.

Additional epidemiological research should focus on collecting and analyzing data on the nature and extent of drug abuse and dependence, drug use patterns, co-occurring drug abuse and psychiatric disorders, and refinement of measurement and analytical tools. Continued and refined epidemiological research will provide the data and analyses necessary for the development of treatment and prevention programs and will inform decisions on future allocation of resources to best address the alcohol, tobacco, and illicit drug abuse problem.

The committee recommends continued epidemiological research to allow for the assessment of a broader range of issues. Those issues may include the extent of drug abuse and dependence; the nature and extent of drug use and abuse among youth; the nature and

extent of co-occurring drug abuse and psychiatric disorders; and improvement in the reliability and validity of the methods for collecting and analyzing the data.

REFERENCES

Anthony JC, Warner LA, Kessler RC. 1994. Comparative epidemiology of dependence on tobacco, alcohol, controlled substances, and inhalants: Basic findings from the National Comorbidity Study. *Experimental and Clinical Psychopharmacology* 2:244–268.

APA (American Psychiatric Association). 1994. *Diagnostic and Statistical Manual of Mental Disorders*. 4th ed. Washington, DC: APA.

Bachman JG, Johnston LD, O'Malley PM, Humphrey RH. 1988. Explaining the recent decline in marijuana use: Differentiating the effects of perceived risks, disapproval, and general lifestyle factors. *Journal of Health and Social Behavior* 29:92–112.

Bachman JG, Johnston LD, O'Malley PM. 1990. Explaining the recent decline in cocaine use among young adults: Further evidence that perceived risks and disapproval lead to reduced drug use. *Journal of Health and Social Behavior* 31:173–184.

Bachman JG, Wallace JM Jr, O'Malley PM, Johnston LD, Kurth CL, Neighbors HW. 1991. Racial/ethnic differences in smoking, drinking, and illicit drug use among American high school seniors, 1976-1989. *American Journal of Public Health* 81:372–377.

Bentler PB, Wu EJC. 1993. *EQS/Windows Users Guide*. Los Angeles: BMDP Statistical Software.

Bray RM, Kroutil LA, Luckey JW, Wheeless SC, Iannacchione VG, Anderson DW, Marsden ME, Dunteman GH. 1992. *1992 Worldwide Survey of Substance Abuse and Health Behaviors Among Military Personnel*. RTI/5154/06-16FR. Research Triangle Park, NC: Research Triangle Institute.

Bray RM, Kroutil LA, Wheeless SC, Marsden ME, Bailey SL, Fairbank JA, Harford TC. 1995. *1995 Department of Defense Survey of Health Related Behaviors Among Military Personnel*. RTI/6019/06FR. Research Triangle Park, NC: Research Triangle Institute.

Chen K, Kandel DB. 1995. The natural history of drug use from adolescence to the mid-thirties in a general population sample. *American Journal of Public Health* 85:41–47.

Collins LM, Graham JW, Rousculp SS, Fidler PL, Pan J, Hansen WB. 1994. Latent transition analysis and how it can address prevention research questions. *NIDA Research Monograph* 142:81–111.

Cone EJ, Welch MJ, Babecki MBG, eds. 1995. *Hair Testing for Drugs of Abuse: International Research on Standards and Technology*. Rockville MD: National Institute on Drug Abuse. NIH Publication No. 95-3727.

Crowley TJ. 1988. Learning and unlearning drug abuse in the real world: Clinical treatment and public policy. *NIDA Research Monograph* 84:100–121.

de Alarcon R. 1969. The spread of heroin abuse in a community. *Bulletin on Narcotics* 21:17–22.

Duncan TE, Duncan SC. 1995. Modeling the processes of development via latent growth curve methodology. *Structural Equation Modeling* 2:187–213.

Eaton WW, Kessler LG, eds. 1985. *Epidemiologic Field Methods in Psychiatry: The NIMH Epidemiologic Catchment Area Program*. Orlando FL: Academic Press.

Glantz MD, Pickens RW, eds. 1992. *Vulnerability to Drug Abuse*. Washington, DC: American Psychological Association.

Graham JW, Hofer SM, Piccinin AM. 1994. Analysis with missing data in drug prevention research. *NIDA Research Monograph* 142:13–63.

Hughes PH, Crawford GA. 1972. A contagious disease model for researching and intervening in heroin epidemics. *Archives of General Psychiatry* 27:149–155.

Johnston LD, O'Malley PM, Bachman JG. 1995. *National Survey Results on Drug Use from the Monitoring the Future Study, 1975–1994. Vol. 1, Secondary School Students*. Ann Arbor, MI: Institute for Social Research, University of Michigan.

Kessler RC, Nelson CB, McGonagle KA, Edlund MJ, Frank RG, Leaf PJ. 1996. The epidemiology of co-occurring addictive and mental disorders in the National Comorbidity Survey: Implications for prevention and service utilization. *American Journal of Orthopsychiatry* 66(1):17–31.

Kozel NJ, Adams EH. 1986. Epidemiology of drug abuse: An overview. *Science* 234:970–974.

Last JM, ed. 1983. *A Dictionary of Epidemiology*. New York: Oxford University Press.

Lillienfeld DE, Stolley PD. 1994. *Foundations of Epidemiology*. 3rd ed. New York: Oxford University Press.

Muthén B. 1993. Latent variable modeling of growth with missing data and multilevel data. In: Cudras CM, Rao CR, eds. *Multivariate Analysis: Future Directions*. New York: North Holland Publishing.

NIDA (National Institute on Drug Abuse). 1976. *Epidemiology of Drug Abuse: Current Issues*. NIDA Research Monograph 10. Rockville, MD: NIDA.

NIDA (National Institute on Drug Abuse). 1994a. *1995 Budget Estimate*. Rockville, MD: NIDA.

NIDA (National Institute on Drug Abuse). 1994b. *Prevalence of Drug Use in the DC Metropolitan Area Household and Nonhousehold Populations: 1991*. Technical Report 8. Rockville, MD: NIDA.

NIDA (National Institute on Drug Abuse). 1995. *Community Epidemiology Work Group, December 1994 Report. Vol. I: Highlights and Executive Summary*. Rockville, MD: NIDA.

NIDA (National Institute on Drug Abuse). 1996. *National Pregnancy and Health Survey: Drug Use Among Women Delivering Livebirths, 1992*. NIH Publication No. 96-3819. Rockville, MD: NIDA.

NIJ (National Institute of Justice). 1994. *Drug Use Forecasting 1993 Annual Report on Adult Arrestees*. NCJ 147411. Washington, DC: NIJ.

NRC (National Research Council). 1995. *Preventing HIV Transmission: The Role of Sterile Needles and Bleach*. Washington, DC: National Academy Press.

ONDCP (Office of National Drug Control Policy). 1995. *Pulse Check: National Trends in Drug Abuse*. Washington, DC: ONDCP.

Regier DA, Farmer ME, Rae DS, Locke BZ, Keith SJ, Judd LL, Goodwin FK. 1990. Comorbidity of mental disorders with alcohol and other drug abuse. Results from the Epidemiologic Catchment Area Study. *Journal of the American Medical Association* 264(19):2511–2518.

Rogers FB, ed. 1965. *Studies in Epidemiology*. New York: Putnam.

Rootman I, Smart RG. 1985. A comparison of alcohol, tobacco, and drug use as determined from household and school surveys. *Drug and Alcohol Dependence* 16:89–94.

SAMHSA (Substance Abuse and Mental Health Services Administration). 1995a. *Annual Medical Examiner Data, 1993. Data from the Drug Abuse Warning Network*. Statistical Series I, Number 13-B. Rockville, MD: SAMHSA.

SAMHSA (Substance Abuse and Mental Health Services Administration). 1995b. *Preliminary Estimates from the Drug Abuse Warning Network: 1994 Preliminary Estimates of Drug-Related Emergency Department Episodes. Advance Report Number 11*. Rockville, MD: SAMHSA.

SAMHSA (Substance Abuse and Mental Health Services Administration). 1995c. *National Household Survey on Drug Abuse: Population Estimates 1994*. Rockville, MD: SAMHSA.

Singer JD, Willett JB. 1994. Designing and analyzing studies of onset, cessation, and relapse: Using survival analysis in drug abuse prevention research. *NIDA Research Monograph* 142:196–263.

Turner CF, Lessler JT, Gfroerer, JC. 1992. Future directions for research and practice. In: Turner CF, Lessler JT, Gfroerer JC, eds. *Survey Measurement of Drug Use: Methodological Studies*. Rockville, MD: NIDA.

Uebersax JS. 1994. Latent class analysis of substance abuse patterns. *NIDA Research Monograph* 142:64–80.

Wallace JM Jr, Bachman JG. 1994. Validity of self-reports in student-based studies on minority populations: Issues and concerns. *NIDA Research Monograph* 130:167–200.

Warner LA, Kessler RC, Hughes M, Anthony JC, Nelson CB. 1995. Prevalence and correlates of drug use and dependence in the United States. Results from the National Comorbidity Survey. *Archives of General Psychiatry* 52:219–229.

5

Etiology

Etiological research focuses primarily on the likely causes and correlates of drug use; it has identified many factors that affect drug use, although no single variable or set of variables explains drug use by an individual. There is no reason to believe that the same factor will affect all individuals in the same way, nor is there any reason to believe that the factors responsible for initiation of drug use are of equal importance in the continuation or escalation of use. Further, there appears to be no consensus as to what factors are involved in all cases of drug use and abuse (OTA, 1994). Generally, etiological studies conducted on population samples have focused on drug use; those conducted on clinical samples, especially those concerned with familial factors, have tended to focus on the etiology of drug abuse and dependence.

Two general categories of variables have been examined—risk factors and protective factors— although research, to date, has focused primarily on risk factors associated with drug use rather than on abuse and dependence. Risk factors are related to the probability of an individual's developing a disease or to vulnerability, which is a predisposition to a specific disease process (IOM, 1994b). Before a factor is labeled a risk factor, it has to satisfy the following conditions: the risk factor must be statistically associated with the disease; the risk factor must precede the onset of disease; and the observed association must not be spurious. There have been several recent reviews of the extensive literature on risk factors for drug use (see Newcomb and Bentler, 1986; Maddahian et al., 1988; Bry,

1989; Kumpfer, 1989; Brook and Brook, 1990; Swaim, 1991; Clayton, 1992; Glantz and Pickens, 1992; Hawkins et al., 1992; Petraitis et al., 1995).

Protective factors are variables that are statistically associated with reduced likelihood of drug use (see Garmezy, 1983; Rutter, 1983; Brook et al., 1986a; Labouvie and McGee, 1986). In statistical terms, a protective factor moderates the relationship between a risk factor and drug use or abuse, or it buffers the impact of risk factors on the individual. When the protective factor is present, it is assumed that there will be considerably less drug use or abuse than would otherwise be expected, given the risk factors that are also present. Recent research has described two types of protective factors that could operate among adolescents (Brook et al., 1990). In the first type of protection (risk-protective), risk factors are attenuated by protective factors in the adolescent's personality. The second type of protection (protective-protective) involves a synergistic interaction whereby one protective factor potentiates the effects of another, so that their joint effect is greater than the sum of either protective factor considered alone.

One of the goals of etiologic research has been to identify variables (such as risk and protective factors) that may be associated with drug use. The underlying interest in such variables is to determine if manipulation of risk and protective factors can moderate drug use outcomes. For either a risk factor or a protective factor to be targeted in intervention efforts, however, it is first necessary to demonstrate that the variable is amenable to manipulation and can be influenced by changes in the environment or by educational or medical interventions. Finally, intervention efforts must be carried out as well-controlled, rigorous experiments for the analysis of results to be meaningful.

ACCOMPLISHMENTS

Over the past 25 years, progress has been made in understanding risk factors associated with drug use, including biological, psychosocial, and contextual (social and environmental) risk factors. Unfortunately less is known about protective factors. The accomplishments noted below are representative of advances in the field and are not meant to document all risk factors or protective factors that have been identified. Finally, this chapter is not meant to be exhaustive, but to illustrate the types of studies that have illuminated knowledge in this field and to highlight opportunities for further study.

Biological Factors

Genetic Vulnerability

Family studies are important for identifying genetic vulnerability for drug abuse; for example, studies that have investigated generational differences in the transmission of drug abuse revealed that drug use or abuse is elevated among siblings of drug abusers and that there is a direct relationship between parental drug use or abuse and offspring use or abuse (Merikangas et al., 1992). A number of studies have focused on the familial aggregation of alcoholism and illicit drug abuse (see reviews by Merikangas, 1990; Glantz and Pickens, 1992; Gordon, 1994). Sons and daughters of alcoholics demonstrate a three- to fourfold risk of developing alcoholism (Cotton, 1979; Schuckit, 1986). Differences in the risk of alcohol and illicit drug use among individuals with a parental history of alcoholism may emerge at the time of transition from late adolescence to early adulthood, which may be a critical period for the expression of drug use vulnerability (Pandina and Johnson, 1989). The high recurrence of alcoholism among offspring of parents with alcoholism demonstrates that family history is one of the most potent predictors of vulnerability to alcohol abuse, which results to some extent from genetic factors (Merikangas, 1990; Pickens et al., 1991). However, the mechanism through which the family confers an increased risk is unknown. In addition to the contributions of genetic and biological factors to individual vulnerability for drug abuse, both transmitted and nontransmitted family factors, as well as unique environmental factors, appear to be involved in the vulnerability for drug abuse (Pickens et al., 1991). Family studies by themselves, however, cannot definitively determine the effect of genetics versus the environment on the development of alcoholism or drug abuse.

Twin Studies A traditional study paradigm used to identify the role of genetic factors in the etiology of a trait or disorder is the study of twins. Typically, a comparison is made between the prevalence of a disorder among twin pairs who possess identical genes (monozygotic or identical twins) and twin pairs who have only half of their genes in common (dizygotic or fraternal twins). For any disease, if the environment has no influence, monozygotic twins would always be concordant (similar) with respect to the disease. However, because both genetic and environmental factors play a role, it is generally not possible to discriminate among the many possible influences. Additionally, monozygotic twins are often raised in similar environments (e.g., they are dressed alike, often share friends, and copy each other's behaviors) and often share environmental factors to a greater extent than dizygotic twins, which makes it difficult to discriminate between genetic and environmental influences (Helzer and Burnam, 1991).

Nonetheless, many twin studies have provided useful insight regarding the possible role that genetic factors play in the familial aggregation of drug abuse (Cloninger et al., 1981; Gurling et al., 1981; Hrubec and Omenn, 1981; Pedersen, 1981; Murray et al., 1983; Pickens et al., 1991). Cloninger and colleagues (1981) and others have found that monozygotic twins are about twice as likely as dizygotic twins (of the same sex) to be concordant for alcoholism. The highest twin correlations, however, were reported for nicotine and caffeine, based on a study of the Swedish twin registry (Pederson et al., 1981). The role of genetic factors in the etiology of drug abuse for monozygotic twins reared apart has been studied (Grove et al., 1990). Researchers examined the concordance for alcoholism, illicit drug abuse, and antisocial personality disorder among monozygotic twin pairs separated at birth and found that the heritability of illicit drug abuse exceeded that of alcoholism. Pickens and colleagues (1991) found that the drug abuse concordance rate was significantly greater for monozygotic twins than for dizygotic twins in males but not in females. Furthermore, illicit drug abuse has been found to be associated with conduct disorder in childhood and with antisocial personality in adulthood (see below). The aggregate of these findings suggests that genetic factors explain some of the variance in the development of drug abuse and that a large proportion of the heritability of drug abuse in adulthood may be attributed to genetic factors that underlie the development of behavior problems in childhood (Cadoret et al., 1980; Grove et al., 1990).

Adoption Studies The optimal study paradigm for discriminating the interaction of genetic and environmental factors in the development of a trait or disorder is cross-adoption studies, in which adoptees with biological vulnerability for drug abuse, for example, are reared in homes of non-drug-abusing adoptive parents, and adoptees whose biological parents lack a history of drug abuse are reared in homes of parents with drug abuse. Cross-adoption studies of children of alcoholics who were raised by nonalcoholic adoptive parents have shown a three- to fourfold increased risk for alcohol abuse and dependence compared to adoptees whose parents were not alcoholics (Schuckit et al., 1972; Goodwin et al., 1973; Cadoret et al., 1980; Bohman et al., 1981; Cloninger et al., 1981).

Physiological Vulnerability

Review of the current state of knowledge of individual differences with regard to physiological effects of illicit drugs is beyond the scope of this chapter. However, such differences (see Chapter 3) are expected to be key factors in the formulation of theories regarding the etiology of drug abuse. Physiological influences that may exacerbate an individual's vulnerability to drug abuse could include neurochemical system impairment and heightened susceptibility to a drug because of biologically determined responsiveness. Although there has been substantial research on individual differences in response to ethanol and nicotine, less is known regarding the effects of the major classes of illicit drugs of abuse, such as opioids, stimulants, and cannabis.

Metabolic Variations There are large interindividual and interethnic variations in the outcome of alcohol use and abuse (Goedde et al., 1992). Studies have demonstrated that, in contrast to Caucasians, many Asians are biologically protected from becoming alcoholics because of the polymorphism of two liver enzymes: aldehyde dehydrogenase (ALDH2) and alcohol dehydrogenase-2 (ADH2). The Asians appear to have a protective factor in the form of inactive ALDH2 and high frequencies of atypical ADH2 (Higuchi et al., 1995), whereas Caucasians primarily have only active ALDH2 and usual ADH2 (Yoshida et al., 1991). The inactive form of ALDH2 is considered protective against alcoholism because it allows high levels of acetaldehyde to accumulate in the blood and causes adverse reactions, known as the flushing response (Thomasson et al., 1991; Yoshida et al., 1991). This increase in acetaldehyde blood levels after ingestion of ethanol appears to have a protective influence on further ingestion and thus appears to lower the rate of alcoholism (Bosron and Li, 1986).

Efficient ethanol metabolism may enhance the risk of alcoholism by allowing ingestion of a sufficient quantity to mediate the addictive potential of alcohol. Studies of the male offspring of alcoholics have demonstrated that the ability to tolerate large quantities of alcohol with fewer subjective effects may be a potent signal of the subsequent development of alcoholism (Schuckit, 1984, 1985). Thus, the inability to metabolize a drug may be a protective influence in continued exposure, whereas efficient metabolism may permit high levels of exposure conducive to the development of abuse and dependence.

Biochemical Markers Monoamine oxidase (MAO) is a widely studied biochemical marker for alcohol abuse. Several studies comparing alcoholics with nonalcoholics have found decreased platelet MAO activity levels among alcohol abusers (von Knorring et al., 1985; Pandey et al., 1988; Tabakoff et al., 1988). MAO is an enzyme that is important in the metabolism of a variety of brain neurotransmitters that affect behavior, including dopamine, norepinephrine, and serotonin. Although other biochemical markers have been investigated, no consistent findings have emerged.

Psychosocial Factors

The majority of studies of psychosocial risk factors focus on adolescents and the initiation of drug use, rather than on the risk of escalating to abuse or dependence. Unfortunately, many of the studies are cross sectional, so that it is difficult to disentangle the risk factors for use from those for abuse and dependence. Additionally, many of these studies fail to control for parental alcoholism, psychiatric disorders, or other risk factors, and many of them do not distinguish between use and abuse. Given those limitations, a selection of studies that demonstrate risk factors contributing to psychological vulnerability for drug use is presented below.

Personality Traits

There is a substantial literature regarding the relationship between personality traits and drug use, particularly in adolescents (Jessor et al., 1973; Jessor and Jessor, 1975; Kandel, 1980; Hawkins et al., 1985; Brook and Brook, 1990; Clayton, 1992). Relatively few studies, however, have examined the specific role of personality traits in the development of drug abuse and dependence. The majority of studies have focused on the characteristics of alcoholics (McCord and McCord, 1960; Robins, 1966; Vaillant and Milofsky, 1982; Cloninger et al., 1988; Tarter et al., 1990). For example, the landmark studies of McCord and McCord (1960) and Robins (1966) revealed that alcoholism in adulthood was associated with antisocial behavior and aggressivity in childhood. Aggressive behavior in the first grade has been found to predict heavy alcohol use in late adolescence (Kellam et al., 1983).

The onset of drinking is signaled by several antecedent personality attributes reflecting lower levels of conventionality, for example, lower values on academic achievement (Jessor and Jessor, 1975; Brook et al., 1986a), lower expectations of academic achievement (Jessor et al., 1972; Jessor and Jessor, 1975), more tolerant attitudes toward deviant behavior (Jessor and Jessor, 1975; Brook et al., 1986a), lower levels of religiosity (Jessor and Jessor, 1975; Webb et al., 1991), less of an orientation to hard work (Brook et al., 1986a), greater rebelliousness (Brook et al., 1986a), rejection of parental authority (Webb et al., 1991), fewer reasons for not drinking or less negative beliefs about the harmfulness of drinking (Jessor et al., 1972; Jessor and Jessor, 1975; Margulies et al., 1977), and greater positive expectancies about the social benefits of drinking (Christiansen et al., 1989; Smith and Goldman, 1994).

Studies of the association between adolescent personality characteristics and illicit drug use found that many of the characteristics that signaled the onset of drinking also predicted drug use. The most powerful predictors of more frequent drug use are the unconventionality variables, including rebelliousness, tolerance of deviance, and low school achievement (Brook et al., 1986a). Similar antecedent personality attributes reflecting lower levels of conventionality and more positive attitudes toward drug use predict the initiation of smoking, drinking, and drug use (Chassin et al., 1984; Krohn et al., 1985; Skinner et al., 1985; Mittelmark et al., 1987). In general, adolescents who start to use marijuana are less conventional in their attitudes and values and have weaker bonds to the conventional institutions of school and religion. This is shown in more tolerant attitudes toward deviance (Jessor et al., 1973; Brook et al., 1980), lower religiosity (Jessor et al., 1973), greater rebelliousness and lower obedience (Smith and Fogg, 1979), lower educational expectations (Brook et al., 1980), greater opposition to authority (Pederson, 1990), and more favorable beliefs about marijuana use (Jessor et al., 1973; Kandel and Andrews, 1987).

Psychopathology

Adult deviant behavior and antisocial behavioral patterns are often preceded by problem behaviors (i.e., rejection of societal rules, goals, and values) in late childhood and early adolescence (Jessor and Jessor, 1977; Robins, 1978). These behaviors coupled with increasing life stresses appear to be risk factors for drug abuse. Conduct disorder has been shown to precede the onset of drug abuse in several studies (Robins, 1966; McCord, 1981; August et al., 1983; Gittelman et al., 1985; Boyle et al., 1992) and to occur conjointly with drug abuse in others (Loeber, 1982; Lilienfeld and Waldman, 1990; Loeber et al., 1995). A prospective longitudinal study by Boyle and colleagues (1992) revealed that an earlier diagnosis of conduct disorder indicated greater risk for the initiation of marijuana and other illicit drug use four years later. It should be noted, however, that the majority of children with problem behaviors or conduct disorders do not become antisocial or drug-abusing adults.

Although studies have observed that early antisocial behaviors and deviance are risk factors for drug abuse (Robins, 1966; Elliott et al., 1985; Kaplan et al., 1986; Robins and McEvoy, 1990), the two most common psychopathologies that have been identified repeatedly are depression and antisocial personality (Cadoret et al., 1980; Alterman et al., 1985; Deykin et al., 1987; Block et al., 1988; Muntaner et al., 1989; Grove et al., 1990).

Studies of clinical and epidemiological samples also have suggested that drug abuse and psychopathology are often linked (Merikangas et al., 1994; Kessler et al., 1996). Inpatient and outpatient surveys reveal that approximately one-third of patients in treatment for psychiatric disorders are drug abusers (Crowley et al., 1974; Fischer et al., 1975; Davis, 1984; Eisen et al., 1987). In these samples, disorders that have been associated with increased risk of alcoholism and drug abuse include conduct and oppositional disorders, especially those manifesting antisocial behavior; attention deficit disorder; and the anxiety disorders, particularly phobic disorders and depression (Weiss et al., 1988; Fergusson et al., 1994; Riggs et al., 1995; Kessler et al., 1996). The commonality of findings across these studies and samples further supports the results, in particular the studies of treated samples, delinquents, general population samples, and samples of different ages, such as adolescents (Riggs et al., 1995) or adults (Kessler et al., 1996). Additionally, a number of reports have shown a high incidence of drug abuse in psychiatric patients (Galanter and Castaneda, 1988; Caton et al., 1989; Drake and Wallach, 1989; Miller et al., 1989), and other studies have shown that many patients entering drug abuse treatment facilities suffer from co-occurring psychiatric disorders (Khantzian and Treece, 1985; Rounsaville and Kleber, 1986; Ross et al., 1988; Weiss et al., 1988). The prevalence of psychiatric disorders in patients entering drug abuse treatment is substantially higher than one would expect to find in the general population (Rounsaville and Kleber, 1986; Ross et al., 1988, see Chapter 3).

High rates of externalizing disorders have been observed in clinical and epidemiological samples of both adult and adolescent drug abusers (Rounsaville and Kleber, 1985, 1986; Helzer and Pryzbeck, 1988; Ross et al., 1988; Weiss et al., 1988). There is a very large degree of overlap between disruptive behavior disorders and drug use in older adolescents, particularly among those with co-occurring conduct disorder (Windle, 1990; Neighbors et al., 1992; Henry et al., 1993; Riggs et al., 1995).

Contextual Factors

Factors external to the individual and arising in the social (family setting or peer group) or broader environment may also affect the level of drug use and abuse (IOM, 1994b). The complex interrelationships among these contextual factors underscore the complexity of the pathways of drug use and abuse.

Familial Factors

A number of family factors may be associated with the development of drug use and abuse. As reviewed in Glantz and Pickens (1992), these may include poor quality of the child–parent relationship, family disruptions (e.g., divorce, acute or chronic stress), poor parenting, parent and/

or sibling drug use, parental attitudes sympathetic to drug use, and social deprivation.

Parents may confer increased risk of drug abuse on their offspring not only through their genes but also by providing negative role models, and especially by using and abusing drugs as a coping mechanism. Through social learning, children and adolescents internalize the values and expectations of their parents and possibly acquire their maladaptive coping techniques. This has been found to be the case with adolescent cigarette smoking (Isralowitz, 1991) and initiation of marijuana use among adolescents (Bailey and Hubbard, 1990). Further, parental attitudes toward use and abuse also play a role (Barnes and Welte, 1986; Brook et al., 1986b). Among Mexican American adolescents, family influence may have a stronger and more direct positive (or protective) effect than is found among white American youth. This may be particularly true for females and seems to be related to the strength of the family's identification with traditional Hispanic culture (Swaim et al., 1993). African American drug abuse and polydrug abuse may be viewed, in part, as contingency reinforcements for the deprivation of stable family and interpersonal relationships (Brunswick et al., 1992). Among young Native Americans, many of whom are physically isolated on reservations, the primary risk factors for alcohol and illicit drug use are socialization links, family problems, and family dysfunction (Swaim et al., 1989).

Finally, although many family-related factors have been identified as possible risk factors for drug abuse, many of these studies have failed to demonstrate the specificity of parental and familial effects because they do not include comparison groups of parents with other chronic disorders.

Peer Factors

The peer environment also makes a substantial contribution to variation in drug use and abuse (Barnes and Welte, 1986; Oetting and Beauvais, 1987a,b, 1990; Oetting and Lynch, in press). Among older adolescents, peers have a greater effect than parents on drug use and abuse among several groups, including whites, African Americans, Asians, and Hispanics (Newcomb and Bentler, 1986). Typically, adolescent drug use takes place within the context of peer clusters that consist of best friends or very close friends (Oetting and Beauvais, 1987a,b). Drug use among friends, deviance, and time spent with drug-using peers are also associated with moderate alcohol and marijuana use (Kandel et al., 1978; Brook et al., 1992). Peer influence on drug use and abuse may occur in a mutually reinforcing pattern based on the tendency for drug-using adolescents to select similar peers (Kandel, 1985). Studies have not yet demonstrated, however, the influence of peers in the transition from drug use to abuse (Kaplan et al., 1986). Further, the contributing effects of peer influences are likely to be different at different stages of development (Glantz and Pickens, 1992).

Sociocultural or Environmental Factors

The sociocultural factors that have an impact on drug use or abuse include community drug use patterns (Robins, 1984) and neighborhood disorganization (Sampson, 1985). Growing up and living in a community with high rates of crime, ready availability of drugs, association with delinquent peers, and acceptance of drug use and abuse are all associated with drug abuse (Clayton and Voss, 1981; Elliott et al., 1985; Brook et al., 1988; Cohen et al., 1990; Robins and McEvoy, 1990). The larger sociocultural environment also has important effects on drug use. The frequency and nature of representation of alcohol, tobacco, and illicit drugs in the media (including advertising and modeling by those in the sports and entertainment industries) may have important effects on the normative climate. In addition, social and legal policies (taxes, restrictions on conditions of purchase and use, legal status, enforcement) may have important effects on use and abuse.

Ethnographic studies have explored various risk factors for drug use and abuse, as well as the impact of drug abuse on the community. The degree of acculturation and assimilation of individuals and their families into the community has been found to be of some importance as a contextual factor. Among Mexican Americans, it has been noted that several risk factors such as low socioeconomic status, higher school dropout rates, and residing in barrios in large cities exacerbate drug use (Padilla et al., 1979; Carter and Wilson, 1991).

In many African American communities, individuals may occupy marginal social positions that prevent access to broader opportunities. This could result in failure to be responsive to dominant social norms. Detachment from conventional norms is expressed in unconventional life-stage roles (Brunswick et al., 1992). In samples of whites, there is typically a termination of drug use in the midtwenties age range, when adult roles of marriage and employment are adopted (Miller et al., 1983; Bachman et al., 1984; Yamaguchi and Kandel, 1985; Kandel et al., 1986). It is not surprising that in some African American populations, drug abuse continues into adulthood since conventional adult roles are not assumed (Brunswick et al., 1992). Yamaguchi and Kandel (1985) found that the African American women in their New York State sample were more likely than white women to continue marijuana use. It has been confirmed (Bennett et al., 1989) that low-income African American women have lower marriage rates than comparable white women. Similarly, young African American men have nearly double the unemployment rate of white men (U.S. Bureau of the Census, 1988).

Native American youth interact on reservations, which are physically isolated from other communities. In these communities, unemployment rates are high and result in conditions in which drug use can flourish (Oetting et al., 1989). Furthermore, among Native American adolescents, school adjustment is a serious problem and dropout rates are high (Chavers, 1991). Additionally, delinquency and crime are strongly linked to drug use, and there is increasing involvement of reservation youth in gangs.

Alternatively, the environment can reinforce a protective sense of self-worth, identity, safety, and environmental mastery. Neighborhood and community factors may also serve to protect individuals from drug use and abuse. For example, restrictions on tobacco use in public places are statements of the preferences of the larger community. Such restrictions also reduce the number of opportunities to use tobacco. Restrictions on smoking in public places reinforce the norm that tobacco use is not acceptable (IOM, 1994a).

RESEARCH OPPORTUNITIES

Drug abuse is the end product of a series of biological, psychosocial, and contextual (social and environmental) factors that have complex interrelationships. Although, there has been substantial progress in identifying the many correlates of drug use, there is a dearth of research on the correlates of abuse and dependence and on the protective factors that are associated with decreased likelihood of abuse and dependence. Additionally, much of the research in the etiology of drug abuse has been conducted within specific disciplines, with little integration across multiple fields. For example, studies of social factors linked to drug abuse often fail to include key biological factors, and studies of the genetics of drug abuse rarely include assessments of the social context in which drug abuse occurs. Therefore, to advance progress in this area of research there is a need for multidisciplinary studies on the variables associated with the development of drug abuse.

Protective Factors

Although risk reduction is the goal of many prevention programs, another approach is to enhance protective factors. At the present time, however, there has been little longitudinal research on protective factors and little, if any, research on the transition from use to abuse and dependence.

Several investigators have noted that protective factors can moderate the effects of risk conditions, thereby reducing vulnerability and enhancing resiliency (Garmezy, 1985; Werner, 1989; Brook et al., 1990; Rutter et al., 1990). Protective factors that have been suggested based on analyses of cross-sectional data include a positive mutual attachment between parent and child (Brook et al., 1990), nondeviant siblings, academic achievement, positive group norms (Hawkins et al., 1992), and dimensions of conventionality such as low rebelliousness and adherence to broad social norms. Moreover, the effect of one parent's drug use can be offset by the nonuse of the other parent. Additional protective factors that have been identified in young adulthood include employment, marriage, and child-rearing responsibilities. It has been noted that several protective factors can ameliorate the negative effects of exposure to extreme stress (Garmezy, 1985). These include the child's temperament, a supportive family, and an external support system that reinforces the child's efforts at coping (Brook et al., 1986a; Labouvie and McGee, 1986). Further research is needed, however, to determine which protective factors are relevant at different developmental stages, and more attention also needs to be given to mechanisms by which protective factors influence the onset and progression of drug abuse.

Additionally, research on drug use has documented substantial racial and ethnic differences in drug use among adolescents, such as lower use of tobacco products among African American adolescents than white adolescents (IOM, 1994a; Johnston et al., 1995). The reason for this particular difference is unclear; influences may include the church, cultural consensus against youth tobacco use, or lack of attention from advertisers (IOM, 1994a). Research should be conducted to enhance understanding of racial and ethnic differences in the acceptability of tobacco use and how these differences may be used in the design of prevention interventions related to other drugs of abuse.

Risk Factors

Numerous longitudinal studies have identified the childhood antecedents of adolescent drug use (e.g., Kellam et al., 1983; Pulkkinen, 1983; Baumrind and Moselle, 1985; Block et al., 1986; Brook et al., 1986a). However, far less research has been done on identifying childhood risk factors associated with drug abuse and dependence that are not associated with behavior problems but with individual vulnerability factors (such as genetic predisposition and emotional disorders). Additionally, there has been little research on exposure to environmental factors that promote exposure to addictive drugs.

Furthermore, there has been little hypothesis-based research to distinguish between causal factors and vulnerability factors for the development of drug abuse and dependence. Prospective longitudinal studies, especially of samples at high risk for drug abuse, would be useful in identifying risk factors and in discriminating between risk factors specifically associated with drug abuse and those that emanate from the broader context of deviant behavior. Additional work is also needed on the role of risk factors and protective factors at discrete developmental stages, particularly the transition from adolescence to adulthood, which has received scant attention.

It is important to obtain a deeper understanding of the complex ways in which family factors affect adolescent drug use, including the role both of parents and of siblings. There is a striking lack of controlled family studies designed to address the role of familial factors that are critical for identifying patterns of expression of drug abuse and co-occurring psychiatric disorders; for testing the classic modes of genetic transmission of drug abuse; for determining the role of sex-specific patterns of transmission of drug abuse; and for elucidating the role of genetic and environmental factors and their interaction. The interaction of individual and familial risk factors in producing vulnerability to drug abuse also requires further study. For example, recent evidence suggests that parent and child psychopathology may occur in a mutually interactive fashion, with maternal depression elicited by offspring with behavior problems (Blanz et al., 1991).

Unique environmental factors may also play significant roles in determining which children within a family are at risk. In other words, one cannot assume that all children within a single family will experience the same environment, including their interactions with significant others. Both transmitted and nontransmitted family factors, as well as unique environmental factors, have been shown to have a major impact on the development of drug abuse (Pickens et al., 1991). Environmental risk factors tend to operate most strongly in children with genetic vulnerability (Rutter et al., 1990). It is therefore critical to identify the joint role of environmental and genetic factors in the etiology of drug abuse.

The genetic epidemiological approach, which focuses on the joint effects of the contributions of host, agent, and environment, provides a powerful paradigm by which to gain an understanding of the interaction of variables for drug abuse. Several cohorts of subjects should be studied, including half-siblings, which would permit identification of nongenetic familial factors that may potentiate underlying vulnerability; fraternal twins, which would provide clues to the environmental risk and protective factors for drug abuse; and migrants, which would provide an opportunity to elucidate the role of cultural factors while controlling for genetic and familial factors. Finally, the continued investigation of cohorts of twins and adoptees, particularly in studies that are designed specifically to reveal the mechanisms through which genes exert their influence on drug abuse vulnerability, are also likely to be fruitful.

A family history of drug abuse is one of the most important risk factors for the development of drug abuse. However, the extent to which the increased risk is attributable to genetic factors involved in the metabolic, physiological, or subjective effects of drugs or to shared environmental factors such as impaired family relationships, negative role modeling, or, indirectly, transmission of psychopathology, should be examined. There is a need for more studies that can discriminate the roles of genetics and social environment, and their interaction in the development of drug abuse. Genetic epidemiological paradigms such as adoption studies, twin studies, migrant studies, multigenerational family studies, and high-risk studies are particularly important methods for identifying the specific sources of familial influences on drug abuse.

Research and treatment programs for drug abuse and psychiatric disorders have generally proceeded independently, with little emphasis on the large overlap between them. Indeed, treatment programs for drug abuse often require cessation of psychotropic medication as an admission requirement. Evidence from retrospective studies of drug abusers, and from a growing number of prospective studies, reveals a link between signs of emotional and behavioral problems beginning in early childhood and the subsequent development of drug abuse. Studies are needed to elucidate the specific mechanisms for the development of drug abuse secondary to psychiatric disorders such as bipolar illness, depression, anxiety disorders, and learning disabilities.

The committee recommends multidisciplinary research to investigate the combined effects of biological, psychosocial, and contextual factors as they relate to the development of drug use, abuse, and dependence. The committee further recommends that studies be of long enough duration to enable follow-up of participants in determining the role of risk and protective factors related to the transition from use to abuse and dependence. Research areas should include the role of the following: family factors in the etiology of drug use and abuse; psychopathology as a precursor to drug use and abuse in adolescents and adults; risk and protective factors related to drug use and abuse, especially during discrete developmental stages; and childhood risk and protective factors that are associated with adult drug abuse and dependence.

Reliable results from those studies would best be accomplished by hypothesis-based prospective longitudinal studies of both representative samples of adolescents and child and adolescent samples at high risk for the development of drug abuse. Information resulting from such studies would be useful to the design of prevention and treatment programs. Efforts should be made to incorporate biological measurements in epidemiological studies of drug use, abuse, and dependence in representative population samples, both to establish the validity of the drug use reports and to identify biological risk markers for dependence.

REFERENCES

Alterman A, Tarter R, BaughmanT, Bober R, Fabian S. 1985. Differentiation of alcoholics high and low in childhood hyperactivity. *Drug and Alcohol Dependence* 15:111–121.

August GJ, Stewart MA, Holmes CS. 1983. A four year follow-up of hyperactive boys with and without conduct disorder. *British Journal of Psychiatry* 143:192–198.

Bachman JG, O'Malley P, Johnston L. 1984. Drug use among young adults: The impacts of role status and social environment. *Journal of Personality and Social Psychology* 47:629–645.

Bailey SL, Hubbard RL. 1990. Developmental variation in the context of marijuana initiation among adolescents. *Journal of Health and Social Behavior* 31:58–70.

Barnes GM, Welte JW. 1986. Patterns and predictors of alcohol use among 7–12th grade students in New York State. *Journal of Studies on Alcohol* 47:53–62.

Baumrind D, Moselle KA. 1985. A developmental perspective on adolescent drug abuse. *Advances in Alcohol and Substance Abuse* 4:41–67.

Bennett NG, Bloom DE, Craig PH. 1989. The divergence of black and white marriage patterns. *American Journal of Sociology* 95:692–722.

Blanz B, Schmidt MH, Esser G. 1991. Familial adversities and child psychiatric disorders. *Journal of Child Psychology and Psychiatry* 32(6):939–950.

Block J, Keyes S, Block JH. 1986. *Childhood Personality and Environmental Antecedents of Drug Use: A Prospective Longitudinal Study.* Paper presented at the meeting of the Society for Life History Research in Psychopathology, Palm Springs, CA.

Block J, Block J, Keyes S. 1988. Longitudinally foretelling drug usage in adolescence: Early childhood personality and environmental precursors. *Child Development* 59:336–355.

Bohman M, Sigvardsson S, Cloninger R. 1981. Maternal inheritance of alcohol abuse: Cross-fostering analysis of adopted women. *Archives of General Psychiatry* 38:965–969.

Bosron WF, Li TK. 1986. Genetic polymorphism of human liver alcohol and aldehyde dehydrogenases and their relationship to alcohol metabolism and alcoholism. *Hepatology* 6:502–510.

Boyle MH, Offord DR, Racine YA, Szatmari P, Fleming JE, Links PS. 1992. Predicting substance use in late adolescence: Results from the Ontario Child Health Study Follow-Up. *American Journal of Psychiatry* 149(6):761–767.

Brook DW, Brook JS. 1990. The etiology and consequences of adolescent drug use. In: Watson RR, ed. *Drug and Alcohol Abuse Prevention.* Clifton NJ: Humana Press. Pp. 339–362.

Brook JS, Lukoff IF, Whiteman M. 1980. Initiation into adolescent marijuana use. *Journal of Genetic Psychology* 137:133–142.

Brook JS, Whiteman M, Gordon AS, Cohen P. 1986a. Dynamics of childhood and adolescent personality traits and adolescent drug use. *Developmental Psychology* 22:403–414.

Brook JS, Gordon AS, Whiteman M, Cohen P. 1986b. Some models and mechanisms for explaining the impact of maternal and adolescent characteristics on adolescent stage of drug use. *Developmental Psychology* 22:460–467.

Brook JS, Whiteman M, Nomura C, Gordon AS, Cohen P. 1988. Personality, family, and ecological influences on adolescent drug use: A developmental analysis. *Journal of Chemical Dependency Treatment* 1:123–161.

Brook JS, Brook DW, Whiteman M, Gordon AS, Cohen P. 1990. The psychosocial etiology of adolescent drug use and abuse. *Genetic, Social and General Psychology Monographs* 116(2).

Brook JS, Cohen P, Whiteman M, Gordon AS. 1992. Psychosocial risk factors in the transition from moderate to heavy use or abuse of drugs. In: Glantz M, Pickens R, eds. *Vulnerability to Drug Abuse*. Washington, DC: American Psychological Association.

Brunswick A, Messeri PA, Titus SP. 1992. Predictive factors in adult substance abuse: A prospective study of African American adolescents. In: Glantz M, Pickens R, eds. *Vulnerability to Drug Abuse*. Washington, DC: American Psychological Association.

Bry B. 1989. The multiple risk factor hypothesis: An integrating concept of the etiology of drug abuse. In: Einstein S, ed. *Drug and Alcohol Use: Issues and Factors*. New York: Plenum Press.

Cadoret RJ, Cain C, Grove W. 1980. Development of alcoholism in adoptees raised apart from alcoholic biologic relatives. *Archives of General Psychiatry* 37:561–563.

Carter DJ, Wilson R. 1991. *Ninth Annual Status Report: Minorities in Higher Education*. Washington, DC: American Council on Education.

Caton CLM, Gralnick A, Bender S, Simon R. 1989. Young chronic patients and substance abuse. *Hospital and Community Psychiatry* 40:1037–1040.

Chassin L, Presson CC, Sherman SJ, Corty E, Olshavsky RW. 1984. Predicting the onset of cigarette smoking in adolescents: A longitudinal study. *Journal of Applied Social Psychology* 14(3):224–243.

Chavers D. 1991. Indian education: Dealing with disaster. *Principal* 70(3):28–29.

Christiansen BA, Smith GT, Roehling PV, Goldman MS. 1989. Using alcohol expectancies to predict adolescent drinking behavior after one year. *Journal of Clincal and Consulting Psychology* 57(1):93–99.

Clayton R. 1992. Transitions in drug use: Risk and protective factors. In: Glantz M, Pickens R, eds. *Vulnerability to Drug Abuse*. Washington DC: American Psychological Association.

Clayton R, Voss H. 1981. *Young Men and Drugs in Manhattan: A Causal Analysis*. NIDA Research Monograph Series 39. Rockville, MD: NIDA.

Cloninger CR, Bohman N, Sigvardsson S. 1981. Inheritance of alcohol abuse: Cross-fostering analysis of adopted men. *Archives of General Psychiatry* 36:861–868.

Cloninger CR, Sigvardsson S, Bohman M. 1988. Childhood personality predicts alcohol abuse in young adults. *Alcoholism: Clinical and Experimental Research* 12:494–505.

Cohen P, Brook J, Cohen J, Velez C, Garcia M. 1990. Common and uncommon pathways to adolescent psychopathology and problem behavior. In: Robins L, Rutter M, eds. *Straight and Devious Pathways from Childhood to Adulthood*. Cambridge, England: Cambridge University Press. Pp. 242–258.

Cotton NS. 1979. The familial incidence of alcoholism. *Journal of Studies on Alcohol* 40:89–116.

Crowley T, Chesluk K, Dilts S, Hart R. 1974. Drug and alcohol abuse among psychiatric admissions. *Archives of General Psychiatry* 30:13–20.

Davis DI. 1984. Differences in the use of substances of abuse by psychiatric patients compared with medical and surgical patients. *Journal of Nervous and Mental Disorders* 172:654–657.

Deykin E, Levy J, Wells V. 1987. Adolescent depression, alcohol, and drug abuse. *American Journal of Public Health* 77:178–192.

Drake RE, Wallach MA. 1989. Substance abuse among the chronically mentally ill. *Hospital and Community Psychiatry* 40:1041–1046.

Eisen SV, Grob MC, Dill DL. 1987. Substance abuse in a generic inpatient population. McLean Hospital Evaluation Service Unit, Report No. 71. As cited in: Miller NS, ed. 1991. *Comprehensive Handbook of Drug and Alcohol Addiction*. New York: Marcel Dekker.

Elliott D, Huizinga D, Menard S. 1985. *Explaining Delinquency and Drug Use*. Beverly Hills, CA: Sage.

Fergusson DM, Horwood LJ, Lynskey M. 1994. The childhood of multiple problem adolescents: A 15–year longitudinal study. *Journal of Child Psychology and Psychiatry* 35(6):1123–1140.

Fischer D, Halikas J, Baker J, Smith J. 1975. Frequency and patterns of drug abuse in psychiatric patterns. *Diseases of the Nervous System* 36:550–553.

Galanter M, Castaneda R. 1988. Substance abuse among general psychiatric patients: Place of presentation, diagnosis and treatment. *American Journal of Drug and Alcohol Abuse* 14:211–235.

Garmezy N. 1983. Stressors of childhood. In: Garmezy N, Rutter M, eds. *Stress, Coping, and Development in Children*. New York: McGraw-Hill. Pp. 43–84.

Garmezy N. 1985. Stress-resistent children: The search for protective factors. *Journal of Child Psychology and Psychiatry* 4: (Book Suppl.):213–233.

Gittelman R, Mannuzza S, Shenker R, Bonagura N. 1985. Hyperactive boys almost grown up: I. Psychiatric status. *Archives of General Psychiatry* 42:937–947.

Glantz M, Pickens R. 1992. *Vulnerability to Drug Abuse*. Washington, DC: American Psychological Press.

Goedde HW, Agarwal DP, Fritze G, Meier-Tackermann D, Singh S, Beckmann G, Bhatia K, Chen LZ, Fang B, Lisker R, et al. 1992. Distribution of ADH2 and ALDH2 genotypes in different populations. *Human Genetics* 88(3):344–346.

Goodwin DW, Schulsinger F, Hermansen L, Guze SB, Winokur G. 1973. Alcohol problems in adoptees raised apart from alcoholic biologic parents. *Archives of General Psychiatry* 28:238–243.

Gordon HW. 1994. Human neuroscience at the National Institute on Drug Abuse: Implications for genetics research. *American Journal of Medical Genetics* 54(4):293–294.

Grove W, Eckert E, Heston L, Bouchard T, Segal N, Lykken D. 1990. Heritability of substance abuse and antisocial behavior: A study of monozygotic twins reared apart. *Biological Psychiatry* 27:1293–1304.

Gurling HMD, Murray RM, Clifford CA. 1981. *Investigations into the Genetics of Alcohol Dependence and into its Effects on Brain Function: Twin Research 3. Epidemiologic Clinical Studies*. New York: Liss.

Hawkins JD, Lishner D, Catalano R, Howard M. 1985. Childhood predictors of adolescent substance abuse: Toward an empirically grounded theory. *Journal of Children in Contemporary Society* 18:11–48.

Hawkins JD, Catalano RF, Miller JY. 1992. Risk and protective factors for alcohol and other drug problems in adolescence and early adulthood: Implications for substance abuse prevention. *Psychological Bulletin* 112(1):64–105.

Helzer JE, Burnam A. 1991. Epidemiology of alcohol addiction: United States. In: Miller NS, ed. *Comprehensive Handbook of Drug and Alcohol Addiction*. New York: Marcel Dekker.

Helzer JE, Pryzbeck TR. 1988. The co-occurence of alcoholism with other psychiatric disorders in the general population and its impact on treatment. *Journal of Studies on Alcohol* 49:219–224.

Henry B, Feehan M, McGee R, Stanton M, Moffitt TE, Silva P. 1993. The importance of conduct problems and depressive symptoms in predicting adolescent substance use. *Journal of Abnormal Child Psychology* 21(5):469–480.

Higuchi S, Matsushita S, Murayama M, Takagi S, Hayashida M. 1995. Alcohol and aldehyde dehydrogenase polymorphisms and the risk for alcoholism. *American Journal of Psychiatry* 152(8):1219–1221.

Hrubec Z, Omenn GS. 1981. Evidence of genetic predisposition to alcoholic cirrhosis and psychosis: Twin concordances from alcohol availability, alcohol consumption, and demographic data. *Journal of Studies on Alcohol* 43:1199–1213.

IOM (Institute of Medicine). 1994a. *Growing Up Tobacco Free*. Washington, DC: National Academy Press.

IOM (Institute of Medicine). 1994b. *Reducing Risks for Mental Disorders: Frontiers for Prevention Intervention Research*. Washington, DC: National Academy Press.

Isralowitz RE. 1991. Licit and illicit drug patterns and problems among kibbutz young adults. *Journal of Adolescent Health* 12(6):421–426.

Jessor R, Jessor SL. 1975. Adolescent development and the onset of drinking: A longitudinal study. *Journal of Studies on Alcohol* 36(1):27–51.

Jessor R, Jessor S. 1977. *Problem Behavior and Psychosocial Development: A Longitudinal Study of Youth*. San Diego: Academic Press.

Jessor R, Collins MI, Jessor SL. 1972. On becoming a drinker: Social-psychological aspects of adolescent transition. *Annals of the New York Academy of Sciences* 197:199–213.

Jessor R, Jessor SL, Finney J. 1973. A social psychology of marijuana use: Longitudinal studies of high school and college youth. *Journal of Personality and Social Psychology* 26(1):1–15.

Johnston LD, O'Malley PM, Bachman JG. 1995. *National Survey Results on Drug Use from the Monitoring the Future Study, 1975–1994. Vol. 1, Secondary School Students*. Ann Arbor, MI: Institute for Social Research, University of Michigan.

Kandel DB. 1980. Drug and drinking behavior among youth. *Annual Review of Sociology* 6:235–285.

Kandel DB. 1985. On processes of peer influence in adolescent drug use: A developmental perspective. *Advances in Alcohol and Substance Abuse* 4:139–163.

Kandel DB, Andrews K. 1987. Processes of adolescent socialization by parents and peers. *International Journal of the Addictions* 22:319–342.

Kandel DB, Kessler RC, Margulies RZ. 1978. Antecedents of adolescent initiation into stages of drug use: A developmental analysis. In: Kandel DB, ed. *Longitudinal Research on Drug Abuse: Empirical Findings and Methodological Issues*. Washington, DC: Hemisphere. Pp. 73–99.

Kandel DB, Davies M, Karus D, Yamaguchi K. 1986. The consequences in young adulthood of adolescent drug involvement. *Archives of General Psychiatry* 43:746–754.

Kaplan HB, Martin SS, Johnson RJ, Robbins CA. 1986. Escalation of marijuana use: Application of a general theory of deviant behavior. *Journal of Health and Social Behavior* 27:44–61.

Kellam SG, Brown C, Rubin B, Ensminger M. 1983. Paths leading to teenage psychiatric symptoms and substance use: Developmental epidemiologic studies in Woodlawn. In: Earls F, Barrett J, eds. *Childhood Psychopathology and Development*. New York: Raven Press. Pp. 17–51.

Kessler RC, Nelson CB, McGonagle KA, Edlund MJ, Frank RG, Leaf PJ. 1996. The epidemiology of co-occuring addictive and mental disorders: Implications for prevention and service utilization. *American Journal of Orthopsychiatry* 66(1):17–30.

Khantzian EJ, Treece C. 1985. DSM-III psychiatric diagnosis of narcotic addicts. *Archives of General Psychiatry* 42:1067–1071.

Krohn MD, Massey JL, Skinner WF, Lauer RM. 1985. Social learning theory and adolescent cigarette smoking: A longitudinal study. *Social Problems* 32(5):455–473.

Kumpfer KL. 1989. Prevention of alcohol and drug abuse: A critical review of risk factors and prevention strategies. In: Shaffer D, Philips I, Enzer NB, eds. *Prevention of Mental Disorders, Alcohol and Other Drug Use in Children and Adolescents.* OSAP Prevention Monograph No. 2. DHHS Publication No. (ADM)90–1646. Rockville MD: Office of Substance Abuse Prevention.

Labouvie E, McGee C. 1986. Relation of personality to alcohol and drug use in adolescence. *Journal of Consulting and Clinical Psychology* 54:289–293.

Lilienfeld SO, Waldman ID. 1990. The relation between childhood attention-deficit hyperactivity disorder and adult antisocial behavior reexamined: The problem of heterogeneity. *Clinical Psychology Review* 10:699–725.

Loeber R. 1982. The stability of antisocial and delinquent child behavior: A review. *Child Development* 53:1431–1446.

Loeber RS, Green S, Keenan K, Lahey BB. 1995. Which boys will fare worse? Early predictors of the onset of conduct disorder in a six year longitudinal study. *Journal of the American Academy of Child and Adolescent Psychiatry* 34(4):499–509.

Maddahian E, Newcomb M, Bentler P. 1988. Risk factors for substance use: Ethnic differences among adolescents. *Journal of Substance Abuse* 1:11–23.

Margulies RZ, Kessler RC, Kandel DB. 1977. A longitudinal study of onset of drinking among high school students. *Journal of Studies on Alcohol* 38(5):897–912.

McCord J. 1981. Alcoholism and criminality. *Journal of Studies on Alcohol* 42:739–748.

McCord W, McCord J. 1960. *Origins of Alcoholism.* Stanford, CA: Stanford University Press.

Merikangas KR. 1990. The genetic epidemiology of alcoholism. *Psychological Medicine* 20:11–22.

Merikangas KR, Rounsaville BJ, Prusoff BA. 1992. Familial factors in vulnerability to substance abuse. In: Glantz M, Pickens R, eds. *Vulnerability to Drug Abuse.* Washington, DC: American Psychological Association.

Merikangas KR, Risch NR, Weissman MM. 1994. Co-morbidity and co-transmission of alcoholism, anxiety and depression. *Psychological Medicine* 24:69–80.

Miller FT, Busch F, Tanebaum JH. 1989. Drug abuse in schizoprenia and bipolar disorder. *American Journal of Drug and Alcohol Abuse* 15:291–295.

Miller J, Cisin L, Gardner-Keaton H, Wirtz P, Abelson H, Fishburne P. 1983. *National Survey on Drug Abuse: Main Findings, 1982.* Rockville, MD: NIDA.

Mittelmark MB, Murray DM, Luepker RV, Pechacek TF, Pirie PL, Pallonen UE. 1987. Predicting experimentation with cigarettes: The Childhood Antecedents of Smoking Study (CASS). *American Journal of Public Health* 77(2):206–208.

Muntaner C, Nagoshi C, Jaffe J, Walte D, Haertzen C, Fishbein D. 1989. Correlates of self-reported early childhood aggression in subjects volunteering for drug studies. *American Journal of Drug and Alcohol Abuse* 15:383–402.

Murray RM, Clifford C, Gurlin HM. 1983. Twin and adoption studies: How good is the evidence for a genetic role? In: Galanter M, ed. *Recent Developments in Alcoholism, Vol. 1.* New York: Gardner Press. Pp. 25–48.

Neighbors B, Kempton T, Forehand R. 1992. Co-occurence of substance abuse with conduct, anxiety, and depression disorders in juvenille delinquents. *Addictive Behaviors* 17(4):379–386.

Newcomb MD, Bentler PM. 1986. Cocaine use among adolescents: Longitudinal association with social context, psychopathology and use of other substances. *Addictive Behavior* 11:263–273.

Oetting ER, Beauvais F. 1987a. Common elements in youth drug abuse: Peer clusters and other psychosocial factors. *Journal of Drug Issues* 17(1,2):133–151.

Oetting ER, Beauvais F. 1987b. Peer cluster theory, socialization characteristics and adolescent drug use: A path analysis. *Journal of Counseling Psychology* 34(2):205–213.

Oetting ER, Beauvais F. 1990. Adolescent drug use: Findings of national and local surveys. *Journal of Consulting and Clinical Psychology* 58(4):385–394.

Oetting ER, Lynch RS. In press. Peers and the prevention of adolescent drug use. In: Bukoski WJ, Amsel Z, eds. *Drug Abuse Prevention*. Westport, CT: Greenwood Publishing Group.

Oetting ER, Swaim RC, Edwards RW, Beauvais F. 1989. Indian and Anglo adolescent alcohol use and emotional distress: Path models. *American Journal of Alcohol and Drug Abuse* 15(2):153–172.

OTA (Office of Technology Assessment). 1994. *Technologies for Understanding and Preventing Substance Abuse and Addiction*. OTA–EHR–597. Washington, DC: U.S. Government Printing Office.

Padilla ER, Padilla AM, Morales AP, Olmedo EL, Ramirez R. 1979. Inhalant, marijuana, and alcohol abuse among barrio children and adolescents. *International Journal of the Addictions* 147(7):945–964.

Pandina RJ, Johnson V. 1989. Familial history as a predictor of alcohol and drug consumption among adolescent children. *Journal of Studies on Alcohol* 50:245–253.

Pandey GN, Fawcett J, Gibbons R, Clark DC, Davis JM. 1988. Platelet monoamine oxidase in alcoholism. *Biologic Psychiatry* 24:15–24.

Pedersen N. 1981. Twin similarity for usage of common drugs. In: Gredda L, Paris P, Nance W, eds. *Twin Research 3: Epidemiological and Clinical Studies*. New York: Liss. Pp. 53–59.

Pederson LL, Baskerville JC, Lefcoe NM. 1981. Multivariate prediction of cigarette smoking among children in grades six, seven and eight. *Journal of Drug Education* 11(3):191–203.

Pederson W. 1990. Adolescents initiating cannabis use: Cultural opposition or poor mental health? *Journal of Adolescence* 13(4):327–339.

Petraitis J, Flay BR, Miller TQ. 1995. Reviewing theories of adolescent substance use: Organizing pieces in the puzzle. *Psychological Bulletin* 117(1):67–86.

Pickens RW, Svikis DS, McGue M, Lykken D, Heston M, Clayton P. 1991. Heterogeneity in the inheritance of alcoholism: A study of male and female twins. *Archives of General Psychiatry* 48:19–28.

Pulkkinen L. 1983. Youthful smoking and drinking in a longitudinal perspective. *Journal of Youth and Adolescence* 12:253–283.

Riggs PD, Baker S, Mikulich SK, Young SE, Crowley TJ. 1995. Depresssion in substance-dependent delinquents. *Journal of the American Academy of Child and Adolescent Psychiatry* 34(6):764–771.

Robins LN. 1966. *Deviant Children Grow Up: A Sociological and Psychiatric Study of Sociopathic Personality*. Baltimore: Williams & Wilkins.

Robins LN. 1978. Sturdy childhood predictors of adult antisocial behavior: Replications from longitudinal studies. *Psychological Medicine* 8:611–622.

Robins LN. 1984. The natural history of adolescent drug use. *American Journal of Public Health* 74:656–657.

Robins LN, McEvoy L. 1990. Conduct problems as predictors of substance abuse. In: Robins L, Rutter M, eds. *Straight and Devious Pathways from Childhood to Adulthood*. Cambridge, England: Cambridge University Press. Pp. 242–258.

Ross HE, Glaser FB, Germanson T. 1988. The prevalence of psychiatric disorders in patients with alcohol and other drug problems. *Archives of General Psychiatry* 45:1023–1032.

Rounsaville BJ, Kleber HD. 1985. Untreated opiate addicts. *Archives of General Psychiatry* 42:1072–1077.

Rounsaville BJ, Kleber HD. 1986. Psychiatric disorders in opiate addicts: Preliminary findings on the course and interaction with program type. In: Meyer RE, ed. *Psychopathology and Addictive Disorders*. New York: Guilford Press. Pp. 140–168.

Rutter M. 1983. Stress, coping, and development: Some issues and some questions. In: Garmezy N, Rutter M, eds. *Stress, Coping, and Development in Children*. New York: McGraw-Hill. Pp. 1–41.

Rutter M, McDonald J, Couteur A, et al. 1990. Genetic factors in child psychiatric disorders. II. Empirical findings. *Journal of Child Psychology and Psychiatry* 31:39–83.

Sampson RJ. 1985. Neighborhood and crime: The structural determinants of personal victimization. *Journal of Research on Crime and Delinquency* 22:7–40.

Schuckit MA. 1984. Subjective responses to alcohol in sons of alcoholics and controls. *Archives of General Psychiatry* 41:879–884.

Schuckit MA. 1985. Ethanol–induced changes in body sway in men at high alcoholism risk. *Archives of General Psychiatry* 42:375–379.

Schuckit MA. 1986. Alcoholism and affective disorders: Genetic and clinical implications. *American Journal of Psychiatry* 143:140–147.

Schuckit MA, Goodwin DA, Winokur GA. 1972. A study of alcoholism in half-siblings. *American Journal of Psychiatry* 128:1132–1136.

Skinner WF, Massey JL, Krohn MD, Lauer RM. 1985. Social influences and constraints on the initiation and cessation of adolescent tobacco use. *Journal of Behavioral Medicine* 8(4):353–376.

Smith GM, Fogg CP. 1979. Psychological antecedents of teen-age drug use. *Research in Community and Mental Health* 1:87–102.

Smith GT, Goldman MS. 1994. Alcohol expectancy theory and the identification of high-risk adolescents. *Journal of Research on Adolescence* 4(2):229–247.

Swaim RC. 1991. Childhood risk factors and adolescent drug and alcohol abuse. *Educational Psychology Review* 3:363–398.

Swaim RC, Oetting ER, Edwards RW, Beauvais F. 1989. The links from emotional distress to adolescent drug use: A path model. *Journal of Cross Cultural Psychology* 15(2):153–172.

Swaim RC, Oetting ER, Thurman PJ, Beauvais F, Edwards R. 1993. American Indian adolescent drug use and socialization characteristics: A cross-cultural comparison. *Journal of Cross Cultural Psychology* 24(1):53–70.

Tabakoff B, Hoffman PL, Lee JM, Saito T, Willard B, De Leon-Jones F. 1988. Differences in platelet enzyme activity between alcoholics and nonalcoholics. *New England Journal of Medicine* 318:134–139.

Tarter R, Laird S, Kabene M, Bukstein O, Kaminer Y. 1990. Drug abuse severity in adolescents is associated with magnitude of deviation in temperament traits. *British Journal of Addiction* 85:1501–1504.

Thomasson HR, Edenberg HJ, Crabb DW, Mai XL, Jerome RE, Li TK, Wang S-P, Lin YT, Lu RB, Yin SJ. 1991. Alcohol and aldehyde dehydrogenase genotypes and alcoholism in Chinese men. *American Journal of Human Genetics* 48:677–681.

U.S. Bureau of the Census. 1988. *Statistical Abstract of the United States*. 109th ed. Washington, DC: U.S. Government Printing Office.

Vaillant G, Milofsky E. 1982. The etiology of alcoholism: A prospective viewpoint. *American Psychologist* 37:494–503.

von Knorring AL, Bohman M, von Knorring L, Oreland L. 1985. Platelet MAO activity as a biological marker in subgroups of alcoholism. *Acta Psychiatrica Scandinavica* 72(52):51–58.

Webb JA, Baer PE, McLaughlin RJ, McKelvey RS, Caid CD. 1991. Risk factors and their relation to initiation of alcohol use among early adolescents. *Journal of the American Academy of Child and Adolescent Psychiatry* 30:563–568.

Weiss RD, Mirin SM, Griffin ML, Michael ML. 1988. Psychopathology in cocaine abusers: Changing trends. *Journal of Nervous and Mental Disease* 176:719–725.

Werner EE. 1989. High-risk children in young adulthood: A longitudinal study from birth to 32 years. *American Journal of Orthopsychiatry* 59:72–81.

Windle M. 1990. A longitudinal study of antisocial behaviors in early adolescence as predictors of late adolescent substance use: Gender and ethnic group differences. *Journal of Abnormal Psychology* 99(1):86–91.

Yamaguchi K, Kandel B. 1985. Dynamic relationships between premarital cohabition and illicit drug use: A life event history analysis of role selection and role socialization. *American Sociological Review* 50:530–546.

Yoshida A, Hsu L, Yasunami M. 1991. Genetics of human alcohol metabolizing enzymes. *Progress in Nucleic Acid Research and Molecular Biology* 40:235–287.

6

Prevention

Drug abuse prevention research parallels recent trends in mental and physical health promotion and the emerging new discipline of prevention science (Coie et al., 1993; IOM, 1994b). This enterprise requires the integration of epidemiological, etiological, and preventive intervention research. As applied to drug abuse, prevention science began in the mid- to late 1970s with attempts to prevent cigarette smoking among adolescents. The early focus was on changing the individual rather than the environment, and interventions usually occurred in schools.

Public health officials categorize preventive interventions based on when the intervention occurs: primary prevention involves intervening before the behavior appears; secondary prevention involves intervening after the onset of the behavior but before it becomes habitual; tertiary prevention involves intervening after the behavior has become habitual, with the goal of reducing or eliminating the behavior. Since 1990, a second model has been used increasingly to supplement these public health categories for preventive interventions: universal (delivered to the general population); selective (targeted at those presumed to be most "at risk"); and indicated (targeted at those who are exhibiting some clinically demonstrable abnormality, though perhaps not the "disease" itself) (Gordon, 1983; IOM, 1994b). In the past 10 to 15 years there has been substantial interest in prevention programs in the United States, particularly school-based intervention. Almost all of these programs can be characterized as "primary" and "universal," where the goal is to reduce the incidence and prevalence of drug use. However, there is an ongoing debate regarding the wisdom of continued emphasis on (and dedication of resources to) primary and universal prevention (focused on prevention of use) at the expense of secondary and selective prevention (focused on prevention of abuse and dependence). As the committee notes throughout this report, more information is needed about the serious problems of drug abuse and dependence.

Experimenting with drugs, particularly alcohol and tobacco products, is woven into the developmental life cycle. Well over half of all youth try these two drugs, which are legal commodities for adults. However, most youth do not regularly use illegal drugs, and most of those who have used them do not make the transition to drug abuse or dependence. Thus, it is unclear whether drug use per se is the most appropriate target of intervention. Moreover, the effects of primary prevention are usually too small to have a significant overall impact on drug abuse and dependence in the society. Given limited resources and shrinking budgets at the federal and state levels, it may be more important to focus on abuse and dependence.

Those who argue for the importance of primary and universal prevention efforts note that all young people are at risk for experimenting with alcohol, tobacco, and illicit drugs. They believe it would be irresponsible not to provide them with preventive interventions, since there can be negative consequences associated with even infrequent use (e.g., alcohol-impaired driving). Further, the etiology of drug use is complex, and targeting prevention to a "select" sample of youth would yield far too many "false positives." Such an approach could lead to inappropriate labeling and the possibility of missing some adolescents who need preventive interventions. Finally, a universal orientation is thought to be more cost-effective and logistically feasible given the structure of school systems (i.e., it is less expensive to provide everyone with the intervention than to selectively recruit those most at risk).

Despite the debate about the relative value of universal and selective interventions, they do not have to be viewed as mutually exclusive. In fact, it is more fruitful to view them as mutually supportive rather than competing alternatives. For example, universal interventions can promote antidrug norms in the larger society, and selective interventions can then build on universal preventive messages. Moreover, preventive intervention messages designed specifically for high-risk youth can be delivered within the context of universal prevention programs, avoiding the risk of harmful labeling. Both universal and targeted interventions have promise for prevention science but require more careful examination.

ACCOMPLISHMENTS

School-Based Interventions

For almost 20 years, researchers in the United States have been systematically evaluating strategies designed to prevent or delay the onset of drug use among youth, mostly through school-based programs. These programs have been organized into five types: (1) information and values clarification, (2) affective education, (3) social influence, (4) comprehensive, and (5) providing alternatives to drug use (see Hansen, 1992).

The scientific basis for understanding how to prevent adolescent drug use has expanded considerably in a very short time, and valuable lessons have been learned. For example, some program types (information and values clarification, affective education, and alternatives to drug use) have virtually no effect on preventing the use of alcohol, tobacco, or illicit drugs (see Tobler, 1992; IOM, 1994a). However, in spite of consistent scientific evidence of minimal impact, such programs are often chosen as prevention interventions for children in schools. A prominent example is D.A.R.E. (Drug Abuse Resistance Education), the most widely disseminated school-based drug abuse prevention program in the United States (Ennett et al., 1994a; Ringwalt et al., 1994). Evaluations of D.A.R.E. consistently show only short-term effects on knowledge, attitudes, and drug use, and these effects decay within a year or so (Ennett et al., 1994b).

The failure of early school-based prevention programming to produce significant long-term effects has led to creative attempts to develop interventions focused on several known risk factors for drug use, including deficits in social and peer resistance skills and misperceptions about the extent of drug use among peers. These social influence programs have been rigorously evaluated scientifically and have been closely tied to psychosocial theoretical models of drug use initiation. School-based social influence programs have shown short-term success in reducing the prevalence of adolescent cigarette smoking (IOM, 1994a; U.S. DHHS, 1994), alcohol use (Dielman et al., 1992), and marijuana use (Ellickson and Bell, 1990, 1992; Hansen and Graham, 1991; Ellickson et al., 1993). However, most program effects lessen with time, and long-term outcomes have been disappointing (Murray et al., 1989; Ellickson et al., 1993). A number of the reasons that program effects may subside have been identified: insufficient dose, insufficient implementation, inappropriate expectations, curriculum limitations, attrition of high-risk students, inappropriate assumptions about age at onset, and inappropriate messages (Resnicow and Botvin, 1993).

Two school-based prevention interventions that have demonstrated long-term success are the Life Skills Training curriculum and the Midwestern Prevention Project. The Life Skills Training curriculum (Botvin et al., 1995a) is administered to seventh-grade students with booster sessions in the eighth and ninth grades. The curriculum was delivered in an interactive format by teachers who received training by videotape or personal training and technical assistance from the developers of the curriculum. Six-year follow-up results showed significant effects on use and heavy use of cigarettes and alcohol (although not on illicit drug use). There were minimal differences in effectiveness as a function of the type of teacher training. Although the findings apply only to white, middle-class students, the study is important for demonstrating long-term effectiveness, highlighting the potential importance of booster sessions, demonstrating the value of quality teacher training, and focusing on students who were exposed to 60 percent or more of the sessions (a so-called high-fidelity sample).

The Midwestern Prevention Project (Pentz et al., 1989a,b) is another social influence prevention intervention that produced significant six-year follow-up effects on the use of cigarettes, alcohol, marijuana, and cocaine for both high- and low-risk students. The primary vehicle for this intervention was a 10-session, school-based, social skills, and peer-resistance skills curriculum. However, the school intervention was supplemented by a parental involvement component, media campaigns, and training of community leaders. This suggests that a coordinated and comprehensive community-wide intervention may be more effective in producing long-term effects than a school-based program alone.

In summary, school-based, universal, primary prevention programs have been the dominant approach to preventing adolescent drug use in the past two decades. Research efforts have shown significant progress in developing, implementing, and evaluating the effects of school-based interventions. Most notably, recent social influence programs have empirically demonstrated short-term effectiveness; fairly consistent research results demonstrate that one can achieve 20 percent or greater net reductions in rates of initiation of drug use from school programs that focus on counteracting social influences to drug use; these include standardized teacher or staff training, multiple class sessions, booster sessions, student peer leaders, and active social learning methods (Pentz, 1994). However, there have been only a few studies showing long-term success of school-based and curriculum-driven prevention interventions.

Research on school-based prevention interventions has contributed important knowledge to the broader field of prevention science. For example, recent social influence programs have strengthened the integral relationship between etiology and prevention (Bandura, 1977a,b, 1985; Hawkins and Weis, 1985; Brook et al., 1992; Brunswick et al., 1992; Glantz and Pickens, 1992; Hawkins et al., 1992a; Cloninger et al., 1993, 1995; Flay and Petraitis 1994a,b). Social influence programs have recognized the importance of constructing theory-based interventions designed to counteract known risk factors for drug use initiation and of identifying the mediating mechanisms through which interventions have their effects (MacKinnon et al., 1991). In this way, preventive interventions enhance basic etiological research, with school-based interventions providing important experimental tests of theories of adolescent drug use and problem behavior (Coie et al., 1993).

Prevention intervention research (led by recent school-based programs) has also stimulated important advances in methodology, including quantitative methods for evaluating program effectiveness. The drug abuse research field in general has been a productive seedbed for innovations in statistical techniques, such as structural equation modeling (Bentler, 1991), latent transition analysis (Collins et al., 1994), mechanisms for dealing with missing data (Graham et al., 1994), managing problems of attrition (Hansen et al., 1985, 1990; Biglan et al., 1991), hazard survival analysis (Yamaguchi, 1991), and measuring mediating mechanisms underlying intervention effects (MacKinnon et al., 1991). School-based prevention research is now benefiting from advances in the analysis of multilevel data, allowing for the study of children nested within classrooms and schools (Laird and Ware, 1982; Bryk and Raudenbusch, 1992; Gibbons and Hedeker, 1994; Hedeker et al., 1994). Important work has also been done in evaluating the validity of self-reported drug use as an outcome measure, including bioassays to detect smoking or alcohol consumption (Harrell, 1988; Rouse et al., 1988) and emergent technologies such as analysis of protein in hair samples.

Family-Based Interventions

Research on risk and protective factors associated with adolescent drug use and abuse provides several rationales for family-based prevention interventions. First, research suggests that parenting characterized by high levels of support, consistent rule enforcement, and monitoring of child behavior is associated with lower rates of drug use (Steinberg 1991; Hawkins et al., 1992a). Thus, interventions to improve parenting practices may lower the risk for adolescent drug use. Second, research suggests that parental drug abuse is a risk factor for drug abuse by offspring (Merikangas et al., 1992), and that disrupted parenting in these families may contribute to the risk (Mayes, 1995). If so, parenting interventions could help to reduce the risk for drug abuse among children of drug-abusing parents. Third, research also shows that impaired parental monitoring, poor contingency management, and coercive discipline are associated with childhood aggression and conduct problems (Reid, 1993).

Because childhood conduct problems (delinquency, aggression, conduct disorder, or oppositional defiant disorder) are important risk factors for drug abuse, they may share common etiological pathways (see Oetting and Beauvais, 1987; Patterson et al., 1989; Gottfredson et al., 1991; Abikoff and Klein, 1992; Moffitt, 1993; Huizinga et al., 1994). Family-based interventions designed to prevent conduct disorder may therefore have important effects on drug abuse and dependence.

Parent education and family support interventions have successfully reduced parental stress, enhanced parental confidence, and reduced child abuse and neglect (Olds et al., 1986; Wolfson et al., 1992). Children whose parents have received these types of interventions exhibit fewer school attendance and academic problems (Seitz et al., 1991). However, family support interventions alone may be insufficient to produce lasting effects on antisocial behavior or drug use. A review of early intervention programs for delinquency prevention suggested that interventions for urban, low-income families that combined high-quality preschool environments with family support interventions, and were delivered for multiple years, had the highest rates of success (Yoshikawa, 1994).

Although parent training programs alone are insufficient to reduce drug abuse in children, parent training interventions that directly teach parents to monitor behavior, use appropriate contingency management, and reduce coercive discipline have been shown to reduce antisocial behavior in children (Kazdin, 1987). Parenting interventions alone are not developmentally appropriate after school entry because they do not influence important risk factors such as peer relationships and school achievement (Reid, 1993). For elementary school children, few controlled studies have examined the effects of interventions in school and family simultaneously. One study that combined modified teaching practices in mainstream classrooms and parent training (designed to be developmentally appropriate as students went from the first through the fourth grades) demonstrated significantly lower rates of alcohol initiation and delinquency initiation in students whose parents received training than in control students (Hawkins et al., 1992b).

Another study is currently evaluating a combination of parent training, home visits and family support, social skills training, anger management training, academic tutoring, and modifications in the classroom environment (Conduct Problems Prevention Research Group, 1992). This program includes both universal components (the school curriculum) and selective interventions (family and social skills components) for children screened in kindergarten who showed high levels of disruptive behaviors. These researchers suggest that effective intervention requires multiple years and that both entry into elementary school and the transition to middle school are particularly important times for intervention (Conduct Problems Prevention Research Group, 1992). Outcome data are not yet available, but other studies have found long-term reductions in adolescent drug use by using a multicomponent program including a school-based social influence intervention, family involvement, media intervention, and community organization (Pentz et al., 1989a,b).

Media-Based Interventions

Media-based interventions, particularly PSAs (public service announcements), are an interesting but understudied channel for drug abuse prevention. The appeal of using media (radio, TV, billboards, and print) is that this can be a relatively cost-effective way to reach a large audience; however, few studies have attempted to demonstrate the successes of media-based drug prevention. In the only widespread attempt to use television for antidrug programming, the Partnership for a Drug-Free America was very successful in obtaining both donated services for preparing antidrug PSAs and donated time to air for them.[1] Unfortunately, rigorous examination of the effects of PSAs on actual drug use and abuse are not available, although they may have important effects on generating and sustaining drug-free norms.

A small number of empirically evaluated media interventions have been used to prevent adolescent cigarette smoking. One evaluation found significant main effects for both classroom training and television programming on knowledge and prevalence estimates, and significant impacts of classroom and television programming on knowledge, disapproval of parental smoking, and efforts at coping (Flay et al., 1995). However, sustained effects on smoking were not observed. An earlier evaluation found that adolescents who received both school-based prevention programs and (independently delivered) radio and TV antismoking messages showed significant reductions in smoking prevalence compared to those who received school-based intervention alone (Flynn et al., 1992). The earlier study is important in showing that a media component can significantly enhance the outcomes of a school-based campaign. Researchers estimated that after a concentrated antismoking campaign, sales of cigarettes in California were reduced by more than 1 billion packs from the third quarter of 1990 through the fourth quarter of 1992, and that approximately 20 percent of this reduction was attributable to the media campaign (the other 80 percent was attributed to a 25-cent increase in the

---

[1]However, between 1989 and 1993 there was an 83 percent reduction in coverage of drug use issues by major network television news and the dollar value of Partnership PSAs declined by 29 percent between 1990 and 1993 (Clayton and Ann Arbor Group, 1994).

sales tax) (Hu et al., 1995). This shows the relative effectiveness of a policy change intervention in conjunction with a media intervention, and the most effective use of media may be in combination with other interventions.

Community-Based Interventions

Since the 1970s, preventive interventions have expanded their focus from the individual to the broader community. In part, this interest in community-wide interventions stems from the realization that it is difficult if not impossible to effect changes in individuals when there are countervailing forces in the larger social environment. For example, school-based interventions alone will be ineffective if they are delivered in a community in which drug use is widespread and normative (e.g., drugs are widely available, and no sanctions are applied against drug use). Typically, community interventions relating to drug use have been implemented in conjunction with political actions that focus on changing laws and policies concerning drug use. Policy goals include strict enforcement of regulations against use, reducing youth access, increasing the costs of legal drugs (e.g., through tobacco taxes), and changing community norms about drug use.

Although there has been substantial activity involving the delivery of community interventions for drug abuse prevention, few programs have been evaluated rigorously. In the field of adolescent smoking, Perry and colleagues (1992) demonstrated that a community intervention improved outcomes above and beyond those of a school-based intervention alone. Moreover, the Midwest Prevention Project (Pentz et al., 1989a), which included a community component, demonstrated long-term reductions in drug use prevalence (although the effects of the community component were not identified separately). Smith and Davis (1993) found that community prevention programs can be successful in poor neighborhoods with substantial technical assistance. Finally, several promising community interventions are currently under way to reduce adolescent alcohol consumption (Wagenaar and Perry, 1994). In general, however, there have been few empirically rigorous demonstrations of success, and the successes that have been recorded have been described as "meager" compared to the effort that has been expended (Susser, 1995).

Reasons for modest demonstrations of success can be found in the complexity of evaluating these community programs (Pirie et al., 1994). First, programs administered on a large scale cannot be as tightly organized as programs administered to small groups, making monitoring of implementation both necessary and challenging. Second, because multiple program components are occurring simultaneously, it is difficult to assess the effects of any one component. Third, the recipients of the programs are located throughout the community and may be poorly identified, making evaluation and data collection complex and expensive. Fourth, most community programs do not occur in a vacuum, but rather coexist with national and local programs, making it difficult to disentangle the effects of the program under consideration from the background of similar programs.

In addition to methodological explanations for the weak effects, community interventions may also fail if the interventions are not sufficiently intense or if they are too brief to achieve enduring behavior change. A challenge for community trials is to sustain the efforts, transferring ownership to ongoing community groups after the research team has ended its involvement (Bracht et al., 1994). Ironically, the effects obtained by community interventions may also appear meager because they are eclipsed by the very same social movements that originally provided the impetus for the intervention (Susser, 1995). For example, the current national movement toward health consciousness may result in declines in drug use and abuse that render it difficult to produce or detect further change through controlled interventions.

At this time, the conclusion that is most appropriate is that community approaches to drug abuse prevention are intuitively appealing, but evidence of effectiveness is relatively weak. This is true because the amount and quality of existing research is limited, not because the evidence is broad based and inconclusive. Thus, rigorous and systematic research on community-based prevention interventions is needed.

GAPS AND NEEDS

School-Based Interventions

Despite important advances in prevention science directly attributable to school-based interventions, many research needs and opportunities remain. Specifically, there is a need both for a better understanding of the role of booster sessions to sustain early gains and methods for improving the long-term maintenance of program effects. The committee has also identified six areas for future research on school-based interventions:

1. *Tailoring interventions to high-risk subgroups within universal school-based interventions*: To date, school-based prevention interventions have been "universal" (directed at the general adolescent population). It is important to learn how segmented groups of students (particularly those at high risk for drug use and abuse) are affected by particular interven-

tions. Subgroups of special interest include those with preexisting conduct problems, chronic absentees or truants, and those with poor academic achievement.

Etiologic research has documented the importance of these individual differences in predicting drug use and abuse (Chapter 5).

2. *The effectiveness of culturally tailored interventions*: In addition to subgroups that vary on known risk factors for drug use, little is known about tailoring preventive interventions to particular ethnic subgroups. One study found that a culturally tailored intervention produced improved outcomes over a generic skills program at two-year follow-up (Botvin et al., 1995b). However, there is a dearth of basic information to provide a rationale for culturally tailored interventions, and little is known about their efficacy.

3. *Evaluating multichannel interventions*: Efforts must be made to incorporate the effects of preventive interventions from other channels into analyses of school-based programs. Recent research suggests that prevention effectiveness is improved by combining school-based programs with family, peer, community, and media interventions (Pentz et al., 1989a,b,c; Botvin, 1990; Hansen et al., 1990; Johnson et al., 1990; Tobler, 1992). Additional research is needed on the outcome effects of the multiple components of comprehensive interventions.

4. *Preventing the transition from drug use to abuse and dependence:* Most school-based programs focus on the prevention of drug use, but research is also needed on effective ways to prevent transitions from drug use to abuse and dependence. This research should identify modifiable risk and protective factors associated with the transition to drug abuse, so that intervention programs can be designed to influence these factors. At the present time, some risk factors have been identified, but many are not easily modifiable through school-based intervention (e.g., parental drug abuse and antisocial behavior, family history of psychopathology and disruption, childhood conduct problems, aggression, difficulties in regulating emotional arousal, sensation seeking, impulsivity, poor school achievement, and difficulties in coping [Glantz and Pickens, 1992]). The extent to which school-based programs can modify these risk factors and influence high-risk youth is an important area for future research. Additionally, school-based programs are targeted primarily at elementary and middle school children, who may or may not be at the stage of onset of drug use, whereas there are fewer prevention interventions targeted at adolescents and young adults, who are in the peak stages of drug use and abuse.

5. *Diffusion as a focus of research*: For the few interventions that have demonstrated enduring success, research on the process of dissemination is warranted. Although some research does exist on the fidelity of pro-

grams that are transferred from controlled research protocols to the community, the evidence is insufficient to justify conclusions at this time. Further, the actual impact of programs that have been transported from researcher to practitioner has not been systematically studied (Botvin, 1990; Butterfoss et al., 1993; Jackson et al., 1994; Leupker, 1994; Pirie et al., 1994). Therefore, research on the diffusion process by which programs are marketed, received, adopted, and transferred from researchers to practitioners, and on the effectiveness of such "transferred" programs, is another area for further study.

6. *Cost–benefit considerations in preventive intervention:* Continued research is needed on the public health impact and cost-effectiveness of school-based prevention programs. Pentz (1994) estimated that for every $1 spent on the Midwestern Prevention Project, $8 in treatment costs was saved for teenagers and $67 in treatment costs for adults. Botvin and colleagues (1995a) estimated the number of potential lives that would be saved from net reductions in cigarette smoking among those who received the Life Skills Training program. These early attempts at cost–benefit and cost-effectiveness analysis would be enhanced by substantially more conceptual clarity and measurement rigor. An assessment of the benefits and cost-effectiveness of school-based prevention interventions should be considered an integral part of program evaluations.

Family-Based Interventions

In general, family-based interventions show promise as prevention strategies because they impact known risk and protective factors associated with adolescent drug use and abuse and because they impact important mediating variables (such as childhood conduct problems) that are known risk factors for later drug abuse and dependence. At the present time, however, there have been too few studies specifically focused on drug use and abuse as outcomes to draw definitive conclusions. Moreover, studies that have evaluated the prevention and treatment of antisocial behavior and delinquency suggest that family interventions alone are inadequate; social skills training, academic tutoring, high-quality school environments, and family support services may be required for significant and sustained outcomes.

These multicomponent programs, although theoretically promising in influencing known risk factors for drug abuse, have important limitations. First, outcome studies have not focused on drug use and abuse, so the efficacy of these programs in preventing drug abuse is unknown. Second, they face challenges to implementation, including the need to actively recruit and retain high-risk families (Conduct Problems Prevention Research Group, 1992). Third, selective interventions focused on high-risk children must include screening methods that minimize false positives and false negatives and also minimize the risk of negative labeling effects. For example, recent data on early elementary school children show high false-positive rates (up to 30 percent) in screening for risk of conduct problems (Lochman and the Conduct Problems Prevention Research Group, 1995). Fourth, recent data raise the possibility of iatrogenic effects produced by selective interventions that concentrate groups of antisocial adolescents in peer group interventions; such a strategy may inadvertently increase adolescent problem behavior (Dishion and Andrews, 1995).

Thus, despite substantial progress in the development, implementation, and evaluation of family-based prevention interventions, there are continuing needs and opportunities for research in the following areas:

• *Family interventions for high-risk groups:* Research is needed on effective family interventions for groups at high risk for drug abuse, including children with conduct problems and children of drug-abusing parents. These are not necessarily independent subgroups; children of drug-abusing parents may be at risk for drug abuse partially because of their conduct problems. Because many of these programs target early elementary school children, longitudinal follow-up is necessary to assess relevant drug use outcomes, although short-term impacts on risk mediators (e.g., problem conduct) might be seen even in the elementary school years. Additionally, greater integration of preventive interventions focused on drug use or abuse, conduct disorders, and delinquency is needed (IOM, 1994b).

Current methods for defining and assessing high-risk groups produce high rates of false positives. It is necessary, therefore, to develop reliable and valid screening and assessment instruments, as well as methods of intervention delivery, designed to minimize the likelihood of negative labeling effects for selective interventions. This might be accomplished by incorporating interventions within existing treatment programs for drug-abusing parents, within existing prevention and treatment services for children with conduct problems, or within existing treatment and prevention programs in the juvenile justice system. In these ways, children would not be further labeled.

• *Developmentally appropriate interventions:* At early ages, high-quality preschool environments and social skills training may be important additions to family-based interventions. At later (adolescent) ages, interventions may also benefit from focusing on communication skills and family management of external stress (Tolan et al., 1995). However, concentrating antisocial adolescents in peer group interventions may have negative effects (Dishion and Andrews, 1995).

Media-Based Interventions

Media interventions are appealing because of their potential to reach a large audience in a cost-effective manner, but few studies have evaluated the utility of media campaigns in preventing drug abuse. Moreover, the challenges of implementing a media intervention include achieving sufficient intensity so that individuals are actually exposed to the message; targeting high-risk subgroups; tailoring messages to the needs and values of those groups; creating messages that are compelling enough to engage the viewer and be remembered; and preventing unintended negative consequences (e.g., inadvertently creating the impression that drug use is widespread and normative; U.S. DHHS, 1994). For legal drugs, media messages must also be powerful enough to counter intensive advertising campaigns. Finally, a media campaign alone is unlikely to be sufficient for prevention and should be combined with school-based or community policy interventions for maximum benefit (Pentz et al., 1989a,b; Flynn et al., 1992). Because there has been little research on the effectiveness of media interventions in the prevention of drug abuse, this area may warrant future research.

Community-Based Interventions

Research on the efficacy of policy-oriented community interventions must overcome several major challenges. A guiding principle of prevention research is that the intervention must effectively manipulate the mediating variables in order to produce change in a desired direction. Unfortunately, mediating variables at the community level are not yet well understood. There is a need for theory-based community interventions in which the theory of change addresses community-level mediating mechanisms in interaction with individual-level risk factors (Holder, 1994). Another challenge for community-based research is to develop effective methods for achieving the desired policy changes (above and beyond the question of whether policy changes actually produce the desired reductions in drug use, abuse, and dependence). Most community interventions involve coalition development, community organization, and a mobilization of community leaders. However, to date the literature on building and maintaining such coalitions can be characterized as "wisdom literature," because it is largely anecdotal and tends to be based on experiences and impressions (Butterfoss et al., 1993).

RESEARCH OPPORTUNITIES

From both a practical and a research perspective, prevention interventions are a core feature of the nation's attempts to reduce the demand for alcohol, tobacco, and illicit drugs among people of all ages and in all settings. As a result of prevention intervention research, however, many intuitively appealing strategies for reducing the demand for alcohol, tobacco, or illicit drugs, particularly among young people, have been found inadequate or even irrelevant. A "magic bullet" is no more likely to be found in prevention than in treatment or drug control. Instead, all modes of intervention must be pursued concurrently in order to maximize their contributions to the overall effort. For this reason, adequate evaluation research should be regarded as an essential feature of any preventive intervention. The committee has identified future research needs within each major area of prevention research, but many of its suggestions and recommendations for future research directions converge on several priorities for the field as a whole, including the following areas:

- *Prevention intervention research should focus more attention on the transition from use to abuse and dependence.* To date, most prevention research has focused on preventing initiation of drug use. Without neglecting initiation, more research is needed on determinants of the transition from drug use to abuse and dependence and on the ways that preventive interventions can influence that transition. This need includes further research on measuring risk for drug abuse and dependence and whether risk measurement is appropriately sensitive and specific to support selective interventions. Within universal prevention programs, there is a need to study program impact on subgroups of subjects at high risk for drug abuse and dependence.
- *Prevention research should be diversified to target populations other than young adolescents.* Until now, drug abuse prevention research has focused on the transition to adolescence because this is the time of drug use initiation. However, prevention research has been relatively neglected at other key points in the life span. Prevention research is needed in the preschool and elementary school years, targeted on preexisting risk factors for drug abuse—particularly the development of conduct problems. Prevention research is also needed during the transition to young adulthood, when drug abuse and dependence disorders are at peak levels. Possible settings for these interventions include colleges, work sites, the military, and settings where school dropouts (high school and college) congregate (Pentz, 1994). Finally, little is known about preventing drug abuse problems in later adulthood (Burton et al., in press).
- *Prevention research should be diversified to reach minority populations.*

Until recently, most prevention research and evaluations of preventive interventions have been limited to white, middle-class populations. Little is known about the effectiveness of prevention interventions on populations segmented on race, ethnicity, and socioeconomic status. Etiological and prevention research should be expanded to reach diverse populations. An important question that requires attention concerns the degree to which preventive intervention programs need to be "culturally specific" in order to be maximally effective.

- *Prevention research should focus on the design and evaluation of multicomponent interventions, especially at the community level.* As noted above, multicomponent interventions show promise for preventing drug use as well as the conduct problems that increase the risk for drug abuse, but more research is needed on the interactions among these components, especially in community-level interventions. Particular attention should be paid to the ways in which various modes of legal intervention can be integrated with traditional modes of prevention. Very little research has been conducted on the relative and synergistic effects of simultaneous supply reduction and demand reduction strategies (Pentz, 1994; Clayton, 1995). As noted in Chapter 10, integrated interventions in drug law enforcement and other community-level channels represent an intriguing opportunity for innovative research.

Additionally, greater attention should be paid to the development and application of models for assessing the benefits and cost-effectiveness of various prevention intervention approaches to drug use, abuse, and dependence. To do so requires an understanding of how to define and measure the units of prevention delivered and received and how to attribute to those exposure units specific outcomes that can also be measured and assigned a value (Plotnick, 1994).

Finally, federal funding agencies should facilitate interagency collaboration and coordination of prevention research. As is evident from the literature on etiology and prevention intervention, drug use prevention is integrally tied to prevention of problems and conditions lying within the province of multiple federal agencies including the National Institute on Drug Abuse (prevention research on drug abuse); the National Institute of Mental Health (prevention research on disorders that precede or are co-occurring with drug abuse); the National Institute on Alcohol Abuse and Alcoholism (prevention research on alcohol abuse and dependence); both the National Cancer Institute and the National Heart, Lung, and Blood Institute (prevention research on nicotine dependence); and the National Institute of Justice (research on the relationship of drug abuse to criminality). For the field of drug prevention science, procedures and structures should be developed to facilitate interagency collaboration and coordination of prevention research (Chapter 1).

> **The committee recommends rigorous evaluation of universal versus targeted prevention intervention programs with regard to effectiveness and cost-effectiveness, with particular focus on the initiation of use and on the transition from use to abuse and dependence. Emphasis should be placed on school-, family-, media-, and community-based interventions; interventions appropriate for high-risk populations; interventions aimed at ethnic subgroups; and multicomponent interventions especially at the community level.**

REFERENCES

Abikoff H, Klein R. 1992. Attention-deficit hyperactivity and conduct disorder: Comorbidity and implications for treatment. *Journal of Consulting and Clinical Psychology* 60:881–892.

Bandura A. 1977a. *Social Learning Theory*. Englewood Cliffs, NJ: Prentice-Hall.

Bandura A. 1977b. Self-efficacy: Toward a unifying theory of behavioral change. *Psychological Review* 84:191–215.

Bandura A. 1985. *Social Foundations of Thought and Action*. Englewood Cliffs, NJ: Prentice-Hall.

Bentler PM. 1991. Modeling of intervention effects. In: Leukefeld CG, Bukoski WJ, eds. *Drug Abuse Prevention Intervention Research: Methodological Issues*. Rockville, MD: NIDA. Pp. 159–182.

Biglan A, Hood D, Brozovsky P, Ochs L, Ary D, Black C. 1991. Subject attrition in prevention research. *NIDA Research Monograph* 107:213–234.

Botvin GJ. 1990. Substance abuse prevention: Theory, practice, and effectiveness. In: Tonry M, Wilson JQ, eds. *Crime and Justice: A Review of Research, Vol. 13*. Chicago: University of Chicago Press. Pp. 461–519.

Botvin GJ, Baker E, Dusenbury L, Botvin EM, Diaz T. 1995a. Long-term follow-up results of a randomized drug abuse prevention trial in a white middle-class population. *Journal of the American Medical Association* 273:1106–1112.

Botvin GJ, Schinke SP, Epstein JA, Diaz T, Botvin EM. 1995b. Effectiveness of culturally focused and generic skills training approaches to alcohol and drug abuse prevention among minority adolescents: Two year follow-up results. *Psychology of Addictive Behaviors* 9:183–194.

Bracht N, Finnegan JR, Rissel C, Weisbrod R, Gleason J, Corbett J, Veblen-Mortenson S. 1994. Community ownership and program continuation following a health demonstration project. *Health Education Research* 9:243–255.

Brook JS, Cohen P, Whiteman M, Gordon AS. 1992. Psychosocial risk factors in the transition from moderate to heavy use or abuse of drugs. In: Glantz MD, Pickins RW, eds. *Vulnerability to Drug Abuse*. Washington, DC: American Psychological Association Press. Pp. 359–388.

Brunswick AF, Messeri PA, Titus SP. 1992. Predictive factors in adult substance abuse: A prospective study of African American adolescents. In: Glantz MD, Pickins RW, eds. *Vulnerability to Drug Abuse*. Washington, DC: American Psychological Association Press. Pp. 419–472.

Bryk A, Raudenbusch S. 1992. *Hierarchical Linear Models: Applications and Data Analysis Methods*. Newbury Park, CA: Sage.

Burton R, Johnson R, Ritter CJ, Clayton RR. In press. The effects of role socialization on the initiation of cocaine use: An event history analysis from adolescence into middle adulthood. *Journal of Health and Social Behavior* 37.

Butterfoss FD, Goodman RM, Wandersman A. 1993. Community coalitions for prevention and health promotion. *Health Education Research* 8:315–330.

Clayton R. 1995. *Marijuana in a Challenging Third-World Region: Appalachia USA*. Denver: Lynne Reinner.

Clayton R, Ann Arbor Group. 1994. *Increase in Use of Selected Drugs: Monitoring the Future Study of 8th, 10th, and 12th Graders*. Ann Arbor, MI: University of Michigan. Report for the Office of National Drug Control Policy.

Cloninger R, Svrakic D, Przybeck T. 1993. A psychobiological model of temperament and character. *Archives of General Psychiatry* 50:975–990.

Cloninger R, Przybeck T, Svrakic D, Wetzel R. 1995. *The Temperament and Character Inventory: A Guide to Its Development and Use*. St. Louis, MO: Center for Psychobiology of Personality.

Coie JD, Norman FW, West SG, Hawkins JD, Asarnow JR, Markman HJ, Ramey SL, Shure MB, Long B. 1993. The science of prevention: A conceptual framework and some directions for a national research program. *American Psychologist* 48:1013–1022.

Collins LM, Graham JW, Rousculp SS, Fidler PL, Pan J, Hansen WB. 1994. Latent transition analysis and how it can address prevention research questions. *NIDA Research Monograph* 142:81–111.

Conduct Problems Prevention Research Group. 1992. A developmental and clinical model for the prevention of conduct disorders: The FAST Track program. *Development and Psychopathology* 4:509–527.

Dielman TE, Kloska D, Leech S, Schulenberg J, Shope JT. 1992. Susceptibility to peer pressure as an explanatory variable for the differential effectiveness of an elementary school-based alcohol misuse prevention program. *Journal of School Health* 62:233–237.

Dishion TJ, Andrews DW. 1995. Preventing escalation in problem behaviors with high-risk young adolescents: Immediate and 1-year outcomes. *Journal of Consulting and Clinical Psychology* 63:538–548.

Ellickson PL, Bell RM. 1990. Drug prevention in junior high: A multi-site longitudinal test. *Science* 247:1299–1305.

Ellickson PL, Bell RM. 1992. Challenges to social experiments: A drug prevention example. *Journal of Research on Crime and Delinquency* 29:79–101.

Ellickson PL, Bell RM, McGuigan K. 1993. Preventing adolescent drug use: Long-term results of a junior high program. *American Journal of Public Health* 83:856–861.

Ennett ST, Rosenbaum DP, Flewelling RL, Bieler GS, Ringwalt CR, Bailey SL. 1994a. Long-term evaluation of Drug Abuse Resistance Education. *Addictive Behaviors* 19:113–125.

Ennett ST, Tobler NS, Ringwalt CL, Flewelling RL. 1994b. How effective is Drug Abuse Resistance Education? A meta-analysis of project DARE outcome evaluations. *American Journal of Public Health* 84(9):1394–1401.

Flay B, Petraitis J. 1994a. The theory of triadic influence: A new theory of health behavior with implications for preventive interventions. *Advances in Medical Sociology* 4:19–44.

Flay B, Petraitis J. 1994b. *A Review of Theory and Prospective Research on the Causes of Adolescent Tobacco Use*. Paper prepared for the Robert Wood Johnson Foundation.

Flay BR, Miller TQ, Hedeker D, Siddiqui O, Britton CF, Brannon BR, Johnson CA, Hansen WB, Sussman S, Dent C. 1995. The Television, School, and Family Smoking Prevention and Cessation Project VIII: Student outcomes and mediating variables. *Preventive Medicine* 24:29–40.

Flynn BS, Worden JK, Secker-Walker RH, Badger GJ, Geller BM, Costanza MC. 1992. Prevention of cigarette smoking through mass media intervention and school programs. *American Journal of Public Health* 82:827–834.

Gibbons RD, Hedeker D. 1994. Application of random-effects probit regression models. *Journal of Consulting and Clinical Psychology* 62:285–296.

Glantz MD, Pickins RW. 1992. Vulnerability to drug abuse: Introduction and overview. In: Glantz MD, Pickins RW, eds. *Vulnerability to Drug Abuse*. Washington, DC: American Psychological Association Press. Pp. 1–14.

Gordon R. 1983. An operational classification of disease prevention. *Public Health Reports* 98:107–109.

Gottfredson D, McNeill R, Gottfredson G. 1991. Social area influences on delinquency: A multilevel analysis. *Journal of Research in Crime and Delinquency* 28:197–226.

Graham JW, Hofer SM, Piccinin AM. 1994. Analysis with missing data in drug prevention research. *NIDA Research Monograph* 142:13–63.

Hansen WB. 1992. School-based substance abuse prevention: A review of the state of the art in curriculum, 1980–1990. *Health Education Research* 7:403–430.

Hansen WB, Graham JW. 1991. Preventing alcohol, marijuana, and cigarette use among adolescents: Peer pressure resistance training versus establishing conservative norms. *Preventive Medicine* 20:414–430.

Hansen WB, Collins LM, Malotte CK, Johnson CA, Fielding JE. 1985. Attrition in prevention research. *Journal of Behavioral Medicine* 8:261–271.

Hansen WB, Tobler NS, Graham JW. 1990. Attrition in substance abuse prevention research: A meta-analysis of 85 longitudinally followed cohorts. *Evaluation Review* 14:677–685.

Harrell AV. 1988. Validation of self-report: The research record. *NIDA Research Monograph* 57:12–21.

Hawkins JD, Weis J. 1985. The social development model: An integrated approach to delinquency prevention. *Journal of Primary Prevention* 6:73–97.

Hawkins JD, Catalano RF, Miller JY. 1992a. Risk and protective factors for alcohol and other drug problems in adolescence and early adulthood: Implications for substance abuse prevention. *Psychological Bulletin* 112:64–105.

Hawkins JD, Catalano RF, Morrison DM, O'Donnell J, Abbott RD, Day LE. 1992b. The Seattle Social Development Project: Effects of the first four years on protective factors and problem behaviors. In: McCord J, Tremblay R, eds. *The Prevention of Antisocial Behavior in Children*. New York: Guilford.

Hedeker D, Gibbons RD, Flay BR. 1994. Random-effects regression models for clustered data with an example from smoking prevention research. *Journal of Consulting and Clinical Psychology* 62:757–765.

Holder HD. 1994. Commentary, Alcohol availability and accessibility as part of the puzzle: Thoughts on alcohol problems and young people. In: Zucker R, Boyd G, Howard J, eds. *The Development of Alcohol Problems: Exploring the Biopsychosocial Matrix of Risk*. Pp. 249–254. NIAAA Research Monograph 26. Rockville, MD: U.S. DHHS.

Hu TW, Sung HY, Keeler TE. 1995. Reducing cigarette consumption in California: Tobacco taxes vs. an anti-smoking media campaign. *American Journal of Public Health* 85(9):1218–1222.

Huizinga D, Loeber R, Thornberry T. 1994. *Urban Delinquency and Substance Abuse: Initial Findings*. Washington, DC: Office of Juvenile Justice and Delinquency Prevention, Department of Justice.

IOM (Institute of Medicine). 1994a. *Growing Up Tobacco Free: Preventing Nicotine Addiction in Children and Youths*. Washington, DC: National Academy of Sciences.

IOM (Institute of Medicine). 1994b. *Reducing Risks for Mental Disorders: Frontiers for Preventive Intervention Research*. Washington, DC: National Academy Press.

Jackson C, Fortmann SP, Flora JA, Melton RJ, Snkider JP, Littlefield D. 1994. The capacity-building approach to intervention maintenance implemented by the Stanford Five City Project. *Health Education Research* 9:385–396.

Johnson C, Pentz M, Weber M, Dwyer J, Baer N, MacKinnon D, Hansen W, Flay B. 1990. Relative effectiveness of comprehensive community programming for drug abuse prevention with high-risk and low-risk adolescents. *Journal of Consulting and Clinical Psychology* 58:447–456.

Kazdin A. 1987. Treatment of antisocial behavior in children: Current status and future directions. *Psychological Bulletin* 102:187–203.

Laird NM, Ware JH. 1982. Random effects models for longitudinal data. *Biometrics* 38:963–974.

Leupker RV. 1994. Community trials. *Preventive Medicine* 23:602–605.

Lochman JE, Conduct Problems Prevention Research Group. 1995. Screening of child behavior problems for prevention programs at school entry. *Journal of Consulting and Clinical Psychology* 63:549–559.

MacKinnon DP, Johnson CA, Pentz MA, Dwyer JH, Hansen WB, Flay BR, Wang E. 1991. Mediating mechanisms in a school-based drug prevention program: First year effects of the Midwestern Prevention Project. *Health Psychology* 10:164–172.

Mayes LC. 1995. Substance abuse and parenting. In: Bornstein MH, ed. *Handbook of Parenting, Vol. 4. Applied and Practical Parenting*. Mahway, NJ: Lawrence Erlbaum Publishers. Pp. 101–125.

Merikangas KR, Rounsaville BJ, Prusoff BA. 1992. Familial factors in vulnerability to substance abuse. In: Glantz MD, Pickins RW, eds. *Vulnerability to Drug Abuse*. Washington, DC: American Psychological Association Press. Pp. 75–98.

Moffitt TE. 1993. Adolescence-limited and life-course-persistent antisocial behavior: A developmental taxonomy. *Psychological Review* 100:674–701.

Murray DM, Pirie P, Luepker RV, Pallonen U. 1989. Five- and six-year follow-up results from four seventh-grade smoking prevention strategies. *Journal of Behavioral Medicine* 12:207–218.

Oetting ER, Beauvais F. 1987. Peer cluster theory, socialization characteristics, and adolescent drug use: A path analysis. *Journal of Consulting Psychology* 34:205–213.

Olds DL, Henderson CR, Chamberlin R, Tatelbaum R. 1986. Preventing child abuse and neglect: A randomized trial of nurse home visitation. *Pediatrics* 78:65–78.

Patterson G, DeBaryshe B, Ramsey E. 1989. A developmental perspective on antisocial behavior. *American Psychologist* 27:329–335.

Pentz MA. 1994. Directions for future research in drug abuse prevention. *Preventive Medicine* 23:646–652.

Pentz MA, MacKinnon D, Flay B, Hansen W, Johnson CA, Dwyer J. 1989a. Primary prevention of chronic diseases in adolescence: Effects of the Midwestern Prevention Project on tobacco use. *American Journal of Epidemiology* 130:713–724.

Pentz MA, Dwyer J, MacKinnon D, Flay BR, Hansen WB, Wang EY, Johnson CA. 1989b. A multicommunity trial for primary prevention of adolescent drug abuse. *Journal of the American Medical Association* 261:3259–3266.

Pentz MA, MacKinnon DP, Dwyer JH, Wang EYI, Hansen WB, Flay BR, Johnson CA. 1989c. Longitudinal effects of the Midwestern Prevention Project on regular experimental smoking in adolescents. *Preventive Medicine* 18:304–321.

Perry CL, Kelder SH, Murray DM, Kepp K-I. 1992. Community-wide smoking prevention: Long-term outcomes of the Minnesota Heart Health Program and the Class of 1989 Study. *American Journal of Public Health* 82:1210–1216.

Pirie PL, Stone EJ, Assaf AR, Flora JA, Maschewsky-Schneider U. 1994. Program evaluation strategies for community-based health promotion programs: Perspectives from the cardiovascular disease community research and demonstration studies. *Health Education Research* 9:23–36.

Plotnick RD. 1994. Applying benefit-cost analysis to substance use prevention programs. *International Journal of the Addictions* 29:339–359.

Reid JB. 1993. Prevention of conduct disorder before and after school entry: Relating interventions to developmental findings. *Development and Psychopathology* 5:243–262.

Resnicow K, Botvin G. 1993. School-based substance use prevention programs: Why do effects decay? *Preventive Medicine* 22:484–490.

Ringwalt C, Greene J, Ennett S, Iachan R, Clayton R, Leukefeld C. 1994. *Past and Future Directions of the D.A.R.E. Program: An Evaluation Review*. Final Report to the National Institute of Justice.

Rouse BA, Kozel NJ, Richards LG. 1988. *Self-Report Methods of Estimating Drug Use: Meeting Current Challenges to Validity*. Rockville, MD: NIDA.

Seitz V, Apfel NH, Rosenbaum LK. 1991. Effects of an intervention program for pregnant adolescents: Educational outcomes at two years postpartum. *American Journal of Community Psychology* 19:911–931.

Smith BE, Davis RC. 1993. Successful community anti-crime programs: What makes them work? In: Davis RC, Lurigio AJ, Rosenbaum DP, eds. *Drugs and the Community: Involving Community Residents in Combatting the Sale of Illegal Drugs*. Springfield, IL: Charles C Thomas. Pp. 123–137.

Steinberg L. 1991. Autonomy, conflict, and harmony in the family relationship. In: Feldman SS, Elliott GR, eds. *At the Threshold: The Developing Adolescent*. Cambridge, MA: Harvard University Press. Pp. 255–276.

Susser M. 1995. The tribulations of trials-intervention in communities. *American Journal of Public Health* 85:156–158.

Tobler NS. 1992. Drug prevention programs can work: Research findings. *Journal of Addictive Diseases* 11:1–28.

Tolan P, Guerra NG, Kendall PC. 1995. A developmental-ecological perspective on antisocial behavior in children and adolescents: Towards a unified risk and intervention framework. *Journal of Consulting and Clinical Psychology* 63:579–584.

U.S. DHHS (U.S. Department of Health and Human Services). 1994. *Preventing Tobacco Use Among Young People: A Report of the Surgeon General*. Atlanta, GA: U.S. DHHS, Public Health Service, Centers for Disease Control and Prevention, National Center for Chronic Disease Prevention and Health Promotion, Office on Smoking and Health.

Wagenaar AC, Perry CL. 1994. Community strategies for the reduction of youth drinking: Theory and application. *Journal of Research on Adolescence* 4:319–345.

Wolfson A, Lacks P, Futterman A. 1992. Effects of parent training on infant sleeping patterns, parents' stress, and perceived parental competence. *Journal of Consulting and Clinical Psychology* 60:41–49.

Yamaguchi K. 1991. *Event History Analysis*. Newbury Park, CA: Sage.

Yoshikawa H. 1994. Prevention as cumulative protection: Effects of early family support and education on chronic delinquency and its risks. *Psychological Bulletin* 115:28–54.

7

Consequences

The ramifications of drug abuse extend far beyond the individual drug abuser, because the health and social consequences of drug abuse—HIV/AIDS (human immunodeficiency virus/acquired immune deficiency syndrome), violence, tuberculosis, fetal effects, crime, and disruptions in family, workplace, and educational environments (Box 7.1)—have devastating impacts on society and exact a cost of billions of dollars annually.[1] Drug abuse is often the result of a constellation of factors including socioeconomic status, educational achievement, co-occurring psychiatric disorders, access to health care, employment status, and numerous other factors present in the lives of drug-abusing individuals (see Chapter 5). Regardless of the factors at work, it is the ultimate goal of the nation's investment in drug abuse research to take more effective measures to prevent drug abuse and to reduce its associated costs and consequences.

A comprehensive assessment of knowledge and research opportunities on the multiple consequences of drug abuse would have far exceeded the committee's allowable time frame and expertise. Consequently, it chose to focus on three areas that involve pronounced social consequences, where the need for strategic interventions are greatest: (1) the transmission and course of HIV infection; (2) fetal and child development; and (3) violent behavior.

---

[1]It should be noted that negative consequences can derive from patterns of problematic use that do not meet the criteria for abuse and dependence as well as from abuse or dependence.

BOX 7.1
Consequences of Drug Abuse

HIV/AIDS

It now appears that injection drug use is the leading risk factor for new human immunodeficiency virus (HIV) infections in the U.S. (Holmberg, 1996). Drug and alcohol abuse heightens the risk for unsafe sexual behavior and is a factor in perinatal transmission of HIV.

TB

Tuberculosis (TB) rates have increased significantly among drug-using populations, especially drug-resistant TB in HIV-infected drug users.

Other diseases and illnesses

Injection drug users (IDUs) are more likely to develop serious infections and illnesses (e.g., viral hepatitis, endocarditis, pneumonia, other bacterial infections) than the non-IDU population due to the harmful effects of drug injection and their infrequent use of primary medical care services. Additionally, some forms of psychiatric disorders may result in part from drug abuse (e.g., alcohol-related depression, PCP-precipitated psychosis).

Fetal and child development

Drug abuse can impact the health of the developing fetus and child. Consequences include retardation of fetal growth, fetal alcohol syndrome, neonatal withdrawal syndrome, and neonatal neurobehavioral affects.

Violence and crime

Violence and crime are linked to illicit drug abuse through the often violent nature of drug sales and distribution. Additionally, some drug addicts resort to theft to support their drug habits. Pharmacological effects of drug abuse associated with violent actions may occur de novo or with predating co-occurring psychiatric disorders.

Public safety

Drug abuse plays a role in numerous transportation or other accidents. For example, the National Highway Traffic Safety Administration estimates that 40.8 percent of traffic fatalities were alcohol related (NHTSA, 1995).

Loss of human capital

Drug abuse can have devastating impacts on an individual's potential (e.g., school delinquency, dropping out of school, involvement in illicit drug selling), thus reducing future educational and job opportunities.

Workplace

Employee drug use, particularly heavy use or abuse, has been found to be associated with increased absenteeism, accidents, job turnover, counterproductive behavior, and job dissatisfaction (NRC, 1994). However, drug abuse does not occur in isolation, and other related life-style behaviors are strongly correlated with employment difficulties.

BOX 7.1
Consequences of Drug Abuse (continued)

Family

Drug abuse leads to reallocation of economic support away from the family; lack of participation in family activities, including caregiving; lack of emotional commitment and support for parents and children; and the inability to provide a reliable and adequate role model for other family members, especially children. This impact on the family affects children's development, learning, and social relations whether or not actual child abuse and neglect occur.

Education

Drug-abusing students may develop cognitive and behavioral difficulties; disrupt classes; have increased psychosocial problems; or be delinquent in attending school or drop out of school (Kandel and Davies, 1996). Additionally, violence increases as buying and selling of drugs occurs at the school site.

HIV/AIDS

Today more than 17 million people worldwide, including an estimated 1 million Americans, are infected with the human immunodeficiency virus (HIV) which causes AIDS. In the United States, according to the Centers for Disease Control and Prevention (CDC), AIDS is now the leading cause of death among 25- to 44-year-olds (Swan, 1995).

It now appears that injection drug use is the leading risk factor for new HIV infection in the United States (Holmberg, 1996). More than one-third of AIDS cases reported through December 1995 were related to injection of illicit drugs through three mechanisms: the sharing of contaminated injection equipment, heterosexual contact with an injection drug user (IDU), or through maternal injection of illicit drugs (Table 7.1) (CDC, 1995a). In women, the percentages of AIDS cases involving injection of illicit drugs are alarmingly high. Of the 71,818 female AIDS cases reported to CDC through December 1995, almost half (33,452 cases) were related to injection of illicit drugs and another 18 percent (13,046 cases) to sex with infected IDU partners (CDC, 1995a).

HIV can be transmitted through direct needle sharing when contaminated blood remains in the syringe and may be released into the next user or through certain injection drug practices during which blood is drawn into the syringe and mixed with the drug. Transmission of the virus can also occur indirectly by the sharing of drug injection equipment such as cotton balls or rinse water (NRC, 1995), and increased frequency of injection and the use of shared equipment increase the risk for seropositivity. HIV risk is also associated with the locations in which drug use occurs.

TABLE 7.1 AIDS Cases Related to Injection of Illicit Drugs (percentage of total cases)

Exposure Category	Cases Reported in 1995		Cumulative Total Reported Through December 1995	
Injection drug use				
Men	14,057	(19)	95,244	(18.5)
Women	5,204	(7)	33,452	(6.5)
Heterosexual contact with an injection drug user				
Men	928	(1.2)	5,664	(1.1)
Women	1,921	(2.6)	13,046	(2.5)
Men who have sex with men and inject drugs	3,425	(4.6)	33,195	(6.5)
Pediatric cases (<13 years old)				
Mother who is an injection drug user	211	(0.3)	2,594	(0.5)
Mother who has sex with an injection drug user	114	(0.2)	1,164	(0.2)
Total cases related to injection drug use	25,860	(34.9)	184,359	(35.8)
Total cases reported	74,180	(100)	513,486	

SOURCE: CDC (1995a).

Injection drug use frequently occurs in "shooting galleries" where users can rent a syringe and needle that is supplied from a common container. The injection equipment may or may not be rinsed, and if rinsed, may be rinsed with infected water.[2]

All drug users, injecting and noninjecting, place themselves at great risk for HIV transmission when engaging in unsafe sexual behavior while under the influence of drugs, such as alcohol and cocaine, or exchanging sex for money or drugs (Edlin et al., 1994; O'Connor et al., 1994). One study found that as many as 80 percent of male IDUs were in a primary

[2]Studies have shown that HIV can survive in tap water for extended periods of time (Resnick et al., 1986).

relationship with women who did not use drugs themselves (Des Jarlais et al., 1984). Since the beginning of the crack cocaine epidemic, that drug has been seen as a sexual stimulant, as well as the cause of high-risk sexual behavior in many users. The disinhibiting effect is stronger than that of depressants such as alcohol or heroin due to the rapid onset of the drug's "high" with a related rapid release of inhibitions (Fullilove and Fullilove, 1989; Chaisson et al., 1991; Edlin et al., 1994). Sex-for-drug exchanges and prostitution—associated with the need to acquire crack cocaine or the money to buy the drug—have resulted in the transmission of HIV to the non-drug-using populations (IOM, 1994).

Maternal–infant transmission of HIV is often an indirect health consequence of injection drug use. Of the 6,948 cases of AIDS in children under 13 years of age reported to CDC through December 1995, 90 percent are attributable to perinatal HIV transmission. Most (54 percent) of the pediatric AIDS cases are associated with injection of illicit drugs—37 percent with maternal injection of drugs and 17 percent with maternal sexual contact with an IDU (CDC, 1995a). Of all infants born to HIV-infected mothers who do not receive antiretroviral therapy (e.g., AZT), an estimated 15–35 percent of those infants become infected (Hardy, 1991; CDC, 1994, 1995b).

As the AIDS epidemic continues to spread, the financial burden of the disease on those affected, the health care system, and society in general will continue to grow. Because data on the use of and expenditures for medical services of persons with AIDS are scarce, the Agency for Health Care Policy and Research (AHCPR) established the AIDS Cost and Service Utilization Survey (ACSUS) in 1989. Estimates in 1992 forecast that the cumulative (national) costs of treating all HIV-infected individuals would surpass $15.2 billion in 1995 (see Table 7.2). That figure, which represents a 48 percent increase from the cost of $10.3 billion in 1992, reflects an increase in the average amount of services used by those infected with HIV as well as the availability of better data on the utilization of medical services (Hellinger, 1992; *Oncology*, 1993).

TABLE 7.2 Estimated Costs of AIDS

Costs	1991	1992	1995
Cost of treating all HIV-infected persons in the United States	$2.3 billion	$10.3 billion	$15.2 billion

SOURCES: Adapted from Scitovsky and Rice (1987), Hellinger (1992), *Oncology* (1993).

Research Opportunities

The United States funds 85 percent of the world's public sector investment in AIDS research, primarily through the National Institutes of Health (NIH) whose AIDS and AIDS-related research portfolio is currently a $1.4 billion effort (OAR, 1996). Research is aimed at all phases of the etiology, prevention, and treatment of the disease. The research accomplishments to date are numerous. This section highlights future research directions related to IDUs and AIDS research. Chapter 8 discusses further research opportunities in the treatment of HIV-infected drug abusers.

HIV Epidemiology

Measuring HIV prevalence (the number of infections at a point in time) and incidence (the number of new infections over time) is crucial to monitoring the course of the epidemic. Statistics on the incidence and prevalence of HIV infection provide a more complete assessment of the magnitude of the epidemic than end-stage statistics of AIDS cases. Efforts to determine HIV prevalence in the drug-abusing population have been based on a range of seroprevalence studies primarily of IDUs. The number of IDUs in the United States has been estimated to range from 1.1 million to 1.8 million (NRC, 1989; OTA, 1990). Estimates of HIV seroprevalence in the IDU population range from 0 to 50 percent depending largely on geographic location. In New York City, HIV seroprevalence was found to be slightly more than 50 percent in a study of injection drug users (Des Jarlais et al., 1994). The Centers for Disease Control and Prevention's HIV/AIDS Surveillance Report provides data on new HIV cases in IDUs. However, these data are not representative of all persons with HIV infection because some states also offer anonymous HIV testing, and the collection of demographic and risk information varies greatly among states (CDC, 1995a).

Because of the difficulties in locating and gaining access to the populations initiating or relapsing into injecting drugs, most of the epidemiological studies to date have focused on long-term, chronic IDUs (IOM, 1994). As a result, little is known about younger, new IDUs who may actually be at increased risk for HIV transmission due to engaging in higher levels of risk behaviors, including needle sharing and use of shooting galleries (Battjes et al., 1992). Additionally, little is known about the extent of HIV transmission that is due to sex-for-drug activities or drug-related prostitution.

Studies are needed to determine the prevalence of HIV infection among vulnerable populations of drug users. Information from such studies may help establish a basis for possible intervention programs directed at preventing further HIV transmission. More extensive epidemiological data regarding HIV incidence in the drug-using population are needed in order for AIDS treatment programs to accurately and adequately meet the needs of those infected.

Prevention and Risk Reduction Strategies

AIDS prevention intervention research is focused mainly on identifying and modifying behaviors known to be associated with HIV transmission; it targets individuals at high risk because of drug use and sexual contact. Education on hygienic injection practices and HIV transmission routes, condom distribution programs, and enrollment in drug abuse treatment are currently the major risk reduction interventions aimed at drug users in the United States. Additionally, there are other programs to prevent HIV infection that have incorporated social interventions to effect change in risky behaviors (Friedman et al., 1992).

Drug abuse treatment has demonstrated varying degrees of success in the reduction of risk factors for HIV among populations of IDUs, primarily through prevention education (Watkins et al., 1992). Studies have shown that drug abuse treatment is associated with reductions in HIV risk behaviors, including reductions in drug use, in risky injection practices, and in the number of sex partners (Ball et al., 1988; Watkins et al., 1992; Longshore et al., 1994; Serpelloni et al., 1994). In general, it has proven to be more difficult to change sexual risk behaviors than to change drug injection behaviors (Des Jarlais, 1992; Battjes et al., 1995).

Recent evidence has shown a decrease in the use of contaminated drug paraphernalia when needle exchange is available (Des Jarlais et al., 1994). For example, the use of contaminated needles declined from 51 percent of injections in 1984 to 7 percent in 1992 in a study of New York City IDUs (Des Jarlais et al., 1994). That work confirms other studies that found HIV risk reduction behaviors among IDUs (Vlahov et al., 1991; Schottenfeld et al., 1993). As noted in a recent National Research Council (NRC, 1995) report, research has also shown that needle exchange programs do not affect the level of drug use among participants and do not appear to recruit new users to injection drugs. Additionally, needle exchange programs can also provide strategic and important sites for the deployment of primary care services and referral for persons with or at risk of HIV infection. Whereas needle exchange programs have been adopted in some European countries and have been associated with a reduction in the incidence of HIV infection (Hart et al., 1989; Hartgers et al., 1989; Ljungberg et al., 1991) and no increase in illicit drug use, such programs have been resisted in the United States.[3] Continued research is needed on the impact of needle exchange programs and on ways to improve their effectiveness along the lines recommended in the NRC report (see also Chapter 10).

Although risk reduction strategies have primarily targeted current injection drug users, it is important for research to focus also on preventing initiation into intravenous drug use. A study by Battjes and colleagues (1992) found that early age of first injection is associated with higher levels of injection and sexual risk behaviors (including needle sharing, frequency of injection, use of shooting galleries, multiple sex partners, and prostitution).

The committee recommends continued and expanded research efforts regarding noninjecting and injecting drug use and HIV transmission. Specifically, epidemiological studies of the prevalence and correlates of HIV infection in vulnerable populations of drug users and IDUs; and studies of effective risk reduction strategies for changing sexual risk behaviors and drug injection behaviors are needed.

IMPACTS ON FETAL, INFANT, AND CHILD DEVELOPMENT

Drug abuse can have a significant impact on the health of children who either are exposed to nicotine, alcohol, or illicit drugs prenatally through maternal drug abuse or grow up in a drug-abusing household. Although it is difficult to estimate the number of children in drug-abusing households, the National Pregnancy and Health Survey, sponsored by the National Institute of Drug Abuse (NIDA), provides nationwide estimates of the use of nicotine, alcohol, and illicit drugs by pregnant women. The survey estimated that in 1992, 20.4 percent of the women (an estimated 820,000 women) smoked cigarettes and 18.8 percent (757,000) used alcohol during pregnancy (NIDA, 1996). The survey also found that 5.5 percent of the women who gave birth (approximately 221,000 women out of 4 million nationally) used one or more illicit drugs during pregnancy; an estimated 119,000 women (2.9 percent) used marijuana, 45,000 (1.1 percent) used cocaine (34,800 of whom used crack cocaine), and 3,600 used heroin during pregnancy (NIDA, 1996).[4]

---

[3]However, a recent survey reported 76 needle exchange programs in 55 U.S. cities (NRC, 1995).

[4]Correlations performed on survey results found that drug use varied by the number of prenatal care visits (mothers with fewer than five prenatal care visits had the highest rates

The economic costs of maternal drug use during pregnancy were estimated to exceed $500 million in 1990 for cocaine-exposed infants and $652 million annually for maternal cigarette smoking (Manning et al., 1989a,b; Phibbs et al., 1991; Frank et al., 1993). Prenatal exposure to these drugs may result in prematurity and low birth weight, which is one of the primary causes of extended hospital stays for drug-exposed infants. For example, a premature cocaine-exposed infant's hospital stay costs an average of $5,200 more than the cost of an unexposed infant (Phibbs et al., 1991). It is more difficult to estimate the cost of other health effects due to prenatal exposure (e.g., HIV infection[5]) or the collateral effects (e.g., homelessness, child abuse, neglect, and malnutrition) of growing up in a drug-abusing household.

The next section provides an overview of the known effects of nicotine, alcohol, heroin, marijuana, and cocaine on fetal development and on later behavior and developmental outcomes. It is followed by a discussion of opportunities for future research on prenatal exposure and on the effects of growing up in a drug-abusing household. Discussion is limited to nicotine, alcohol, heroin, marijuana, and cocaine because those drugs appear to be the most widely used during pregnancy, with the possible exception of caffeine. Before describing the accomplishments, however, the methodological difficulties associated with conducting research on prenatal exposure are discussed.

Methodological Issues

Nicotine, alcohol, heroin, marijuana, and cocaine readily cross the placenta and the blood–brain barrier, creating a potentially increased risk of adverse biological consequences to overall fetal development and specifically to fetal brain development. In most instances, however, demonstrating links between prenatal exposure and immediate or later outcomes is complicated by issues such as interactions with associated conditions

---

of illicit drug use), income level (women with a household income level greater than $50,000 had lower rates of illicit drug or cigarette use but the highest rates of alcohol use), and hospital size (hospitals with 3,000 or more births annually and urban metropolitan hospitals had the highest rates of illicit drug use) (NIDA, 1996).

[5]Vertical transmission of HIV from mother to child may be a consequence of maternal injection drug use or maternal sexual contact with an HIV-infected person. As discussed in the previous section on AIDS, of the 6,948 cases of AIDS in children under 13 years of age reported to CDC through December 1995, 90 percent are attributable to perinatal HIV transmission and 54 percent of those cases are associated with injection of illicit drugs (CDC, 1995a). Additionally, maternal drug abuse is a risk factor for congenital syphilis and transmission of hepatitis (Weintrub et al., 1991; Frank et al., 1993; Webber et al., 1993).

(e.g., poor nutrition, parental stress and psychiatric illness, sexually transmitted diseases) that may also impact on development (Frank et al., 1993; Finnegan, 1994). Further, the majority of women who use heroin, marijuana, or crack cocaine also use varying amounts of alcohol and/or nicotine and may use one or more illicit drugs in combination. Thus, rarely is it possible to speak, for example, of a "pure" crack cocaine effect.

Additionally, longitudinal studies of the developmental outcome of prenatal drug exposure in human infants face four methodological issues that cut across the specific agent of abuse and exposure (reviews by Jacobson and Jacobson, 1995; Neuspiel, 1995; Olson et al., 1995). First, there are difficulties in ascertaining the amount, frequency, and duration of drug abuse during pregnancy due to inaccuracies of maternal self-report and limitations of current biological markers of exposure (Coles, 1992; Kidwell, 1992). Second, the high rate of attrition is a problem in studies of drug-abusing populations (Mayes and Cicchetti, 1995). Third, there are difficulties in choosing the appropriate comparison group (e.g., determining whether the comparison group is drug free or free only of the primary drug of interest, choosing appropriate demographic comparison cohorts). Fourth, determining the appropriate time (developmentally) and length of time to assess infants is another crucial issue. Traditional models of behavioral teratology presume effects that are present at least early in infancy but may or may not persist through childhood. Less frequently discussed are drug-related effects that are not apparent until later in development, when central nervous system processing of information or social skills are required, or during periods of major central nervous system reorganization (e.g, between age 4 and 5 years or during puberty) (see Weiss, 1995).

Animal models provide some basis for comparison because the amount of exposure and environmental conditions may be controlled. Animal models have been particularly useful for studies of the effects of prenatal exposures and for modeling drug-related effects on brain development at the structural, cellular, and functional levels. Neurobehavioral data from animal models should be viewed carefully, however, when extrapolating results from animal models to the complex developmental capacities found in higher primates and humans (e.g., language, complex problem-solving tasks, and neuropsychological functions such as certain domains of memory) (see Stanton and Spear, 1990).

Accomplishments

Prenatal Nicotine Exposure

Nicotine acts as a vasoconstrictor, reducing placental blood flow and the amount of oxygen and nutrients available to the fetus through several mechanisms. Additionally, smoking reduces the mother's appetite, and carbon monoxide from cigarette smoke crosses the placenta, increasing fetal carboxyhemoglobin levels (Werler et al., 1985). Those mechanisms are associated with retarding intrauterine growth in an apparent dose-response relationship; the more cigarettes smoked, the lower is the birth weight (Zuckerman, 1991).[6] Maternal cigarette smoking is also linked to higher rates of negative outcomes, including spontaneous abortions (Risch et al., 1988), stillbirths and perinatal death (Cnattingius et al., 1988; Malloy et al., 1988), and sudden infant death syndrome (SIDS) (Werler et al., 1985; Kandall and Gaines, 1991; Fried, 1992). Additionally, other toxins in cigarettes, including cadmium, lead, and thiocyanate, may also have adverse effects on the developing fetus (Kuhnert, 1991).

Nicotine may affect fetal brain development both indirectly (through nicotine-associated hypoxia) and directly (through specific nicotinic receptors) (Slotkin, 1992). In animal models, it appears that there is a lower dose threshold for adverse effects of fetal nicotine exposure on neuronal development than on overall growth (Slotkin, 1992). The literature regarding later neuro-behavioral outcomes in nicotine-exposed infants and children is not as extensive or as conclusive as those studies regarding pregnancy and birth outcomes (Fried, 1992). One study has found that maternal smoking during pregnancy, when postnatal smoking was controlled, selectively increased the probability that female children would smoke as adolescents and would continue to smoke (Kandel et al., 1994). There is suggestive evidence of a relationship between maternal smoking and later adverse developmental outcomes, including effects on attention and auditory responsiveness (Fried and Watkinson, 1988, 1990). However, those effects, if any, have a small attributable risk.

Prenatal Alcohol Exposure

Alcohol in high doses is a potentially potent teratogen associated with a range of consequences, including congenital anomalies and neurodevelopmental impairments (reviewed in IOM, 1995). In high doses, alcohol acts as a direct neuroteratogen, affecting all aspects of fetal growth (including brain growth, structure, and function) through mechanisms

---

[6]Intrauterine growth retardation (IUGR) can be caused by a number of factors including undernutrition and is associated postnatally with impaired neuromotor performance, including decreased motor maturity, poor state control, and abnormal reflexes (Tronick and Beeghly, 1992). Studies have reported long-term consequences of IUGR, including language delay and poor academic performance, but a direct cause–effect relationship for long-term effects is still considered inconclusive.

that have not yet been elucidated (Schenker et al., 1990; Goodlett and West, 1992).

Studies of gestational ethanol exposure in nonhuman primates have explored dose–response relationships (e.g., Clarren et al., 1988, 1992). Fetal alcohol syndrome (FAS) is caused by prenatal exposure to high levels of alcohol and is characterized by intrauterine growth retardation with concomitant poor growth in fetal weight and/or height; a pattern of specific minor physical anomalies that include a characteristic facial appearance; and central nervous system deficits including microcephaly, delayed development, hyperactivity, attention deficits, intellectual delays, and learning disabilities (Clarren and Smith, 1978; Smith, 1982). Even in the absence of signs of FAS, infants born to alcoholic mothers show an increased incidence of intellectual impairment, congenital anomalies, and decreased birth weight (Sokol et al., 1980; Day, 1992; Aronson et al., 1985). Some children exposed prenatally to alcohol may show delayed development in their first two to three years (e.g., Jacobson et al., 1993; Day and Richardson, 1994) while others do not exhibit this tendency (Greene et al., 1990; Boyd et al., 1991).

Prenatal Opiate Exposure

Newborns who have been exposed prenatally to opiates (heroin or methadone), taken by the mother chronically during the pregnancy, are born passively dependent on the drug and may exhibit withdrawal symptoms in the first days to weeks after delivery (Desmond and Wilson, 1975). The withdrawal symptoms are characterized by hyperirritability, tremors, diarrhea, vomiting, and tachypnea (Finnegan, 1986). Prenatal opioid exposure increases the risk of reduced birth weight and head circumference (e.g., Zagon and McLaughlin, 1984; Doberczak et al., 1987) and of SIDS (e.g., Finnegan, 1979; Kandall et al., 1993). Similar findings in animal models that control for exposure to other drugs, such as alcohol and tobacco, and for poor maternal health support these findings on the effect of opiates on fetal growth (Zagon and McLaughlin, 1984).

Neurobehavioral assessments in the newborn period find that opiate-exposed infants are more easily aroused, are more irritable, and have poor motor control (Strauss et al., 1976; Marcus and Hans, 1982; Jeremy and Hans, 1985). Such neurobehavioral abnormalities generally diminish over the first month of life (Jeremy and Hans, 1985) and thus are assumed to reflect the transitory symptoms of narcotic withdrawal rather than evidence of permanent neurological dysfunction (Hans, 1992).

Follow-up studies of opiate-exposed and non-opiate-exposed children have continued to report few to no differences in developmental and cognitive performance in comparison to social class–matched controls, although there is some indication of problems with motor coordination (Strauss et al., 1976). There are fewer studies of the long-term effects in school-age children of prenatal opiate exposure, and those available usually lack a nonexposed control group or are not based on a longitudinal design (Hans, 1992).

Prenatal Marijuana Exposure

Tetrahydrocannabinol (THC), a psychoactive compound in marijuana, readily crosses the placenta and, in heavy users, it is also concentrated in breast milk (Blackard and Tennes, 1984; Levy and Koren, 1992). Marijuana has an indirect effect on fetal oxygenation through the high level of carbon monoxide found in marijuana smoke, which in turn results in fetal hypoxia. THC during pregnancy has adverse effects (in animals and humans) on pituitary and ovarian function, prolactin secretion, and uterine contractility (Harclerode, 1980). However, studies on the relationship between marijuana use and length of gestation or birth weight have conflicting results (Fried et al., 1983; Zuckerman et al., 1989b).

Studies on marijuana's neurobehavioral affects are inconclusive; some studies have reported that human neonates exposed to maternal marijuana use exhibit increased tremors, higher-pitched cries, and disturbances in sleep patterns (Fried, 1980, 1982; Fried and Makin, 1987; Scher et al., 1988). The paucity of long-term follow-up studies makes it difficult to conclude whether or not prenatal marijuana exposure has a direct effect on later developmental functions such as memory, attention, or impulse control, and/or whether such effects cannot be identified until later in development.

Prenatal Cocaine Exposure

The effect of cocaine on fetal growth may be due to the norepinephrine- and serotonin-related effects of cocaine on vascular tone, which decreases uteroplacental blood flow and contributes to uteroplacental insufficiency (acute and chronic), maternal hypertension, and fetal vasoconstriction (Moore et al., 1986; Woods et al., 1987), in turn resulting in a relative state of fetal hypoxia. Reduced placental blood flow probably contributes to the relation between cocaine and poor fetal growth (low birth weight and microcephaly) (Oro and Dixon, 1987; Chouteau et al., 1988; Zuckerman et al., 1989b; Handler et al., 1991). Other cocaine-associated perinatal effects in pregnant women include premature birth, placenta previa, abruptio placentae, and neonatal cerebrovascular hemorrhage; however, the results to date are inconsistent (Zuckerman and Bresnahan, 1991; Frank et al., 1993; Holzman and Paneth, 1994). Additionally, cocaine has effects on overall adult nutrition, maternal appetite, and compliance with prenatal care, as well as associations with polydrug use such as alcohol, tobacco, and opiate use (Frank et al., 1988; Amaro et al., 1989).

Further, there is some evidence that cocaine may alter the neurotransmitter systems, thus possibly modifying a number of critical processes in brain development. Human infants exposed to cocaine prenatally have exhibited increased norepinephrine and dopamine metabolite levels in cerebrospinal fluid and blood in early infancy (Mirochnick et al., 1991; Needlman et al., 1993). In animal models of prenatal cocaine exposure, significant changes in monoaminergic activity are noted compared to controls (Dow-Edwards et al., 1988; Dow-Edwards, 1989; Seidler and Slotkin, 1992).

Findings on neurobehavioral effects in the newborn period are inconsistent (Anday et al., 1989; Spear et al., 1989a,b; Magnano et al., 1992; Alessandri et al., 1993; Mayes et al., 1993). On general measures of developmental competency, such as the Bayley Scales of Infant Development, few differences are apparent between cocaine-exposed and nonexposed infants (Chasnoff et al., 1992). However, such measures may not be sensitive to subtle effects resulting from prenatal cocaine exposure. Preliminary evidence is beginning to accumulate about impairment of specific functions, such as neonatal habituation, attention or arousal regulation, reactivity to novelty, and conditioned learning. Longer-term follow-up of cocaine-exposed children into school age is necessary in order to explore the potential implications of prenatal exposure for later learning and development.

Research Opportunities

Research to date has begun to elucidate many of the biological mechanisms and health consequences of maternal drug abuse on the fetus and neonate. Additionally, the impact on the child's development of growing up in a drug-abusing household is a growing area of research. However, many unanswered questions still need to be addressed.

Windows of Biological Vulnerability

Critical stages exist throughout gestational development during which the fetus is particularly vulnerable to chemical exposure; consequently, the impact of maternal drug abuse on the fetus will vary depending on the stage of fetal development. The brain develops during the entire course of pregnancy and on into infancy, making it especially vulnerable to developmental toxins.[7] Important data regarding dose–response curves and the relation of developmental outcomes to the severity of exposure in humans are essentially unavailable and, realistically, may be most adequately addressed through animal models. Research is needed to clarify how different drug-using patterns (amount, frequency, duration, method of drug taking) and the timing of drug exposure affect fetal development in order to refine models of teratogenesis for specific drugs of abuse.

Effects of Multiple Drug Use

As already noted, most illicit drug abusers also abuse nicotine and alcohol and frequently abuse more than one illicit drug. These drugs interact in the body, potentially causing additive, synergistic, or antagonistic effects. For example, studies have shown that the presence of cocaine and ethanol in the liver produces cocaethylene, a compound that is more cardiotoxic than cocaine and has a longer half-life (Hearn et al., 1991a,b). Additionally, the effects of opiate–cocaine interactions have not been studied beyond the newborn period. Studies of the consequences of maternal polydrug use on the developing fetus are needed to clarify areas and extent of drug interactions.

Self-Reports and Biological Markers of Exposure

Objective quantification of dose exposure is problematic, particularly for drug exposure during the first trimester when pregnancy may not be recognized. Maternal self-reports of drug use can be inaccurate in the report both of actual use and of amount and frequency. One study found that 12 percent of marijuana use and 35 percent of cocaine use during pregnancy were not reported (Zuckerman et al., 1989c). One contributing factor to underreporting is fear of the legal consequences of disclosure (see Chapter 10). Continued efforts are required to develop drug abuse interviews that are appropriate for pregnant women.

Development of biological markers of exposure will assist in verification of self-reports of drug use. Advances in drug testing, of both fetal hair and meconium, can improve the detection of the presence or absence of drug exposure and may provide an approximation of cumulative dose

[7] Areas of the brain develop at different rates. For example, dopamine receptors are more prevalent in certain areas of the brain early in development. Exposure to dopamine-related compounds, such as cocaine, may have a selective impact on these parts of the brain when exposure to the drug occurs early in pregnancy, while other parts of the brain that have not yet developed dopamine receptors may not be affected.

(see Ostrea, 1995). There is currently no biological marker for quantifying a peak dose (a binge equivalent), however, that may be physiologically critical. Biological markers are needed to develop dose–response analyses to determine if there is a linear correlation between amount of exposure and severity of effect or if a threshold level exists.

Effects of Paternal Drug Use

Drug use and abuse are higher in men than in women, but there has been little research on the biological consequences to the fetus of paternal drug use or on the developmental effects of drug-abusing fathers as caregivers or as partners of drug-abusing mothers. Cocaine binds to human sperm in vitro, and studies have shown that extended use of cocaine increases the risk of lower sperm motility, lower sperm concentration, and higher proportion of morphologically abnormal sperm (Bracken et al., 1990; Yazigi et al., 1991). Thus, research is needed on the biological consequences, developmental outcomes, and psychological effects associated with parenting by a drug-abusing father.

Longitudinal Studies

Ongoing longitudinal research across geographic and sociodemographic ranges should be promoted to identify the health and developmental problems and delays caused by prenatal drug exposure or a drug-abusing environment. As suggested earlier, the possibility of drug-related effects appearing either later in development or under stressful conditions later in life requires carefully maintained longitudinal cohorts. Studies to date have focused primarily on drug-abusing mothers in poor urban areas; the focus must be expanded to cover a wider geographic and socioeconomic range. Longitudinal studies also provide some modeling of the contribution of environmental disruption to the developmental course of apparent drug effects.

Studies of responsive caregiving in a stimulating social environment have shown the plasticity of neurobehavioral development and the potential that premature neonates have to catch up developmentally with full-term children (Beckwith and Parmalee, 1986; Kronstadt, 1991). Research is needed to study whether this plasticity is applicable to drug-exposed infants because it will have important implications for preventive interventions and treatment efforts.

A major issue in neurotoxicology in general, as well as drug abuse research in particular, is how to measure noncognitive neurobehavioral outcomes (e.g., attention, affect regulation, social cognition) across the life span. Studies begun in the 1980s, during the height of crack cocaine use, are just beginning to yield longitudinal data. This type of long-term research is critical for providing public and private programs with necessary data on the needs for treatment and prevention services.

Effects of Parental Drug Abuse

When an infant is born, parental abuse of illicit drugs or alcohol may continue, often resulting in a chaotic life-style and an environment with increased incidence of child neglect, child abuse, and a lack of social interaction or responsive caregiving (Mayes, 1995). Children without prenatal exposure may also suffer collateral health effects due to growing up in a drug-abusing household.[8] There is strong correlation between parental drug abuse and child abuse and neglect (Kelleher et al., 1994; Dore et al., 1995). Additionally, children may be exposed to drugs and nicotine by accidental ingestion, breast-feeding, or passive inhalation. Children's exposure to environmental tobacco smoke increases the risk of respiratory infections (e.g., bronchitis, pneumonia), increases the severity of asthma symptoms, and is a risk factor for new cases of asthma in children (U.S. DHHS, 1993). As with research on prenatal exposure, many variables can be identified that affect the child's development (e.g., poor nutrition, lead exposure), making it difficult to isolate the effects due to drug abuse.

Numerous correlative findings suggest that drug abuse impairs parenting capacities (Mayes, 1995). These include the association of parental drug abuse with (1) other psychiatric disorders, including depression and antisocial personality; (2) multigenerational transmission of both drug abuse patterns and psychiatric disorders; (3) a high incidence of violence, both between adults and toward children; (4) an increased risk of abandonment and neglect; and (5) a generally poor sense of competence as a parent and a poor understanding of the needs of children. How those factors combine to influence an adult's interactive capacities with a child, and how child characteristics influence these patterns of adult interactiveness, are questions that are only now being studied systematically. It is likely that impairments in parenting (the withdrawn or excessively intrusive behaviors seen in observational studies of drug-abusing adults) are not related solely to drug abuse per se but are a cumulative reflection of the many psychological risk factors that accompany drug abuse. Many drug abusers also suffer from co-occurring psychiatric disorders such as depression, which adds to the potential for dysfunctional parenting (Burns et al., 1985; Zuckerman et al., 1989a).

[8]Other members of the household may also suffer collateral health effects from living with a drug abuser. This area is only beginning to be explored.

The committee recommends continued research on the magnitude and extent of the effects of maternal drug abuse on the prenatally exposed infant and child over time and the effects on children of growing up in a drug-abusing household.

DRUG ABUSE AND VIOLENCE

Violence is a leading public concern in American society and is recognized as a major public health problem (Rosenberg and Fenley, 1991). The public health model—emphasizing prevention, research, and education—is being brought to bear on this devastating issue, and the CDC has made the prevention of violence one of its highest priorities (Rosenberg et al., 1992).

The complex and intertwined relationship between drug abuse and violence involves three primary links—systemic, economic, and pharmacological (Goldstein, 1985). It is noteworthy that different forms of violence are linked to different types of abused drugs. The systemic link, the most prevalent form of cocaine- and heroin-related violence, is the result of the violent nature of illicit drug selling and distribution (Goldstein, 1985; see Chapter 10). Illicit drug traffickers use violent acts or the threat of violence to protect and expand markets and to deal with competitors, buyers, or sellers suspected of cheating or with witnesses (BJS, 1992). A recent study of gun use found that it is predominantly sellers of illicit drugs, not users, who employ guns in their activities (Butterfield, 1995). Drug sales and crime are more strongly related than drug use and crime (Chaiken and Chaiken, 1990).

It is difficult to estimate the extent of systemic violence in the illicit drug trade. Police departments have reported that noticeable increases in violent crimes are associated with the sale and distribution of cocaine (Fagan and Chin, 1989). A 1987 study found that cocaine was involved in one-fifth of homicides in San Diego County (Bailey and Shaw, 1989). A 1993 National Research Council study estimated that crimes related to illicit drugs accounted for 10 percent of all homicides nationwide, more than 30 percent of homicides in certain cities, and more than 70 percent of homicides in high-risk areas of certain cities (NRC, 1993).

Income-generating crime is the indirect economic link between illicit drugs and violence. Drug-dependent individuals, particularly those dependent on heroin or cocaine, need substantial amounts of cash to support their drug habits, and some resort to robbery, motor vehicle theft, or other means of illegal and sometimes violently obtained income. In a 1991 survey of state prison inmates, 27 percent of those incarcerated for robbery reported committing the crime to obtain money to buy drugs

(BJS, 1993). However, the majority of crimes committed by drug users are of a nonviolent nature (e.g., shoplifting, prostitution) (Goldstein, 1985).

Pharmacological Effects of Drugs and Violence

One of the most complex and controversial links between drug abuse and violence has been the potential relationship between the pharmacological effects of alcohol or illicit drugs and violence. Individuals initially use alcohol or illicit drugs because they produce some noticeable change in mood or emotional state; the extent and nature of that change varies depending on the specific drug or drug combination and the individual. However, it is difficult to determine a simple cause–effect relationship between the pharmacological actions of alcohol or illicit drugs and an individual's violent behavior because of the many interacting physiological, psychological, and social variables, each of which can have an impact on the drug–violence connection (NRC, 1993). At the biological level, differences between individuals include the amount and chronicity of drug use as well as individual variations in endocrine mechanisms (e.g., modulation of aggression by androgens), neurotransmitter activity, and genetic interactions (Miczek et al., 1994a). At the psychosocial level, risk factors correlated with an increase in aggressive or violent behavior associated with alcohol and illicit drug use include gender (which may involve biological, expectational, and social factors) childhood aggression (associated with alcohol and violent behavior) and co-occurring psychiatric disorders (discussed in more detail below) (NRC, 1993). Macrosocial factors also play a determining role in the link between violence and drug abuse. There are striking cultural and subcultural differences associated particularly with alcohol use and violence (Miczek et al., 1994b). The drug user's expectations and the situation or environment in which drug use takes place are additional macrosocial factors. Research on the link between drug abuse and violence is also complicated by the difficulties inherent in replicating realistic conditions or precursors of violence in laboratory studies on animals or humans (see Chapter 2).

The following sections present an overview of current knowledge on the pharmacological links between drug abuse and violence, followed by a discussion on directions for future research. This overview draws heavily from recent comprehensive reviews of the literature (NRC, 1993; Miczek et al., 1994b).

Alcohol

Alcohol is the drug most studied and most closely associated with violence, although a simple cause–effect relationship has not been established (see Gottheil, 1983; Brain, 1986; NRC, 1993). Studies have shown that chronic or problem drinkers have more frequent histories of violence and more previous arrests for violent crimes than comparable samples (Fagan, 1993; NRC, 1993). Alcohol use is a significant risk factor in domestic violence and sexual assault; studies have reported that 25–68 percent of batterers use alcohol and that the severity of abuse is correlated positively with alcohol use by the assailant (Rosenberg et al., 1992; Fagan and Browne, 1994). It is important to note, however, that most drinking events do not result in interpersonal violence.

Although there are wide individual differences, studies have shown arousing and aggression-heightening effects in the early phases of acute alcohol use in both animal and human studies (Miczek et al., 1994b). Chronic alcohol use and alcoholism also have symptoms associated with aggression, including depression, despair, insomnia, anxiety, and irritability. The neurobiological mechanism for alcohol's aggressive effects is currently being studied; proposed mechanisms have focused on brain serotonin metabolism and the $GABA_A$ receptor complex in the brain (Miczek et al., 1994b). Research has shown that alcoholism has a genetic component (see Chapter 5), although the nature of any genetic influence on alcohol-related violence has not been studied. Additionally, other psychiatric disorders may impact on the aggressive actions of alcohol abusers (Miczek et al., 1994b). Individuals with diagnosed antisocial personality disorder who abuse alcohol have increased prevalence of violent actions (Linnoila et al., 1983; NRC, 1993).

Opiates

Opiates have a high abuse liability because they initially produce analgesia and a sense of tranquility or well-being. However, chronic use of opiates can lead to hostility, suspicion, and confusion. Withdrawal is characterized by depression and by heightened aggressive or defensive actions (Meyer and Mirin, 1979). The primary link between opiates and violence, however, has been reported in association with the need to support an expensive drug habit. Criminal activity significantly increases during times of narcotic dependence; although, crimes by heroin abusers are largely nonviolent property crimes (McGlothin, 1979; Miczek et al., 1994b).

Cocaine

Cocaine has a stimulant effect on the central nervous system, and users initially experience an increased sense of energy and sensory awareness. However, the crash that follows can result in irritability, fatigue, depression, and/or anxiety (Gawin et al., 1994). Use of smokable crack cocaine produces a rapid and intense onset of euphoria (inhaled cocaine reaches the brain about eight seconds after smoking) (U.S. DHHS, 1991). Animal studies have shown that acute use of cocaine increased defensive reactions to stress but disrupted aggressive behavior and that chronic cocaine intake did not result in aggressive behavior (Moore and Thompson, 1978; Emley and Hutchinson, 1983). Chronic cocaine use in humans has been associated in a small number of cases with triggering a paranoid or psychotic state leading to aggressive or violent behavior (APA, 1994). As mentioned above, the cocaine drug trade is reported to be the most violent of all illicit drug trafficking.

Hallucinogens

Most studies of the pharmacological effects of lysergic acid diethylamide (LSD) and its relationship to violence were conducted in the 1960s and 1970s during the height of LSD use in the United States. Studies in humans show that LSD use is infrequently correlated with violence, but in cases where psychopathology predates LSD use, violent outbursts can be exacerbated (Miczek et al., 1994b).

Phencyclidine (PCP) use has been reported in some cases to be associated with violent behavior. However, it has been found that such individuals generally use PCP in conjunction with alcohol and other drugs (Miczek et al., 1994b). Animal studies have shown acute intake of PCP to be associated with inappropriate social signals, provocative actions, and hyperactivity which could be precursors of aggression (Tyler and Miczek, 1982; Schlemmer and Davis, 1983).

Marijuana users have been reported to have decreased aggression compared with nonusers (Cherek and Steinberg, 1987; Miczek et al., 1994b). Animal studies show that acute doses of THC, the psychoactive ingredient in marijuana, can inhibit attack or threat behavior (Miczek et al., 1994b). Large-scale studies of incarcerated adolescents found that marijuana was the drug least likely to be associated with sexual or assaultive crimes (Tinklenberg et al., 1976).

As noted, it is difficult to isolate the independent effect of the drug's pharmacology on an individual's violent behavior. Drugs may act as a cause, response, moderator, and/or mediator of violence (Fagan, 1993). Research is needed to determine the relationship between violence and the pharmacological effects of alcohol and illicit drugs in order to develop effective preventive interventions and treatment strategies, including research on patterns of alcohol and drug abuse involved in violent behavior and events in the early life history that are associated with violent behavior related to alcohol or drug abuse.

Although laboratory models should be developed to distinguish between the many confounding variables influencing the relationship between drug abuse and violence (Chapter 2), the difficulties inherent in replicating realistic conditions or precursory violence in the laboratory make this a formidable endeavor.

Violence, Drug Abuse, and Co-Occurring Psychiatric Disorders

There is evidence of a complex linkage among violence, drug abuse, and co-occurring psychiatric disorders. As discussed in Chapter 4, illicit drug and alcohol abuse are significantly more prevalent among persons who suffer from psychiatric disorders (e.g., schizophrenia, bipolar disorder, and depression) than among persons without psychiatric disorders and are particularly common among those with personality disorders[9] (Regier et al., 1990). Those individuals with co-occurring psychiatric disorders and drug abuse who are also at risk for violent behavior tend to manifest poor outcomes in standard treatment programs and often receive no treatment at all. Thus, they pose a special challenge to the treatment system, as well as to the criminal justice system (Drake and Wallach, 1989; Bartels et al., 1993; Drake et al., 1993; Narrow et al., 1993; Regier et al., 1993). It also has been found that personality disorders often precede the onset of drug abuse and other psychopathologies in persons who become violent criminals (Robins et al., 1991; Hien and Levin, 1994; Kessler and Magee, 1994; North et al., 1994; Widiger and Trull, 1994). Contextual factors—including race, gender, age, discrimination, poverty, homelessness, stressful life events, the characteristics of social networks, and the quality of living environments—are all likely to exert significant moderating effects on the relationships among victimization, co-occurring psychiatric disorders, and violent behavior (Pianta and Egeland, 1994; Hiday, 1995).

Studies have shown that the co-occurrence of psychiatric disorders with alcohol or drug abuse is associated with significantly increased risk for violent behavior in adults (Lindqvist and Allebeck, 1989; Swanson et al., 1990; Swanson, 1993; Mulvey, 1994). Although persons with co-occurring psychiatric disorders and drug abuse comprise only about 3.3 percent of the population (Regier et al., 1993), a recent study found that 7 percent of those diagnosed for depression (without a drug abuse diagnosis) had a history of violence, compared with 21 percent if comorbid for

---

[9]Victims of early-life trauma, abuse, neglect, and violence are more likely as adults to develop personality disorders (e.g., borderline and antisocial personality disorder), as well as addictive disorders and mental illnesses (e.g., depression).

drug abuse and depression (Monahan, 1995). Of those with bipolar disorder (without drug abuse), 5 percent had a history of violence, compared to more than 12 percent of those comorbid for drug abuse and bipolar disorder.

Some of the most important findings regarding the co-occurrence of psychiatric illness, drug abuse, and violence in the general population come from the Epidemiologic Catchment Area (ECA) surveys. This study of more than 20,000 community and institutional residents in five metropolitan areas found lifetime rates of drug abuse or dependence disorders to be as high as 47 percent among respondents with schizophrenia, 32 percent for those with major depressive illness, 56 percent for persons with bipolar affective disorder, and 87 percent for those with antisocial personality disorder (Regier et al., 1990). In data pooled from three ECA sites, about 2 percent of respondents with no disorder reported some violent behavior occurring within a one-year period. By comparison, the violence rates were 7 percent among those with a major psychiatric disorder only (schizophrenia or affective disorder) and 22 percent among those with co-occurring psychiatric and drug abuse disorders.

In multivariable models that controlled for age, sex, race, socioeconomic status, and marital status, the co-occurrence of psychiatric and drug abuse disorders emerged as one of the strongest predictors of violence toward others. Certain demographic covariates also increased the risk of violence among respondents with co-occurring disorders; among younger adult males of lower socioeconomic status, who reported a history of arrest and hospitalization, the predicted probability of violent acts within one year was 64 percent (Swanson, 1994).

Four mechanisms have been proposed to explain the underlying relationship between co-occurring drug abuse and psychiatric disorders and violence (Smith and Hucker, 1994). The first hypothesis is that violence in this group is linked primarily to the chemical effects of psychoactive drugs (e.g., cocaine may stimulate impulsive and aggressive behavior; alcohol may have a disinhibiting effect, possibly reducing tolerance for frustrating situations). Such effects may occur at lower doses for people with underlying psychiatric disorders (Drake et al., 1990). Antisocial personality traits often underlie both drug abuse and violence, and those antisocial traits may co-occur with psychotic disorders or other major psychiatric disorders as well. A third proposed mechanism is that drug use may exacerbate psychiatric symptoms, such as paranoid delusional beliefs, which can lead to violent actions in response to perceived threats. Finally, it has been proposed that social and economic factors—such as poverty and crime in the surrounding environment—largely account for the increased risk of violence among persons with co-occurring psychiatric and drug abuse disorders (Hiday, 1995). Limited evidence exists for each of those hypotheses individually; however, no studies to date have adequately assessed all of those factors together in an effort to examine their relative and interacting effects over time on interpersonal violence.

Although a sizable body of research has accumulated on selected aspects of violence, drug abuse, and co-occurring psychiatric disorders, key questions remain. They include the underlying mechanisms, developmental framework, and social context, as well as the long-term effectiveness of interventions that may be appropriate for this population. Thus, the committee urges a more comprehensive understanding of the risk factors associated with co-occurring psychiatric disorders and drug abuse and violence. Additionally, a more complete understanding of the types of interventions that may prove successful is needed.

The committee recommends research on violence, drug abuse, and co-occurring psychiatric disorders. Particular emphasis should be placed on the mechanisms underlying comorbidity and violent behavior and on developing effective prevention and treatment interventions.

REFERENCES

Alessandri SM, Sullivan MW, Imaizumi S, Lewis M. 1993. Learning and emotional responsivity in cocaine-exposed infants. *Developmental Psychology* 29:989–997.

Amaro H, Zuckerman B, Cabral H. 1989. Drug use among adolescent mothers: Profile of risk. *Pediatrics* 84:144–151.

Anday EK, Cohen ME, Kelley NE, Leitner DS. 1989. Effect of in utero cocaine exposure on startle and its modification. *Developmental Pharmacology and Therapeutics* 12(3):137–145.

APA (American Psychiatric Association). 1994. *Diagnostic and Statistical Manual of Mental Disorders.* 4th ed. Washington, DC: APA.

Aronson M, Kyllerman M, Sabel KG, Sandin B, Olegard R. 1985. Children of alcoholic mothers: Developmental, perceptual, and behavioral characteristics as compared to matched controls. *Acta Paediatrica Scandinavica* 74:27–35.

Bailey DN, Shaw RF. 1989. Cocaine and methamphetamine-related deaths in San Diego County (1987): Homicides and accidental overdoses. *Journal of Forensic Sciences* 34:407–422.

Ball JC, Lange WR, Myers CP, Friedman SR. 1988. Reducing the risk of AIDS through methadone maintenance treatment. *Journal of Health and Social Behavior* 29(3):214–226.

Bartels SJ, Teague G, Drake RE, Clark RE, Bush PW, Noordsy DL. 1993. Substance abuse in schizophrenia: Service utilization and costs. *Journal of Nervous and Mental Disease* 181:227–232.

Battjes RJ, Leukefeld CG, Pickens RW. 1992. Age at first injection and HIV risk among intravenous drug users. *American Journal of Drug and Alcohol Abuse* 18(3):263–273.

Battjes RJ, Pickens RW, Brown LS Jr. 1995. HIV infection and AIDS risk behaviors among injecting drug users entering methadone treatment: An update. *Journal of Acquired Immune Deficiency Syndromes and Human Retroviology* 10(1):90–96.

Beckwith K, Parmalee A. 1986. EEG patterns in preterm infants, home environment, and later I.Q. *Child Development* 57:777–789.

BJS (Bureau of Justice Statistics). 1992. *Drugs, Crime, and the Justice System*. NCJ 1335652. Washington, DC: U.S. Government Printing Office.

BJS (Bureau of Justice Statistics). 1993. *Survey of State Prison Inmates, 1991*. NCJ 136949. Washington, DC: BJS.

Blackard C, Tennes K. 1984. Human placental transfer of cannabinoids. *New England Journal of Medicine* 311:797.

Boyd TA, Ernhart CB, Greene TH, Sokol RJ, Martier S. 1991. Prenatal alcohol exposure and sustained attention in the preschool years. *Neurotoxicology and Teratology* 13(1):49–55.

Bracken MB, Eskenazi B, Sachse K, McSharry JE, Hellenbrand K, Leo-Summers L. 1990. Association of cocaine use with sperm concentration, motility, and morphology. *Fertility and Sterility* 53:315–322.

Brain PF. 1986. *Alcohol and Aggression*. London: Croom Helm.

Burns K, Melamed J, Burns W, Chasnoff I, Hatcher R. 1985. Chemical dependence and clinical depression. *Journal of Clinical Psychology* 41:851–854.

Butterfield F. 1995. Study discounts the role of drug use in gun-related crime. *New York Times* October 8:36.

CDC (Centers for Disease Control and Prevention). 1994. Birth outcomes following zidovudine therapy in pregnant women. *Morbidity and Mortality Weekly Report* 43(22):409–416.

CDC (Centers for Disease Control and Prevention). 1995a. *HIV/AIDS Surveillance Report* 7(2).

CDC (Centers for Disease Control and Prevention). 1995b. Recommendations of the U.S. Public Health Service task force on the use of zidovudine to reduce perinatal transmission of human immunodeficiency virus. *Morbidity and Mortality Weekly Report* 43(RR-11):1–20.

Chaiken JM, Chaiken MR. 1990. Drugs and predatory crime. In: Tonry M, Wilson JQ, eds. *Drugs and Crime. Vol. 13, Crime and Justice: A Review of the Literature*. Chicago: University of Chicago Press. Pp. 203–239.

Chaisson RE, Taylor E, Vlahov D, et al. 1991. *Immune Serum Markers and CD4 Counts in HIV Infected IV Drug Users*. Paper presented at the VIIth International Conference on AIDS, Florence, Italy. Abstract W.B. 2435.

Chasnoff IJ, Griffith DR, Freier C, Murray J. 1992. Cocaine/polydrug use in pregnancy: Two year follow-up. *Pediatrics* 89(2):284–289.

Cherek DR, Steinberg JL. 1987. Effects of drugs on human behavior. In: Burrows GD, Werry JS, eds. *Advances in Human Psychopharmacology*. Greenwich, CT: JAI Press. Pp. 239–290.

Chouteau M, Namerow PB, Leppert P. 1988. The effect of cocaine abuse on birth weight and gestational age. *Obstetrics and Gynecology* 72:351–354.

Clarren SK, Smith DW. 1978. The fetal alcohol syndrome. *New England Journal of Medicine* 298:1063–1067.

Clarren SK, Astley SJ, Bowden DM. 1988. Physical anomalies and developmental delays in nonhuman primates exposed to weekly doses of ethanol during gestation. *Teratology* 37(6):561–569.

Clarren SK, Astley SJ, Gunderson VM, Spellman D. 1992. Cognitive and behavioral deficits in nonhuman primates associated with very early embryonic binge exposure to ethanol. *Journal of Pediatrics* 121(5 Part 1):780–796.

Cnattingius S, Haglund B, Meirik O. 1988. Cigarette smoking as risk factor for late fetal and early neonatal death. *British Journal of Medicine* 297:258–261.

Coles CD. 1992. Measurement issues in the study of effects of substance abuse in pregnancy. *NIDA Research Monograph* 117:248–258.

Day NL. 1992. Effects of prenatal alcohol exposure. In: Zagon IS, Slotkin TA, eds. *Maternal Substance Abuse and the Developing Nervous System*. Boston: Academic Press. Pp. 27–44.

Day NL, Richardson GA. 1994. Prenatal alcohol exposure: A continuum of effects. *Seminars in Perinatology* 15(4):271–279.

Des Jarlais DC. 1992. The first and second decades of AIDS among injecting drug users. *British Journal of Addiction* 87(3):347–353.

Des Jarlais DC, Chamberland ME, Yancovitz SR, Weinberg P, Friedman SR. 1984. Heterosexual partners: A large risk group for AIDS. *Lancet* 2:1346–1347.

Des Jarlais DC, Friedman SR, Sotheran JL, Wenston J, Marmor M, Yancovitz SR, Frank B, Beatrice S, Mildvan D. 1994. Continuity and change within an HIV epidemic: Injecting drug users in New York City, 1984 through 1992. *Journal of the American Medical Association* 271(2):121–127.

Desmond MM, Wilson GS. 1975. Neonatal abstinence syndrome: Recognition and diagnosis. *Addictive Diseases* 2:113–121.

Doberczak TM, Thornton JC, Bernstein J, Kandall SR. 1987. Impact of maternal drug dependency on birth weight and head circumference of offspring. *American Journal of Diseases of Children* 141:1163–1167.

Dore MM, Doris JM, Wright P. 1995. Identifying substance abuse in maltreating families: A child welfare challenge. *Child Abuse and Neglect* 19(5):531–543.

Dow-Edwards D. 1989. Long-term neurochemical and neurobehavioral consequences of cocaine use during pregnancy. *Annals of the New York Academy of Sciences* 562:280–289.

Dow-Edwards D, Freed LA, Milhorat TH. 1988. Stimulation of brain metabolism by perinatal cocaine exposure. *Brain Research* 470:137–141.

Drake RE, Wallach MA. 1989. Substance abuse among the chronically mentally ill. *Hospital and Community Psychiatry* 40:1041–1046.

Drake RE, Osher FC, Noordsy DL, Hurlbut SC, Teague GB, Beaudett MS. 1990. Diagnosis of alcohol use disorders in schizophrenia. *Schizophrenia Bulletin* 16(1):57–67.

Drake RE, McHugo GJ, Noordsy DL. 1993. Treatment of alcoholism among schizophrenic outpatients: 4 year outcomes. *American Journal of Psychiatry* 150:328–329.

Edlin BR, Irwin KL, Faruque S, McCoy CB, Word C, Serrano Y, Inciardi JA, Bowser BP, Schilling RF, Holmberg SD. 1994. Intersecting epidemics—Crack cocaine use and HIV infection among inner-city young adults. *New England Journal of Medicine* 331(21):1422–1427.

Emley GS, Hutchinson RR. 1983. Unique influences of ten drugs upon post-shock biting attack and pre-shock manual responding. *Pharmacology, Biochemistry and Behavior* 19:5–12.

Fagan J. 1993. Interactions among drugs, alcohol, and violence. *Health Affairs* 12(4):65–79.

Fagan J, Browne A. 1994. Violence between spouses and intimates: Physical aggression between women and men in intimate relationships. In: Reiss AJ Jr, Roth JA, eds. *Understanding and Preventing Violence. Vol. 3, Social Influences*. Washington, DC: National Academy Press.

Fagan J, Chin KL. 1989. Initiation into crack and powdered cocaine: A tale of two epidemics. *Contemporary Drug Problems* 16:579–618.

Finnegan LP. 1979. In utero opiate dependence and sudden infant death syndrome. *Clinics in Perinatology* 6:163–180.

Finnegan LP. 1986. Neonatal abstinence syndrome: Assessment and pharmacology. In: Rubaltelli FF, Granati B, eds. *Neonatal Therapy: An Update*. Amsterdam: Excerpta Medica. Pp. 122–146.

Finnegan LP. 1994. Perinatal morbidity and mortality in substance using families: Effects and intervention strategies. *Bulletin on Narcotics* 46:19–43.

Frank DA, Zuckerman BS, Amaro H, Aboagye K, Bauchner H, Cabral H, Fried L, Hignson R, Kayne H, Levenson SM, et al. 1988. Cocaine use during pregnancy: Prevalence and correlates. *Pediatrics* 82:888–895.

Frank DA, Bresnahan K, Zuckerman BS. 1993. Maternal cocaine use: Impact on child health and development. *Advances in Pediatrics* 40:65–99.

Fried PA. 1980. Marijuana use by pregnant women: Neurobehavioral effects in neonates. *Drug and Alcohol Dependence* 6:415–424.

Fried PA. 1982. Marijuana use by pregnant women and effects on offspring: An update. *Neurobehavioral Toxicology and Teratology* 4:451–454.

Fried PA. 1992. Clinical implications of smoking: Determining longterm teratogenicity. In: Zagon IS, Slotkin TA, eds. *Maternal Substance Abuse and the Developing Nervous System*. Boston: Academic Press. Pp. 77–96.

Fried PA, Makin JE. 1987. Neonatal behavioral correlates of prenatal exposure to marijuana, cigarettes, and alcohol in a low risk population. *Neurobehavioral Toxicology and Teratology* 9:1–7.

Fried PA, Watkinson B. 1988. 12- and 24-month neurobehavioral follow-up of children prenatally exposed to marijuana, cigarettes, and alcohol. *Neurotoxicology and Teratology* 10:305–313.

Fried PA, Watkinson B. 1990. 36- and 48-month neurobehavioral follow-up of children prenatally exposed to marijuana, cigarettes, and alcohol. *Journal of Developmental and Behavioral Pediatrics* 11:49–58.

Fried PA, Buckingham M, Von Kulmitz P. 1983. Marijuana use during pregnancy and perinatal risk factor. *American Journal of Obstetrics and Gynecology* 144:922–924.

Friedman SR, Neaigus A, Des Jarlais DC, Sotheran JL, Woods J, Sufian M, Stepherson B, Sterk C. 1992. Social intervention against AIDS among injecting drug users. *British Journal of Addiction* 87(3):393–404.

Fullilove M, Fullilove R. 1989. Intersecting epidemics: Black teen crack use and sexually transmitted disease. *Journal of the American Women's Medical Association* 44:146–153.

Gawin FH, Khalsa ME, Ellinwood E Jr. 1994. Stimulants. In: Galanter M, Kleber H, eds. *The American Psychiatric Press Textbook of Substance Abuse Treatment*. Washington, DC: American Psychiatric Press.

Goldstein PJ. 1985. The drugs-violence nexus: A tri-partite conceptual framework. *Journal of Drug Issues* 15:493–506.

Goodlet CR, West JR. 1992. Alcohol exposure during brain growth spurt. In: Zagon IS, Slotkin TA, eds. *Maternal Substance Abuse and the Developing Nervous System*. Boston: Academic Press. Pp. 45–75.

Gottheil EL, ed. 1983. *Alcohol, Drug Abuse, and Aggression*. Springfield, IL: Charles C Thomas.

Greene T, Ernhart CB, Martier S, Sokol R, Ager J. 1990. Prenatal alcohol exposure and language development. *Alcoholism: Clinical and Experimental Research* 14(6):937–945.

Handler A, Kistin N, Davis F, Ferre C. 1991. Cocaine use during pregnancy: Perinatal outcomes. *American Journal of Epidemiology* 133:818–825.

Hans SL. 1992. Maternal opioid use and child development. In: Zagon IS, Slotkin TA, eds. *Maternal Substance Abuse and the Developing Nervous System*. Boston: Academic Press. Pp. 177–214.

Harclerode J. 1980. *The Effect of Marijuana on Reproduction and Development*. NIDA Monograph No. 31. Rockville, MD: NIDA.

Hardy LM. 1991. *HIV Screening of Pregnant Women and Newborns*. Washington, DC: National Academy Press.

Hart GJ, Carvell AL, Woodward N, Johnson AM, Williams P, Parry JV. 1989. Evaluation of needle exchange in central London: Behavior change and anti-HIV status over one year. *AIDS* 3(5):261–265.

Hartgers CE, Buning C, van Santen GW, Verster AD, Coutinho RA. 1989. The impact of the needle and syringe exchange programme in Amsterdam on injecting risk behavior. *AIDS* 3:571–576.

Hearn WL, Flynn DD, Hime GW, Rose S, Cofino JC, Mantero-Atienza E, Wetli CV, Mash DC. 1991a. Cocaethylene: A unique cocaine metabolite displays high affinity for the dopamine transporter. *Journal of Neurochemistry* 56:698–701.

Hearn WL, Rose S, Wagner J, Ciarleglio A, Mash DC. 1991b. Cocaethylene is more potent than cocaine in mediating lethality. *Pharmacology, Biochemistry and Behavior* 39:531–533.

Hellinger FJ. 1992. Forecasts of the costs of medical care for persons with HIV: 1992–1995. *Inquiry* 29:356–365.

Hiday VA. 1995. The social context of mental illness and violence. *Journal of Health and Social Behavior* 36:122–137.

Hien D, Levin FR. 1994. Trauma and trauma-related disorders for women on methadone: Prevalence and treatment considerations. *Journal of Psychoactive Drugs* 26:421–429.

Holmberg SD. 1996. The estimated prevalence and incidence of HIV in 96 large U.S. metropolitan areas. *American Journal of Public Health* 86(5):642–654.

Holzman C, Paneth N. 1994. Maternal cocaine use during pregnancy and perinatal outcomes. *Epidemiologic Reviews* 16(2):315–334.

IOM (Institute of Medicine). 1994. *AIDS and Behavior: An Integrated Approach*. Washington, DC: National Academy Press.

IOM (Institute of Medicine). 1995. *Fetal Alcohol Syndrome: Diagnosis, Epidemiology, Prevention, and Treatment*. Washington, DC: National Academy Press.

Jacobson JL, Jacobson SW. 1995. Strategies for detecting the effects of prenatal drug exposure: Lessons from research on alcohol. In: Lewis M, Bendersky M, eds. *Mothers, Babies, and Cocaine: The Role of Toxins in Development*. Hillsdale, NJ: Erlbaum. Pp. 111–128.

Jacobson JL, Jacobson SW, Sokol RJ, Martier SS, Ager JW, Kaplan-Estrin MG. 1993. Teratogenic effects of alcohol on infant development. *Alcoholism: Clinical and Experimental Research* 17:174–183.

Jeremy RJ, Hans SL. 1985. Behavior of neonates exposed in utero to methadone as assessed on the Brazelton scale. *Infant Behavior and Development* 8:323–336.

Kandall SR, Gaines J. 1991. Maternal substance abuse and subsequent sudden infant death syndrome (SIDS) in offspring. *Neurotoxicology and Teratology* 13:235–240.

Kandall SR, Gaines J, Habel L, Davidson G, Jessop D. 1993. Relationship of maternal substance abuse to subsequent sudden infant death syndrome in offspring. *Journal of Pediatrics* 123:120–126.

Kandel DB, Davies M. 1996. High school students who use crack and other drugs. *Archives of General Psychiatry* 53:71–80.

Kandel DB, Wu P, Davies M. 1994. Maternal smoking during pregnancy and smoking by adolescent daughters. *American Journal of Public Health* 84:1407–1413.

Kelleher K, Chaffin M, Hollenberg J, Fischer E. 1994. Alcohol and drug disorders among physically abusive and neglectful parents in a community-based sample. *American Journal of Public Health* 84:1586–1590.

Kessler RC, Magee WJ. 1994. Childhood family violence and adult recurrent depression. *Journal of Health and Social Behavior* 35:13–27.

Kidwell DA. 1992. Caveats in testing for drugs of abuse. *NIDA Research Monograph* 117:98–120.

Kronstadt D. 1991. Complex developmental issues of prenatal drug exposure. *Future of Children* 1:36–49.

Kuhnert BR. 1991. Drug exposure to the fetus: The effect of smoking. *NIDA Research Monograph* 114:1–17.

Levy M, Koren G. 1992. Clinical toxicology of the neonate. *Seminars in Perinatology* 16:63–75.

Lindqvist P, Allebeck P. 1989. Schizophrenia and assaultive behavior: The role of alcohol and drug abuse. *Acta Psychiatrica Scandinavica* 82:191–195.

Linnoila M, Virkkunen M, Scheinin M, Nuutila A, Rimon R, Goodwin FK. 1983. Low cerebrospinal fluid 5-hydroxyindoleacetic acid concentration differentiates impulsive from nonimpulsive violent behavior. *Life Science* 33:2609–2614.

Ljungberg B, Christensson B, Tunving K, Andersson B, Landvall B, Lundberg M, Zall-Friberg AC. 1991. HIV prevention among injecting drug users: Three years of experience from a syringe exchange program in Sweden. *Journal of Acquired Immune Deficiency Syndromes* 4(9):890–895.

Longshore D, Hsieh S-C, Anglin MD. 1994. Reducing HIV risk behavior among injection drug users: Effects of methadone maintenance treatment on number of sex partners. *International Journal of the Addictions* 29(6):741–757.

Magnano CL, Gardner JM, Karmel BZ. 1992. Differences in salivary cortisol levels in cocaine-exposed and noncocaine-exposed NICU infants. *Developmental Psychobiology* 25(2):93–103.

Malloy MH, Kleinman JC, Land GH, Schramm WF. 1988. The association of maternal smoking with age and cause of infant death. *American Journal of Epidemiology* 128:46–55.

Manning WG, Keeler EB, Newhouse JP, Sloss EM, Wasserman J. 1989a. The taxes of sin: Do smokers and drinkers pay their way? *Journal of the American Medical Association* 261:1604–1609.

Manning WG, Keeler EB, Newhouse JP, Sloss EM, Wasserman J. 1989b. The taxes of sin: Do smokers and drinkers pay their way? (letter) *Journal of the American Medical Association* 262:901.

Marcus J, Hans SL. 1982. Electromyographic assessment of neonatal muscletone. *Psychiatric Research* 6:31–40.

Mayes LC. 1995. Substance abuse and parenting. In: Bornstein MH, ed. *The Handbook of Parenting*. Mahwah, NJ: Erlbaum. Pp. 101–125.

Mayes LC, Cicchetti D. 1995. Prenatal cocaine exposure and neurobehavioral development: How subjects lost to follow-up bias study results. *Child Neuropsychology* 1:128–139.

Mayes LC, Granger RH, Frank MA, Schottenfeld R, Bornstein MH. 1993. Neurobehavioral profiles of neonates exposed to cocaine prenatally. *Pediatrics* 91(4):778–783.

McGlothin WH. 1979. Drugs and crime. In: DuPont RI, Goldstein A, O'Donnell J, eds. *Handbook on Drug Abuse*. Washington, DC: U.S. Government Printing Office.

Meyer RE, Mirin SE, eds. 1979. *The Heroin Stimulus: Implications for a Theory of Addiction*. New York: Plenum Medical Books.

Miczek KA, Mirsky AF, Carey G, DeBold J, Raine A. 1994a. An overview of biological influences on violent behavior. *Understanding and Preventing Violence, Vol. 2*. Washington, DC: National Academy Press. Pp. 1–20.

Miczek KA, DeBold JF, Haney M, Tidey J, Vivian J, Weerts EM. 1994b. In: Reiss AJ Jr, Roth JA, eds. *Understanding and Preventing Violence. Vol. 3, Social Influences*. Washington, DC: National Academy Press. Pp. 377–570.

Mirochnik M, Meyer J, Cole J, Herren T, Zuckerman B. 1991. Circulating catecholamine concentrations in cocaine-exposed neonates: A pilot study. *Pediatrics* 88:481–485.

Monahan J. 1995. Presentation by John Monahan to APA's Institute on Psychiatric Services, Boston. *Psychiatric News*, December.

Moore MS, Thompson DM. 1978. Acute and chronic effects of cocaine on extinction-induced aggression. *Journal of the Experimental Analysis of Behavior* 29:309–318.

Moore TR, Sorg J, Miller L, Key T, Resnik R. 1986. Hemodynamic effects of intravenous cocaine on the pregnant ewe and fetus. *American Journal of Obstetrics and Gynecology* 155:883–888.

Mulvey E. 1994. Assessing the evidence of a link between mental illness and violence. *Hospital and Community Psychiatry* 45:663–668.

Narrow WE, Regier DA, Rae DS, Manderscheid RW, Locke BZ. 1993. Use of services by persons with mental and addictive disorders: Findings from the National Institute of Mental Health Epidemiologic Area Catchment Program. *Archives of General Psychiatry* 50:95–107.

Needlman R, Zuckerman B, Anderson GM, Mirochnick M, Cohen DJ. 1993. Cerebrospinal fluid monoamine precursors and metabolites in human neonates following in utero cocaine exposure: A preliminary study. *Pediatrics* 92(1):55–60.

Neuspiel D. 1995. The problem of confounding in research on prenatal cocaine effects on behavior and development. In: Lewis M, Bendersky M, eds. *Mothers, Babies, and Cocaine: The Role of Toxins in Development*. Hillsdale, NJ: Erlbaum. Pp. 95–110.

NHTSA (National Highway Traffic Safety Administration). 1995. *Traffic Safety Facts, 1994*. Washington, DC: NHTSA.

NIDA (National Institute on Drug Abuse). 1996. *National Pregnancy and Health Survey: Drug Use Among Women Delivering Livebirths, 1992*. NIH Publication No. 96–3819. Rockville, MD: NIDA.

North CS, Smith EM, Spitznagel EL. 1994. Violence and the homeless: An epidemiologic study of victimization and aggression. *Journal of Traumatic Stress* 7(1):95–110.

NRC (National Research Council). 1989. *AIDS, Sexual Behavior, and Intravenous Drug Use*. Washington, DC: National Academy Press.

NRC (National Research Council). 1993. *Understanding and Preventing Violence*. Washington, DC: National Academy Press.

NRC (National Research Council). 1994. *Under the Influence? Drugs and the American Work Force*. Washington, DC: National Academy Press.

NRC (National Research Council). 1995. *Preventing HIV Transmission: The Role of Sterile Needles and Bleach*. Washington, DC: National Academy Press.

OAR (Office of AIDS Research). 1996. *Report of the NIH AIDS Research Program Evaluation Working Group of the Office of AIDS Research Advisory Council*. Bethesda, MD: OAR, NIH.

O'Connor PG, Selwyn PA, Schottenfeld RS. 1994. Medical care for injection-drug users with human immunodeficiency virus infection. *New England Journal of Medicine* 331(7):450–459.

Olson HC, Grant TM, Martin JC, Streissguth AP. 1995. A cohort study of prenatal cocaine exposure: Addressing methodological concerns. In: Lewis M, Bendersky M, eds. *Mothers, Babies, and Cocaine: The Role of Toxins in Development*. Hillsdale, NJ: Erlbaum. Pp. 129–162.

Oncology. 1993. Cost of HIV care to reach $15 billion by 1995. *Oncology* 7(5):90.

Oro AS, Dixon SD. 1987. Perinatal cocaine and methamphetamine exposure: Maternal and neonatal correlates. *Journal of Pediatrics* 111:571–578.

Ostrea EM. 1995. Meconium drug analysis. In: Lewis M, Bendersky M, eds. *Mothers, Babies, and Cocaine: The Role of Toxins in Development*. Hillsdale, NJ: Erlbaum. Pp. 178–203.

OTA (Office of Technology Assessment). 1990. *The Effectiveness of Drug Abuse Treatment: Implications for Controlling AIDS/HIV Infection*. OTA-BP-H-73. AIDS Related Issues Background Paper 6. Washington, DC: OTA.

Phibbs CS, Bateman DA, Schwartz RM. 1991. The neonatal costs of maternal cocaine use. *Journal of the American Medical Association* 266(11):1521–1526.

Pianta RC, Egeland B. 1994. Relation between depressive symptoms and stressful life events in a sample of disadvantaged mothers. *Journal of Consulting and Clinical Psychology* 62(6):229–234.

Regier D, Farmer M, Rae D, Locke BZ, Keith SJ, Judd LL, Goodwin FK. 1990. Comorbidity of mental disorders with alcohol and other drug abuse: Results from the Epidemiologic Catchment Area (ECA) Study. *Journal of the American Medical Association* 264:2511–2518.

Regier DA, Narrow WE, Rae DS, Manderscheid RW, Locke BZ, Goodwin FK. 1993. The de facto U.S. mental and addictive disorders service system: Epidemiologic Catchment Area prospective 1-year prevalence rates of disorders and services. *Archives of General Psychiatry* 50:85–94.

Resnick L, Veren S, Salahuddin S, Tondreau S, Markham PD. 1986. Stability and inactivation of HTLV-III/LAV under clinical and laboratory environments. *Journal of the American Medical Association* 255:1887–1891.

Risch HA, Weiss NS, Clarke EA, Miller AB. 1988. Risk factors for spontaneous abortion and its recurrence. *American Journal of Epidemiology* 128:420–430.

Robins LN, Tipp J, Przybeck T. 1991. Antisocial personality. In: Robins LN, Regier DA, eds. *Psychiatric Disorders in the Americas: Epidemiologic Catchment Area Study*. New York: Free Press. Pp. 258–290.

Rosenberg ML, Fenley MA. 1991. *Violence in America: A Public Health Approach*. New York: Oxford University Press.

Rosenberg ML, O'Carroll PW, Powell KE. 1992. Let's be clear, violence is a public health problem. *Journal of the American Medical Association* 267:3071–3072.

Schenker S, Becker HC, Randall CL, Phillips DK, Baskin GS, Henderson GL. 1990. Fetal alcohol syndrome: Current status of pathogenesis. *Alcoholism, Clinical and Experimental Research* 14:635–647.

Scher MS, Richardson GA, Coble PA, Day NL, Stoffer DS. 1988. The effects of prenatal alcohol and marijuana exposure: Disturbances in neonatal sleepcycling and arousal. *Pediatric Research* 24:101–105.

Schlemmer RF, Davis JM. 1983. A comparison of three psychomimetic-induced models of psychosis in non-human primate social colonies. In: Miczek KA, ed. *Ethopharmacology: Primate Models of Neuropsychiatric Disorders*. New York: Alan R. Liss. Pp. 33–78.

Schottenfeld RS, O'Malley S, Abdul-Salaam K, O'Connor PG. 1993. Decline in intravenous drug use among treatment-seeking opiate users. *Journal of Substance Abuse Treatment* 10(1):5–10.

Scitovsky AA, Rice DP. 1987. Estimates of the direct and indirect costs of acquired immunodeficiency syndrome in the United States, 1985, 1986, and 1991. *Public Health Reports* 102(1):5–17.

Seidler FJ, Slotkin TA. 1992. Fetal cocaine exposure causes persistent noradrenergic hyperactivity in rat brain regions: Effects on neurotransmitter turnover and receptors. *Journal of Pharmacology and Experimental Therapeutics* 263(2):413–421.

Serpelloni G, Carrieri MP, Rezza G, Morganti S, Gomma M, Binkin N. 1994. Methadone treatment as a determinant of HIV risk reduction among injecting drug users: A nested case-control study. *AIDS Care* 6(2):215–220.

Slotkin T. 1992. Prenatal exposure to nicotine: What can we learn from animal models? In: Zagon IS, Slotkin TA, eds. *Maternal Substance Abuse and the Developing Nervous System*. Boston: Academic Press. Pp. 97–124.

Smith DW. 1982. *Recognizable Patterns of Human Malformation: Genetic, Embryologic, and Clinical Aspects*. 3rd ed. Philadelphia: W.B. Saunders.

Smith J, Hucker S. 1994. Schizophrenia and substance abuse. *British Journal of Psychiatry*, 165:13–21.

Sokol RJ, Miller S, Reed G. 1980. Alcohol abuse during pregnancy: An epidemiological study. *Alcoholism, Clinical and Experimental Research* 4:135–145.

Spear LP, Kirstein CL, Bell J, Yoottanasumpun V, Greenbaum R, O'Shea J, Hoffmann H, Spear NE. 1989a. Effects of prenatal cocaine exposure on behavior during the early postnatal period. *Neurotoxicology and Teratology* 11(1):57–63.

Spear LP, Kirstein CL, Frambes NA, Moody CA. 1989b. Neurobehavioral teratogenicity of gestational cocaine exposure. *NIDA Research Monograph* 95:232–238.

Stanton ME, Spear LP. 1990. Workshop on the qualitative and quantitative comparability of human and animal developmental neurotoxicity. Work group I report: Comparability of measures of developmental neurotoxicity in humans and laboratory animals. *Neurotoxicology and Teratology* 12:261–267.

Strauss ME, Starr RH, Ostrea EM Jr, Chavez CJ, Stryker JC. 1976. Behavioral concomitants of prenatal addiction to narcotics. *Journal of Pediatrics* 89:842–846.

Swan N. 1995. Treatment and outreach research on AIDS: Identifying and treating those at risk. *NIDA Notes* 10(3):9,11,15.

Swanson JW. 1993. Alcohol abuse, mental disorder, and violent behavior: An epidemiologic inquiry. *Alcohol Health and Research World* 17:123–132.

Swanson JW. 1994. Mental disorder, substance abuse, and community violence: An epidemiological approach. In: Monohan J, Steadman H, eds. *Violence and Mental Disorder: Developments in Risk Assessment.* Chicago: University of Chicago Press. Pp. 101–136.

Swanson JW, Holzer CE, Ganju VK, Jono RT. 1990. Violence and psychiatric disorder in the community: Evidence from the Epidemiologic Catchment Area surveys. *Hospital and Community Psychiatry* 41:761–770.

Tinklenberg JR, Roth WT, Kopell BS, Murphy P. 1976. Cannabis and alcohol effects in assaultiveness in adolescent delinquents. *Annals of the New York Academy of Sciences* 282:85–94.

Tronick EZ, Beeghly M. 1992. Effects of prenatal exposure on newborn behavior and development: A critical review. In: U.S. Department of Health and Human Services, Alcohol, Drug Abuse, and Mental Health Administration, Office of Substance Abuse Prevention. *Identifying the Needs of Drug-Affected Children: Public Policy Issues*. DHHS Publication No. (ADM)921814. Rockville, MD: U.S. DHHS.

Tyler CB, Miczek KA. 1982. Effects of phencyclidine on aggressive behavior in mice. *Pharmacology, Biochemistry and Behavior* 17:503–510.

U.S. DHHS (Department of Health and Human Services). 1991. *Drug Abuse and Drug Abuse Research. The Third Triennial Report to Congress.* DHHS Publication No. (ADM)91-1704. Rockville, MD: DHHS.

U.S. DHHS (Department of Health and Human Services). 1993. *Respiratory Health Effects of Passive Smoking: Lung Cancer and Other Disorders.* Bethesda, MD: NIH Publication No. 93-3605.

Vlahov D, Munoz A, Celentano DD, Cohn S, Anthony JC, Chilcoat H, Nelson KE. 1991. HIV seroconversion and disinfection of injection equipment among intravenous drug users, Baltimore, Maryland. *Epidemiology* 2(6):444–446.

Watkins KE, Metzger D, Woody G, McLellan AT. 1992. High-risk sexual behaviors of intravenous drug users in- and out-of-treatment: Implications for the spread of HIV infection. *American Journal of Drug and Alcohol Abuse* 18(4):389–398.

Webber MP, Lambert G, Bateman DA, Hauser WA. 1993. Maternal risk factors for congenital syphilis: A case-control study. *American Journal of Epidemiology* 137(4):415–422.

Weintrub P, Veereman-Wauters G, Cowan MJ, Thaler MM. 1991. Hepatitis C virus infection in infants whose mothers took street drugs intravenously. *Journal of Pediatrics* 119(6):869–874.

Weiss B. 1995. Incipient hazards of cocaine: Lessons from environmental toxicology. In: Lewis M, Bendersky M, eds. *Mothers, Babies, and Cocaine: The Role of Toxins in Development.* Hillsdale, NJ: Erlbaum. Pp. 41–56.

Werler MM, Pober BR, Holmes LB. 1985. Smoking and pregnancy. *Teratology* 32(3):473–481.

Widiger TA, Trull TJ. 1994. Personality disorders and violence. In: Monohan J, Steadman H, eds. *Violence and Mental Disorder: Developments in Risk Assessment*. Chicago: University of Chicago Press. Pp. 203–226.

Woods JR, Plessinger MA, Clark KE. 1987. Effect of cocaine on uterine blood flow and fetal oxygenation. *Journal of the American Medical Association* 257:957–961.

Yazigi RA, Odem RR, Polakoski KL. 1991. Demonstration of specific binding of cocaine to human spermatozoa. *Journal of the American Medical Association* 266:1956–1959.

Zagon IS, McLaughlin P. 1984. An overview of the neurobehavioral sequelae of perinatal opioid exposure. In: Yanai J, ed. *Neurobehavioral Teratology*. Amsterdam: Elsevier. Pp. 197–233.

Zuckerman B. 1991. Drug-exposed infants: Understanding the medical risk. *Future of Children* 1:28–35.

Zuckerman B, Bresnahan K. 1991. Developmental and behavioral consequences of prenatal drug and alcohol exposure. *Pediatric Clinics of North America* 38:1387–1406.

Zuckerman B, Amaro H, Bauchner H, Cabral H. 1989a. Depressive symptoms during pregnancy: Relationship to poor health behaviors. *American Journal of Obstetrics and Gynecology* 160:1107–1111.

Zuckerman B, Frank DA, Hingson R, Amaro H, Levenson SM, Kayne H, Parker S, Vinci R, Aboagye K, Fried LE, Cabral H, Timperi R, Bauchner H. 1989b. Effects of maternal marijuana and cocaine use on fetal growth. *New England Journal of Medicine* 320:762–769.

Zuckerman B, Amaro H, Cabral H. 1989c. Validity of self-reporting of marijuana and cocaine use among pregnant adolescents. *Journal of Pediatrics* 115(5 Part 1):812–815.

8

Treatment

Substantial progress has been made in our knowledge of drug abuse treatment. Much of the treatment research was made possible by expansion of research funding by the National Institute on Drug Abuse (NIDA). Research has shown that drug abuse treatment is both effective and cost-effective in reducing not only drug consumption but also the associated health and social consequences. This chapter begins with a discussion of the need for treatment and then presents the many accomplishments in drug abuse treatment including the range of treatment options available (e.g., pharmacotherapies and psychosocial treatments), treatment effectiveness, the cost-effectiveness of treatment, and the development of tools and techniques for clinical assessment and diagnostic differentiation. The remainder of the chapter discusses opportunities for future research on medications development, treatment of HIV–infected drug abusers, matching patients to treatment options, treatment of patients with co-occurring psychiatric disorders and drug abuse, and treatment of drug abuse in special populations.

OVERVIEW OF DRUG ABUSE TREATMENT

Treatment is clearly indicated for individuals diagnosed with drug dependence, the most serious of the three levels of drug consumption—use, abuse, and dependence (see definitions in Chapter 1). Drug dependence occurs when a person has met three or more of the seven DSM-IV criteria items for dependence within the last year (see Appendix C for

DSM-IV criteria) (APA, 1994). As a consequence of compulsive drug-seeking behavior and loss of control over consumption, drug dependence is usually a chronically relapsing disorder (i.e., one that may persist indefinitely and is prone to recur even after periods of remission). A diagnosis of drug abuse may also require treatment, but most clients in treatment have the more serious diagnosis of dependence.

The number of heavy drug users, using at least once a week, is difficult to determine. It has been estimated that in 1993, there were 2.1 million heavy cocaine users and 444,000–600,000 heavy heroin users (Rhodes et al., 1995). Although cocaine and heroin represent the major drugs of abuse for a large proportion of individuals who seek treatment, most patients abuse more than one drug. In addition, others seek help for abuse of marijuana, phencyclidine, benzodiazepines, other sedatives, or abuse of multiple drugs. It was estimated that in 1994, 3.6 million people in the U.S. had drug problems severe enough to need drug treatment services (ONDCP, 1996). The actual number of clients in treatment falls far short of this estimate. For example, the National Drug and Alcoholism Treatment Unit Survey (NDATUS) reported that almost 1.0 million people in 1993 were in private and public drug abuse treatment programs; approximately 20 percent of those in treatment were enrolled mainly for illicit drug abuse, 45 percent for alcohol, and 35 percent for combined alcohol and other drug dependencies (SAMHSA, 1995a). Although the figures are not comparable or definitive, the magnitude of the gap between the need for treatment and the use of treatment services is clear.

There are many reasons for the inadequate number of clients in treatment, including insufficient public funding for drug abuse treatment, cutbacks in treatment availability in the private sector, an unwillingness of many clients to seek treatment, and the deterrent effect of being placed on a waiting list for treatment (IOM, 1990b). Treatment should be available to all who request it, and long waiting lists are counterproductive (Goldstein and Kalant, 1990). That is particularly true given recent studies (cited later in this chapter and elsewhere) that demonstrate the effectiveness and cost-effectiveness of treatment.

ACCOMPLISHMENTS

Clearly, the development of varied treatment modalities and interventions discussed below are major accomplishments of drug abuse research. They include treatment options (e.g., pharmacotherapies and/or psychosocial), treatment effectiveness, cost-effectiveness, and the development of tools and techniques for clinical assessment and diagnostic differentiation.

Treatment Options

Treatment is provided in a variety of settings, and within each treatment setting a range of interventions may be available (e.g., pharmacotherapy, education, psychosocial treatment) (IOM, 1990a,b). Structured treatment programs are generally classified according to four major treatment modalities: methadone maintenance, outpatient drug-free programs, therapeutic communities, and chemical dependency programs. Methadone maintenance with counseling is the primary treatment option for opiate addiction (McLellan et al., 1993). Methadone maintenance treatment is provided in tightly regulated programs or clinics, which are almost universally located in outpatient facilities. Outpatient drug-free programs serve the largest share of patients in drug abuse treatment. The programs provide counseling as the predominant form of treatment, but there is great variation in the array and intensity of counseling services, the quality and training of treatment staff, and the composition of patients. Therapeutic communities are highly structured long-term residential programs lasting up to 18 months and tailored primarily to the hardcore user. Chemical dependency programs are short-term residential programs patterned after the 12-step model of treatment (for more detailed descriptions, see IOM, 1990b). Commonalities across all treatment settings include a combination of individual and group counseling, education, and/or pharmacotherapy. Additionally, treatment providers generally recommend that formal therapy be combined with participation in self-help groups such as Alcoholics Anonymous. Furthermore, patients are usually encouraged to continue self-help group participation after leaving formal treatment to reinforce abstinence and a healthy life-style, because relapse to dependence after periods of remission is common (Woody and Cacciola, 1994).

The following sections separate pharmacotherapeutic and psychosocial treatment options, it should be understood, however, that those approaches are combined in most clinical settings. The utility of that approach has been demonstrated, and it has been shown that methadone alone for the treatment of opiate dependence was not as effective as a combined regimen of methadone and psychosocial services as a more comprehensive approach to treatment (McLellan et al., 1993).

Pharmacotherapy

Pharmacotherapies have been developed or are being tested for the full spectrum of clinical needs: overdose, detoxification,[1] dependence,

[1]Medications, including methadone and clonidine, are often used to detoxify drug abuse patients and to manage withdrawal symptoms.

and relapse prevention. NIDA's Medications Development Division has made important contributions in the development of pharmacotherapies for drug addiction and has served as a catalyst in promoting drug development (IOM, 1995b). Medications development for the treatment of heroin and cocaine addictions is discussed more fully in a recent Institute of Medicine report (IOM, 1995b).

Two opiate agonist medications, methadone and LAAM (*levo*-alpha-acetylmethadol), have been approved for the treatment of opiate addiction. Agonists act by substituting at the opioid receptor site, thereby blocking the euphoria of subsequently administered opiates (via cross-tolerance) and inhibiting the symptoms of acute and chronic abstinence. Methadone was approved for use in 1972, and there are currently an estimated 650 methadone maintenance programs throughout the United States (IOM, 1995a,b). The data supporting the efficacy of methadone maintenance have been reviewed extensively (e.g., Ball and Ross, 1991; Kreek, 1992). In 1993, LAAM was approved for use in treating opiate dependence; this medication has the advantage of requiring three doses per week rather than daily doses, thus freeing subjects from daily clinic attendance. Clinical guidelines for the use of each of these medications have recently been published by the Substance Abuse and Mental Health Services Administration (SAMHSA, 1993, 1995c).

Naltrexone, an orally effective and long-acting opiate antagonist, has been shown effective in preventing relapse to opiate dependence in highly motivated patients (e.g., probationers, parolees, health care providers) who are under strong external pressure to remain opiate free (Brahen et al., 1978). Naltrexone has also been found to reduce relapse to alcohol dependence (Volpicelli et al., 1992). A newer opiate antagonist, nalmafene, which is currently undergoing testing, appears to have positive effects similar to those of naltrexone (Mason et al., 1994). Opiate antagonist medications work by binding to the opioid receptor site, preventing receptor activation by the abused drug and thereby blocking the drug's euphorigenic and dependence-producing effects. This blockade represents competitive antagonism, and thus its clinical efficacy can be modified by the dose of the antagonist, the time elapsed since the antagonist was taken, and the dose of the abused drug.

Buprenorphine is a partial opiate agonist that produces less physiological dependence than methadone or LAAM and is currently in clinical trials (Bicket and Amass, 1995; Cowan and Lewis, 1995). It has been shown to be effective in maintenance therapy, in retaining patients in treatment, and in facilitating abstinence from illicit opiates (Johnson et al., 1992; Kosten et al., 1993). Buprenorphine is currently being tested in combination with naloxone in a sublingual preparation to reduce its abuse liability. The eventual goal is to develop a pharmacotherapy that avoids the strict scheduling controls that have been applied to methadone and LAAM. Fewer scheduling requirements would expand use to a wider range of settings (see IOM, 1995b).

Psychosocial Treatments

Psychosocial treatments include counseling, psychotherapy, and cognitive skills development. Counseling attempts to identify specific problems in the patient's life and to provide support, deliver concrete services, encourage abstinence, foster compliance with clinic rules, identify emergent problems, and refer the patient to more specialized services when needed (Woody et al., 1983). A series of well-designed studies has shown that drug counseling can produce substantial reductions in drug use and in the severity of problems that are associated with dependence. Those studies have been carried out in methadone programs (McLellan et al., 1982, 1988, 1993) and, more recently, in programs treating patients with cocaine and/or alcohol dependence (Rawson et al., 1993; Alterman et al., 1994, 1996; Shopshaw et al., 1995). In some instances, counseling may be provided by individuals who are recovering from drug dependencies and who have little formal education in health-related fields.

Unlike counseling, which focuses mainly on concrete, external factors, psychotherapy strives to identify and modify maladaptive interpersonal processes. There are many types of psychotherapy and they differ according to their theoretical basis and focus. For example, cognitive-behavioral psychotherapy aims to identify and change false beliefs and their associated behaviors (Beck et al., 1990). Supportive-expressive psychotherapy attempts to identify and change repetitive and problematic relationships and behaviors (Luborsky, 1984; Luborsky et al., 1995). Interpersonal psychotherapy tries to identify and change current maladaptive interpersonal problems. Motivational enhancement therapy may be more appropriate for an individual in the precontemplative stage of drug abuse (see Prochaska and DiClemente, 1983, 1986 below). Two prospective studies done in methadone programs using random assignment and a range of measures have shown that these psychotherapies can provide additional benefits to patients with moderate to high levels of psychiatric symptoms (Woody et al., 1984, 1995b).

An interesting area of research is contingency contracting, which applies behavioral methods of reinforcement to the treatment of drug abuse (Chapter 2). Contingency contracting involves the use of graduated rewards, which are given to patients when they meet specific treatment goals such as keeping appointments, seeking work, or providing drug-free urine samples. Rewards may include objects such as a lottery ticket or vouchers for the purchase of valued goods and services, methadone take-home doses, or other socially appropriate rewards. Studies using this approach have found reductions in drug use among patients with heroin (Stitzer et al., 1992; Kidorf et al., 1994) or cocaine dependence (Higgins et al., 1993, 1994). The principles used in those studies have evolved from behavioral research, as summarized in Chapter 2. Most behavioral interventions have the advantage of being easily integrated within existing modalities.

Treatment Effectiveness

The effectiveness of treatment for drug addictions has been reviewed extensively (see Simpson and Sells, 1982, 1990; IOM, 1990b, 1995a,b; Prendergast et al., in press). Treatment gains are typically found in reduced intravenous and other drug use, reduced criminality, and enhanced health and productivity. The largest multisite studies, which are described below and cover multiple treatment modalities, provide strong evidence of long-term treatment effectiveness, usually based on comparisons between client behaviors before, during, and after treatment. The length of time in treatment consistently has been found to be an important determinant of both short- and long-term improvement. It is important to note, however, that most study results include the effects of patient self-selection in their preferred type of treatment modality. Although random assignment of patients to a treatment modality is preferred, it is difficult to achieve because of regulatory constraints, treatment facility capacities, study design, and ethical considerations.

Three comprehensive studies of drug abuse treatment effectiveness are discussed. The first study, the Drug Abuse Reporting Program (DARP), included more than 44,000 clients entering more than 50 treatment programs from 1969 to 1973 (Simpson and Sells, 1982, 1990). A subset of the cohort was studied 6 and 12 years after treatment. The second study is the Treatment Outcome Prospective Study (TOPS), which included almost 12,000 clients in 41 treatment programs (Hubbard et al., 1989). Clients were followed up to five years after treatment. The final study, which is still in progress, is the Drug Abuse Treatment Outcome Study (DATOS).

The first two studies, DARP and TOPS, both found evidence of treatment effectiveness for methadone maintenance, outpatient drug-free programs, and residential treatment (in therapeutic communities). Posttreatment outcomes were associated directly with the duration of treatment, with three months as the minimum time in treatment to observe an effect. Both DARP and TOPS found major reductions in the use of drugs and in criminal activity. TOPS also found modest improvements in productivity. In DARP, for example, the long-lasting nature of improvement was in evidence 12 years after treatment, but most of the improvement was attained in the first 3 years after treatment. The results of these and other studies collectively indicate that 30–50 percent of patients are able to remain abstinent one year after the completion of treatment (McLellan et al., in press, a).

These gains are comparable to those seen in treatment for other chronic, relapsing disorders. Studies that compared compliance of patients in drug treatment with that of patients being treated for hypertension, adult onset diabetes, and asthma found that to remain symptom-free, each of these medical conditions requires patients to undergo major changes in life-style, often accompanied by medication (O'Brien and McLellan, 1996; McLellan et al., in press, a). Less than 30 percent of patients being treated for diabetes and hypertension were found to comply with dietary and other behavioral recommendations, and less than 30 percent of those with hypertension or asthma comply with their medication schedules.

DATOS, the final large-scale treatment outcome study begun in the early 1990s, enrolled 10,000 clients, one-third of whom were women, to determine the effectiveness of about 99 programs throughout the country. Four major modalities are under investigation: methadone maintenance, outpatient drug-free, long-term residential, and short-term inpatient programs (R. Hubbard, Research Triangle Institute, personal communication, 1995).

Treatment Cost–Benefit and Cost-Effectiveness

Drug abuse treatment is a judicious public investment and is less expensive than the alternatives (Figure 8.1). TOPS, cited above, performed a cost–benefit analysis[2] by comparing the cost of treatment with the benefits (i.e., cost savings) of reduced crime and increased productivity during treatment and one year afterward. The ratio of benefits to costs for each treatment modality ranged from 4:1 to 1:1, depending on which of two complex scenarios was used to calculate societal benefits (Hubbard et al., 1989).

The economic benefits of reduced crime, enhanced productivity, and lower health care utilization were captured in a more recent study (Gerstein et al., 1994). This study, the first cost–benefit study to include the benefit of lower health care utilization, was undertaken by the State of California on 3,000 clients discharged from treatment programs in 1992.

---

[2]A cost–benefit analysis assigns monetary values to all of the costs and benefits of a program or policy to determine whether the benefits outweigh the costs.

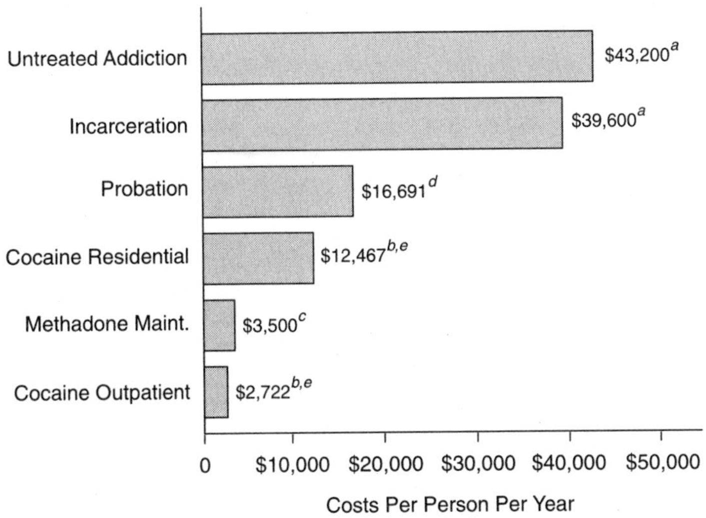

FIGURE 8.1 Treatment is less expensive than alternatives. NOTE: [a]1991 dollars; [b]1992 dollars; [c]1993 dollars; [d]1992 dollars, inflation adjusted from 1983 data; [e]the average cost per admission is much lower than this figure because most patients are in treatment less than one year. SOURCES: Lewin-VHI, unpublished estimates; McLellan et al. (1994); Rydell and Everingham (1994); SAMHSA (1994a).

The study group consisted of a random sample of 150,000 clients in treatment programs throughout the state. By comparing the one-year period before treatment with the one-year period after, substantial benefits were realized relative to the cost of treatment. According to two different benefit measures, the ratio of benefits to costs was about 7:1 or 2:1 when all treatment modalities were combined. Health care costs for the sample were lowered after treatment by 23.5 percent; these savings alone offset about 55 percent of the cost of a treatment episode. Most of the economic benefits from both the TOPS and the California studies came in the form of reduced crime-related costs.

The cost-effectiveness[3] of treatment has also been assessed in comparison with other drug control strategies (Everingham and Rydell, 1994; Rydell and Everingham, 1994). Investigators found treatment programs to be far more cost-effective than a range of drug control strategies in reducing cocaine use. The study analyzed the costs required by four different strategies—treatment, domestic enforcement, interdiction, and

[3]A cost-effectiveness analysis strives to identify which of the different programs can attain a desired objective at the lowest cost (Center of Alcohol Studies, 1993).

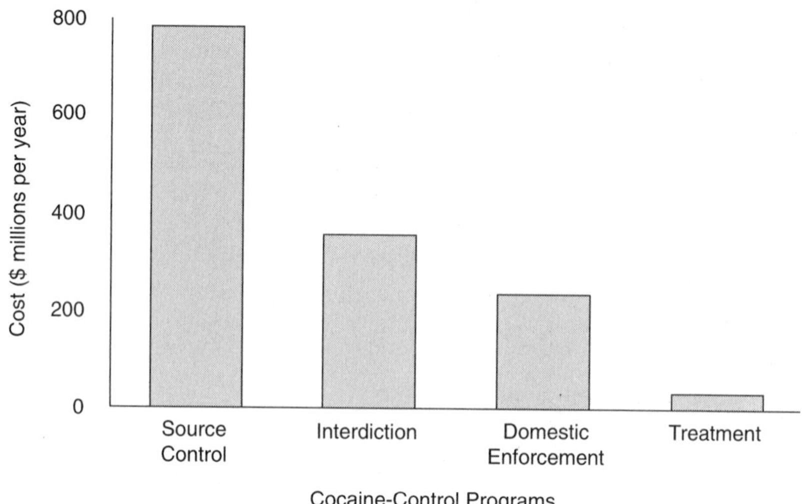

FIGURE 8.2 Effectiveness of cocaine control strategies. The RAND study compared treatment (a demand control strategy) and three supply control strategies: source country control, interdiction, and domestic enforcement. It calculated the cost required for each strategy to acheive a common measure of effectiveness—a reduction in cocaine consumption by 1 percent of current annual consumption. To meet this objective, researchers found that the additional cost of treatment would be $34 million, an amount 7.3 times less than that needed for the next most effective strategy, domestic enforcement, and 23 times less expensive than source country control. SOURCE: Rydell and Everingham (1994).

source country control—to achieve a 1 percent reduction in cocaine consumption. Treatment cost the least ($34 million) to achieve the objective, whereas other strategies cost between $250 million and $800 million (Figure 8.2). Thus, treatment was determined to be 7.3 times less costly than the least expensive alternative and more than 20 times less costly than the most expensive strategy, source country control.

It should be pointed out that all of these cost–benefit studies examined "effectiveness" from a societal point of view and found treatment to be a wise public investment. However, studies did not address critical questions facing providers regarding the most cost-effective treatments. There are only a few studies comparing the relative cost-effectiveness of different treatments. That information gap is discussed in Chapter 9.

Clinical Assessment and Diagnostic Differentiation

Research advances in diagnosis have made it possible to conduct detailed assessments of clients in treatment. Among these advances has been the development of instruments that reliably assess drug abuse and dependence and co-occurring psychiatric disorders according to the criteria of the *Diagnostic and Statistical Manual of Mental Disorders, Fourth Edition* (DSM-IV; APA, 1994) and the International Classification of Diseases (ICD-10; WHO, 1992). Some of the most commonly used instruments are the Composite International Diagnostic Interview (CIDI); the Substance Abuse Module of the CIDI (the CIDI-SAM); the Diagnostic Interview Schedule (DIS); and the Structured Clinical Interview for DSM-IV (SCID). Work is currently under way to modify them to improve the distinctions between primary psychiatric disorders and drug-produced psychiatric syndromes in order to further improve treatment (D. Hasin, 1995 New York State Psychiatric Institute, personal communication).

Other instruments have been developed to assess the severity of patients' problems and their need for treatment across a wider range of areas. Among these, the most widely used is the Addiction Severity Index (ASI), which was developed in the early 1980s with research funds from both NIDA and the Department of Veterans Affairs (VA). ASI measures the degree of impairment and the need for treatment in each of seven areas commonly affected by drug abuse: drug and alcohol use, medical, family or social, employment, legal, and psychiatric (McLellan et al., 1980). The ASI has been found to be reliable and applicable within a wide range of settings, provided that appropriate training has been given to those who administer it. Unlike CIDI, DIS, and SCID, ASI does not make diagnoses but rather quantifies the degree to which impairment exists (and treatment is needed) in each of the seven areas. It is often used in clinical practice for evaluation and treatment planning.

One immediate positive effect of newer assessment techniques is the development of improved descriptions of patients. A very consistent finding, from a large number of studies using one or more of these assessment measures, is that the patient population is often engaged in polydrug use (i.e., use of a variety of illicit drugs and alcohol) and has other serious current or past problems in addition to drug abuse (e.g., psychiatric, employment, family/social problems) (Rounsaville et al., 1982; McLellan et al., 1994). These findings have been useful in developing treatment matching strategies (discussed below).

Advances in diagnosis have also led to comprehensive and accurate methods for assessing outcomes. The ASI has been particularly useful because it can measure degrees of improvement when administered on repeated occasions before, during, and after treatment. In treatment outcome studies, the ASI is usually supplemented with other measures such as urinalysis, breath alcohol tests, structured interviews for assessing psychiatric disorders, measures of psychiatric symptoms, arrest and employment records, and interviews with family members.

A newer assessment instrument that derives from the ASI is the Treatment Services Review (TSR). It is administered by a trained technician at periodic intervals during an episode of treatment, and it measures the services actually delivered in each of the areas assessed by ASI (McLellan et al., 1992). By using the TSR along with the ASI, treatment outcome can be measured against services actually received. Early studies using ASI and TSR show that patients generally improve if they receive the services they need and usually do not improve if services are not tailored to their needs (McLellan et al., 1994). Thus, programs may also be assessed on how effectively they have addressed the needs of patients.

RESEARCH OPPORTUNITIES

The continued research challenge will be to develop more effective and cost-effective pharmacotherapeutic and psychosocial treatments that address the specific needs of individual patients and to refine the tools and techniques for clinical assessment and diagnostic differentiation. Questions remain regarding the different outcomes among programs using the same treatment modality; studies are needed to evaluate those program characteristics that produce the most efficacious results (e.g., the degree to which programs are willing to retain patients with persistent "dirty" urines or other signs of less than optimal progress, or the degree to which difficult patients are accepted into treatment). Furthermore, while long-term methadone maintenance has proven to be effective (Ball and Ross, 1991), questions remain regarding the length of time patients remain in treatment. Studies consistently have demonstrated that as long as patients are in methadone maintenance treatment there is a reduction in drug abuse. However, relapse to prior drug use occurs when treatment is terminated (IOM, 1990b; Ball and Ross, 1991). These findings have serious implications for HIV transmission as current data show that HIV infection is more likely among those who leave treatment than those who remain in treatment (e.g., Metzger and coworkers [1993] found that 4 percent of injection drug users who remained in treatment for the first 18 months became HIV infected, as compared with 22 percent of those not in treatment).

Additionally, research in medications development, HIV/AIDS and injection drug use, treating patients with co-occurring psychiatric disorders and drug abuse, and treating special populations of drug abusers is critical to fully meet the treatment needs of this population and to reduce the associated social and health consequences to society. These issues are discussed more fully below.

Medications Development

NIDA, through its Medications Development Division, is actively supporting the development of antiaddiction medications (see IOM, 1995b). The development of medications to treat drug addictions is tied closely to advances in basic research. The behavioral sciences (discussed in Chapter 2) have provided the foundation for objectively measuring drug-taking behaviors, for understanding many of the basic biobehavioral mechanisms underlying addiction, and for evaluating the abuse liability of new drugs. Neuroscientists have identified neural circuits in the brain that mediate the acute reinforcing effects of drugs, specific changes in the brain that are associated with withdrawal and sensitization, and specific neurotransmitter receptors and receptor subtypes for mediating reinforcement actions that may provide a molecular basis for long-term changes in the brain associated with relapse and vulnerability (see Chapter 3). The wealth of scientific information and understanding of opiate addiction, ranging from the clinical to the molecular level, that has been obtained over the last several decades has led to the development of several medications. Studies of methadone, LAAM, naltrexone, and buprenorphine have demonstrated the potential effectiveness of these medications as treatment approaches.

While basic research has shown that addictive drugs reinforce voluntary drug taking in humans and laboratory animals (see Chapters 2 and 3) and that the reinforcing effects of opiates and cocaine can be reduced by medications that alter their ability to activate the brain's reward system, there has not been a medication developed to treat cocaine addiction. Although recent work has provided information on the molecular basis of acute cocaine action and on the several neurotransmitter systems, including those mediated by dopamine, serotonin, and norepinephrine, that play a role in cocaine's effect on the brain reward system, there are gaps in knowledge about cocaine addiction.

Cocaine addiction differs importantly from opiate addiction (see Chapter 3), and the complexity of cocaine's mechanism of action, coupled with gaps in knowledge, has resulted in difficulty in developing an effective pharmacotherapy. Although an effective medication to treat cocaine addiction has not been developed, a wide range of medications continues to be tested that may affect the euphoria, craving, or withdrawal associated with cocaine dependence (Kleber, 1992). Some data suggest that tricyclic antidepressants may be useful for selected patients with intranasal use of cocaine or with co-occurring depression, but further studies are needed to confirm that observation (Nunes et al., 1995).

Despite advances in slow-release formulations of many medications, there are no slow-release, depot preparations or implantable pumps for the treatment of drug abuse. Those methods are ideal for noncompliant and difficult patient populations. The one notable exception has been the work to develop depot naltrexone for alcohol and opiate dependence, but no clinically usable product has emerged thus far. Polydrug abuse poses another challenge to medications development because many opiate and cocaine abusers also abuse alcohol, tobacco, and other illicit drugs.

A few current pharmacotherapeutic agents are useful in the treatment of drug dependence. More are useful in the treatment of co-occurring psychiatric disorders or withdrawal. Treatment providers require additional pharmacotherapies to assist them in treating the range of behavioral and physiological manifestations of drug addiction. Thus, it is critical to continue support of basic research in the behavioral and neurosciences to provide the foundation for medications development.

HIV/AIDS

Drug users with HIV infection pose many challenges for both the drug abuse and the primary care treatment systems. As discussed in Chapter 7, it now appears that injection drug use is the leading risk factor for new HIV infection in the United States (Holmberg, 1996). This section does not attempt to review the large volume of HIV/AIDS treatment research (other Institute of Medicine [IOM] and National Research Council [NRC] reports on HIV/AIDS include IOM, 1994; NRC, 1989, 1990, 1993, 1995), rather, it highlights research opportunities unique to the treatment of HIV-infected drug abusers and focuses specifically on medical complications and health care delivery issues.

Medical Complications

Although injection drug users (IDUs) display the host of typical HIV-related illnesses and complications, there are some unique differences from non-drug-using HIV-infected populations. The complications listed in Table 8.1 are common adverse consequences of HIV infection, drug use, or both that seem to appear more often among IDUs with HIV infection than among non-drug users (O'Connor et al., 1994). Thus, distinctive clinical characteristics of IDUs with HIV infection include increased rates of endocarditis, cellulitis or abscess, and other infections including bacterial pneumonia, sepsis, hepatitis, and tuberculosis (O'Connor et al., 1994). Kaposi's sarcoma, although common among male homosexuals with AIDS, is uncommon among drug users (Beral et al., 1990; Des Jarlais, 1991). The differences in the medical complications of HIV infection seen in the drug-abusing population are important both as predictors of progression to AIDS and as a source of HIV-related morbidity and mortality

TABLE 8.1 Spectrum of HIV-Related Disease in Injection Drug Users

Bacterial infections
Pneumonia
Endocarditis or sepsis
Tuberculosis
Sexually transmitted diseases (e.g., syphilis, human papillomavirus)
Hepatitis
Cancer

SOURCE: O'Connor et al. (1994).

before AIDS (Selwyn et al., 1992; Selwyn and O'Connor, 1992). Preliminary data suggest that certain clinical conditions (e.g., tuberculosis) may hasten disease progression in HIV-infected drug users (Farizo et al., 1992; Mientjes et al., 1992; IOM, 1994); and it has been hypothesized that the immunosuppressive or immunostimulatory effects of psychoactive drugs may influence HIV disease progression (Des Jarlais, 1991). Further research is needed to determine the possible impact of cofactors in HIV disease progression among drug abusers.

Understanding the natural history of HIV among IDUs and the increased risk of certain infections and complications is important for developing and providing effective treatment strategies for drug users. The medical complications of injection drug use may mimic, obscure, mask, or coexist with HIV-related infection and conditions, resulting in difficulties in diagnosis and more costly interventions. Research is needed to examine the effects of antiretroviral and other HIV medications on the occurrence of bacterial infections in drug users and to explore possible interactions of HIV medications with abused psychoactive drugs. Without proper knowledge of the etiological relationship between drug abuse and the course and progression of HIV disease, efforts at preventing transmission will continue to fall short of addressing the epidemic adequately.

Health Care Services

As research continues to address the best treatment modalities for HIV-infected drug abusers, studies are needed on the issues of access and utilization of treatment that are unique to that population. Research has established that drug abuse treatment is associated with a reduction in HIV transmission or related risk behaviors (see Chapter 7).

The link between the need to treat both AIDS and drug abuse has heightened awareness of drug abuse treatment—a significant step toward the integration of drug abuse treatment into mainstream medical education and practice (National Commission on AIDS, 1991). However, of populations with HIV, drug users are the group least likely to have consistent contact with the health care system, especially primary care or preventive services. This may be due in part to fear of criminal sanctions (Chapter 10). HIV-infected drug abusers are more likely to rely on acute care through sporadic use of emergency rooms for medical complications from injecting drugs and acute HIV-related illnesses (O'Connor et al., 1992). Most of the therapies used to treat HIV and related illnesses (e.g., tuberculosis) require long-term treatment and compliance with treatment regimens. The effective treatment of this population of drug abusers is important for the patient and the general public, as in the case of tuberculosis.[4] Therefore, access to and utilization of health care services for this population are critical.

When HIV-infected drug abusers enter drug abuse treatment programs, they typically are referred to medical clinics for diagnosis and treatment of HIV-related medical problems (Umbricht-Schneiter et al., 1994). Instead of referring them to other sites, however, drug abuse treatment programs may serve as ideal places for primary care (Selwyn et al., 1989a; Haverkos, 1991). Some of the primary care and preventive interventions for HIV-infected drug abusers include monitoring of immune function (e.g., CD4 count), administration of vaccines and antituberculosis therapy, skin testing for tuberculosis, and serologic testing and treatment for sexually transmitted diseases (O'Connor et al., 1994). With appropriate resources, the drug abuse treatment program could perform the following medical functions: assessment and diagnosis, referral to specialty care, coordination and monitoring, counseling, and primary care.

Several paradigms have been developed specifically targeted to the needs of drug users including on-site services in methadone programs and prisons, special hospital-based services, and outpatient programs (e.g., mobile vans linked to needle exchange programs) (Selwyn et al., 1989b; O'Connor et al., 1992). A randomized study of methadone patients found that those who received medical care on-site were far more likely to receive treatment than those whose care was referred off-site. It has been demonstrated that more than 90 percent of methadone patients received medical treatment if it was available on-site whereas only 35 percent received treatment when referred to a nearby location (Umbricht-Schneiter et al., 1994). The actual number of HIV-infected drug abusers

[4]Directly observed therapy for tuberculosis is the most effective means of ensuring compliance and preventing the spread of tuberculosis (Bayer and Wilkinson, 1995; Chaulk et al., 1995).

included in the study was small because the study was targeted to a variety of medical conditions.

There is a plethora of research opportunities to investigate the potential benefits of delivering primary care in drug abuse treatment programs. One major benefit is likely to be the frequent and long-term contact; daily methadone dosing could be combined with daily supervised treatment or prophylaxis for tuberculosis and HIV. Drug treatment programs also are likely to be familiar with some of the unique medical characteristics of HIV infection in drug abusers and with patients' psychosocial needs (Sorensen and Batki, 1992). There is also the possibility of lower costs—if patients' primary care needs are fulfilled, costly hospitalizations may be avoided. Studies demonstrating the cost-effectiveness of the delivery of primary care through drug treatment programs might encourage legislators and public health agencies to provide funding for the expansion of services, including outreach to the community to encourage drug abusers to seek treatment. It is also important for the clinician outside of the drug abuse treatment system to be familiar with the full spectrum of HIV-related diseases and medical complications in this population.

Research is needed to study barriers and access to medical care among the drug-using population, given that this population has high levels of medical needs and historically poor engagement with the health care system. Further, research is needed to explore and evaluate alternative health care delivery systems for drug users who are not well served by mainstream systems of care.

Matching Patients to Treatments

Matching patients to treatments means tailoring treatments to patient needs in an effort to improve outcomes, in contrast to giving the same treatment to all patients with the same diagnosis. Matching can take place on many levels: drug-free versus pharmacotherapy, inpatient versus outpatient, treating or not treating psychiatric or medical disorders in the context of the drug-abuse program, using different types of counseling or psychotherapy, choosing various behavioral contingencies, matching the personality or background of the therapist with the patient, combining legal pressure with treatment in a therapeutic community versus a less intensive and briefer rehabilitation program, and many others. Patients will self-select a treatment modality if given the opportunity. It is critical to the implementation of patient matching strategies that cost-cutting not be the overriding criterion for matching a patient to a given treatment modality.

To conduct patient matching, three elements are needed: comprehensive assessment tools to identify patient problems and needs; placement criteria to ensure placement in the appropriate level (setting), phase (detoxification, rehabilitation, etc.), and intensity of care; and a means of facilitating movement through a continuum of treatment services (SAMHSA, 1995b). Ideally, all three elements are incorporated into patient placement criteria.

There is, however, no national consensus about the most appropriate patient placement criteria, mainly because of the dearth of research, methodological limitations in its conduct, and the inconsistency of some studies (SAMHSA, 1995b). Few managed care companies publish their patient placement criteria. The American Society of Addiction Medicine (ASAM) is one of the first organizations to have developed placement criteria, and the most widely used. The few studies that have evaluated the validity of ASAM criteria have failed to demonstrate effects on patient outcome (McKay et al., 1992); another large-scale study is in progress (D. Gastfriend, Massachusetts General Hospital, personal communication, 1995). Assessing the clinical validity of existing patient placement criteria is a vital area for research attention. This task is complex because there are a range of treatment settings and other options for matching, and most phases of treatment can be delivered in more than one setting (Hayashida et al., 1989; Washton, 1989; Alterman et al., 1994; McKay et al., 1994; Mattick and Hall, 1996).

In addition to decisions about treatment phase, setting, and services for associated problems, providers are faced with other decisions about program characteristics (e.g., intensity, duration, structure, and philosophy) and therapy characteristics (e.g., therapeutic approach, group versus individual therapy, and therapist characteristics) (Hser, 1995). A particularly important element of matching is identifying how patient characteristics interact with different types of treatments and treatment programs. Patients who have psychiatric, medical, family, and/or legal problems are likely to need highly trained staff with special training in complex interventions.

Two studies of matching patients strictly with drug dependencies to treatment settings that addressed particular needs demonstrated better treatment outcomes than treatment settings that did not address specific needs (McLellan et al., 1983, in press, b). Both studies were prospective in nature, however, assignments were not random.

A newer paradigm for matching patients to treatment stems from the concept of "stages of change" (Prochaska and DiClemente, 1983, 1986). This concept was developed from clinical observations that patients with drug abuse disorders have varying levels of motivation to alter their behavior. Six stages have been described: precontemplation, contemplation, determination, action, maintenance, and relapse. Those stages are seen as making up a circle around which patients move in their attempts to stop drug abuse. In studies of smokers, they found that most went through the six stages three to seven times before achieving sustained remission (Prochaska and DiClemente, 1983). This model implies that a therapist should develop different approaches according to the patient's stage. For example, motivational enhancement may be the only approach possible for someone who is a "precontemplator," whereas relapse prevention would be more appropriate for one who is in the action or maintenance phase. Research on how best to measure the stage of change and on developing interventions that address specific changes is currently under way and may provide a mechanism for improving treatment.

However, there has been limited independent research on the costs and benefits of patient matching, and managed care providers and others are matching patients to treatments without empirical evidence that the matching they perform yields the most cost-effective outcomes (Hser, 1995). Further, there is limited research on the optimal, most cost-effective configuration of services for different groups of patients. Yet some managed care contracts place severe limits on the addiction-focused services (e.g., not allowing more than three days for detoxification), whereas others "carve out" drug abuse-focused treatments from treatment services that are related to the psychiatric, medical, and other problems associated with abuse and dependence (see Chapter 9). In some cases, state guidelines require separate licensing for drug abuse and mental health services and separate administration of drug abuse treatment from psychiatric, medical, family, and other related services. The result of these practices can be less service delivery (McLellan et al., in press, a) and poorer outcomes (T. McLellan, University of Pennsylvania, personal communication, 1995) and may defeat the principle of matching patients to the most effective treatments.

Treatment of Patients with Co-Occurring Psychiatric Disorders and Drug Abuse

A related issue is treatment of patients with co-occurring psychiatric disorders and drug abuse.[5] About 64 percent of those seeking treatment for drug abuse have one or more co-occurring psychiatric disorders. The prevalence of co-occurring disorders is much higher in this population than in the general population (Regier et al., 1990; Kessler et al., 1994). These patients are an important population because they are more expensive to treat, they usually require more complex and costly interventions, and they relapse more frequently (Garnick et al., in press).

Assessment and Diagnosis

A long-standing problem has been the difficulty in correctly identifying psychiatric disorders that occur in drug abusers. Drug-produced psychiatric disorders can result from acute drug effects, chronic intoxication, drug withdrawal, or effects that persist for months or years after detoxification has been completed (Woody et al., 1995a). Examples of psychopathology resulting from acute drug effects are alcohol-induced depression, stimulant-induced psychoses, or withdrawal-induced depression and anxiety. Examples of persistent drug effects are dementia associated with chronic alcohol, sedative, or inhalant dependence, or "flashbacks" from hallucinogens such as lysergic acid diethylamide (LSD) (APA, 1994).

Research has clearly demonstrated that drug-produced psychiatric disorders can appear identical to primary, independent psychiatric disorders. Differentiation on the basis of presenting signs and symptoms alone is often impossible (APA, 1994). Correct identification is critical because it has important treatment implications. Primary psychiatric disorders tend to run a long-term course and require extended treatment. Drug-produced psychiatric disorders tend to follow the course of the drug abuse; usually resolve when the drug abuse remits; and often need only observation, supportive counseling, or short-term pharmacotherapy. Additional study of persistent drug-produced psychiatric disorders (e.g., potential long-term effects of dependence on stimulants such as cocaine) is important both in prevention and for the design and implementation of treatment programs.

Pharmacotherapy

Among persons with drug abuse or dependence, the rates of depression reach 26 percent, a higher rate than that found in the general population (Regier et al., 1990; Kessler et al., 1994). Progress has been made in the treatment of depression in clients with opioid or alcohol dependence. Some of this depression may be drug induced and resolve with sustained abstinence (Schuckit, 1994). Several well-controlled studies have shown that antidepressant pharmacotherapies, such as desipramine or imipramine, can be very helpful with carefully selected depressed patients who are drug dependent (Nunes et al., 1995; Mason et al., 1996). However, due to the possible contribution of the drug abuse to the development of depression, there has been some controversy about the conditions under which antidepressants and other pharmacotherapies should be used in this population.

Few studies, however, have been performed on the use of pharmacotherapies and psychotherapies for other co-occurring psychiatric disorders. One controversial group of pharmacotherapies for anxiety disorders among patients with drug abuse has been benzodiazepines. They are generally considered safe and effective for a range of anxiety disorders and are among the most widely used pharmacotherapies (Tyrer, 1984). However, there is clear evidence that some benzodiazepines have a significant abuse liability (Sellers et al., 1993). Consequently, the use of benzodiazepines in patients with a history of drug abuse or dependence is often judged to be contraindicated. However, not all benzodiazepines are equally prone to abuse. Medications such as oxazepam, clorazepate, or others with longer duration to onset of peak effect not only might be useful in treating patients with co-occurring anxiety, but may have little risk of abuse when taken orally. Studies to determine the usefulness of benzodiazepines with slow onset to peak effects for patients with drug abuse and anxiety disorders would be helpful in providing data on this issue.

Additionally, since U.S. drug abusers often abuse multiple drugs, studies are needed to determine the interactions among drugs of abuse, medications used to treat drug dependence, and medications used to treat comorbid psychiatric and medical disorders. For example, a medication intended to prevent relapse to cocaine dependence should be tested for adverse consequences when used in combination with alcohol or opiates since these drugs are commonly used together. This is an area in which the behavioral models discussed in Chapter 2 could make significant contributions.

Further, pharmacokinetic studies of medications are typically carried out in healthy individuals, whereas many drug abusers have multiple health problems. Thus, the interactions among abused drugs, medications for drug abuse or dependence, and medications for psychiatric and medical problems may be altered in drug abusers. To optimize treatment strategies and to prevent adverse health outcomes, pharmacokinetic studies are needed to determine these possible interactions. Additionally, comparative studies of pharmacotherapies and psychotherapies for specific, well-defined depressive or anxiety disorders with this population (drug abuse and psychiatric disorders) could provide important data about the most appropriate therapies.

Special Populations

There is a dearth of research on drug-abusing women, prisoners, and adolescents. For reasons discussed below, it is extremely important for those populations to gain access to, enter, and remain in treatment. Most of the research opportunities center on treatment access, retention, and effectiveness. There are large gaps in our knowledge of these areas, much of which is attributable to methodological difficulties.

Women

The health consequences of drug abuse can be more serious for women than for men, in spite of the fact that fewer women abuse drugs. Women can contract HIV through injection drug use or prostitution to purchase drugs. Maternal drug use can result in transmitting the disease to their fetus, premature delivery with serious complications, and impairments in parenting. Yet research has documented more barriers to treatment entry for female than for male alcoholics (Weisner and Schmidt, 1992; Schmidt and Weisner, 1995). Some of the obstacles for women are the cost of treatment, the possible loss of custody of their children, and the lack of child care (Beckman, 1994). Similar barriers to treatment may be operating for male drug abusers, but the extent of the problem is unknown.

A recent study of more than 12,000 clients in treatment found that women tended to drop out of treatment at higher rates than men (Mammo and Weinbaum, 1993). It is possible that women have difficulty making child care arrangements, fear retribution, or feel uncomfortable talking about their problems when being treated in programs that are predominantly male. Some programs, in an attempt to overcome these barriers, have experimented with women-only groups and with on-site facilities for child care.

Studies have also shown that women with drug abuse disorders typically have more psychiatric disorders (including depression and anxiety) than males (Blume, 1992). Many drug- dependent women have been sexually abused as children, suffer from posttraumatic stress disorder, and have significant problems forming healthy relationships with males (SAMHSA, 1994b). Abusive relationships with drug-abusing males are common, sometimes characterized by situations in which the male exerts control by providing drugs. These complex issues indicate that psychiatric assessment and treatment constitute a particularly important aspect of drug abuse treatment for women. Few studies have been done to examine the effect of integrating psychiatric treatment into the ongoing services of programs that treat drug-abusing women.

In spite of those problems, research shows that when women remain in treatment, they benefit just as much as men do (Sanchez-Craig et al., 1989; Ball and Ross, 1991; Finnegan, 1991). Methadone maintenance programs for pregnant women are the best studied, but outcomes in many other settings indicate that women benefit at least as much as men from the range of treatments that are currently available (Hubbard et al., 1989;

IOM, 1990a). There is a dearth of studies on programs that deliver services tailored to women's needs.

Problems continue to be greatest for pregnant women. In the past, many treatment programs automatically excluded pregnant women because of liability concerns or concerns about lack of expertise with medical complications of pregnancy. Some areas of the country have enacted laws that classify drug abuse during pregnancy as a form of child abuse, which would lead to the placement of children in foster care. These laws do not seem to reduce drug abuse, but they may have the negative effect of discouraging pregnant drug users from seeking treatment (see Chapter 10). Exclusion of pregnant women from treatment programs is beginning to diminish, however. A recent survey of 294 drug treatment programs in five cities revealed that the majority of programs (70–83 percent) accepted pregnant women. Fewer programs, however, accepted women who were Medicaid recipients, and even fewer programs provided child care (Breitbart et al., 1994).

When pregnant women succeed in gaining access to treatment, they face yet another hurdle—the lack of pharmacotherapies specifically approved for use in pregnancy (IOM, 1995b). This problem is true for medications of all kinds, not just for those used in drug abuse treatment. Pharmaceutical firms rarely, if ever, seek Food and Drug Administration (FDA) approval for use of their products in pregnancy, mostly because of liability concerns. When pregnant heroin drug users, for example, need treatment to reduce drug use and the risk of HIV transmission to themselves and their unborn, their doctors are strongly discouraged by federal treatment regulations and by the manufacturer from prescribing LAAM. According to federal treatment regulations, pregnant women are offered methadone, which is not formally approved by the FDA for use in pregnancy. FDA has drafted guidelines recommending that future studies of antiaddiction medications include women, but the guidelines do not provide advice for a mechanism dealing with increased risk for product liability (Woody et al., 1996).

Prisoners

Treatment programs have recently become more prominent in some correctional settings, with therapeutic communities among the most common modalities. The therapeutic community provides a total treatment environment isolated from the rest of the prison population—separated from the drugs, the violence, and the norms and values that mitigate against treatment, habilitation, and rehabilitation. Treatment programs based in correctional settings sometimes include aftercare in the community after release from prison. Although therapeutic communities appear to be the most visible drug abuse treatment programs in correctional settings, there are numerous other modalities, many of which are grounded in individual and group counseling and 12-step approaches. However, there is limited information about these programs in the drug abuse literature. There are virtually no methadone maintenance programs offered in correctional settings, which is most likely a result of policies to eliminate the availability of a medication that is itself a controlled drug.

Most treatment of drug-involved offenders takes place in community-based settings as a condition of parole or probation or in lieu of prison. Treatment in the community is made possible through programs that link the criminal justice system with specialty drug abuse treatment programs. The most prominent example is Treatment Alternatives to Street Crime (TASC), whose programs are found in more than 25 states (Inciardi and McBride, 1991). Evaluation data indicate that TASC-referred clients remain in treatment longer than non-TASC clients (court referrals to treatment without TASC services). Other programs linking treatment to parole and probation have experienced favorable results (Chavaria, 1992; Van Stelle et al., 1994).

Although there are extensive studies of drug-involved offenders who are treated effectively in community settings, there is a dearth of information about drug treatment programs in prisons or about the best means of treating drug abusers in these settings. What is known is that for the few prisoners who succeed in gaining access to a limited number of prison-based therapeutic communities, treatment is effective. Many in the drug treatment community believe that prisoners have the most profound treatment system needs in light of the pervasive violence and widespread availability of illicit drugs within the prison system. The co-occurrence of addictive and severe psychiatric disorders is also highest in the prison population (Regier et al., 1990).

Adolescents

Adolescents are also vulnerable to the consequences of drug abuse, including health effects, accidents and injuries, involvement with violence resulting from illegal activities, and the transmission of HIV (Czechowicz, 1991). Adolescent drug abusers differ from adult drug abusers in several ways that are significant for treatment. The majority of adolescent drug abusers have a shorter history of drug abuse; have less severe symptoms of tolerance, craving, and withdrawal; and usually do not have the long-term physical effects of drug abuse (Kaminer, 1994). However, they are at the greatest risk for developing lifelong patterns of drug abuse (Dusenbury et al., 1992).

Adolescents accounted for about 11.1 percent of all patients in specialty drug abuse treatment programs in 1993 (SAMHSA, 1995a), down from 16.9 percent in 1987, although their proportion appears to be rising again (SAMHSA, 1995a). There is increasing recognition of the need to implement and evaluate treatment programs designed specifically for adolescents (IOM, 1990b). A new study of treatment effectiveness for 3,000 adolescents enrolled in standard treatment programs is under way, with findings to be reported in 1997 (R. Hubbard, Research Triangle Institute, personal communication, 1995). There are additional opportunities to design and evaluate the effectiveness of special programs with services tailored to adolescents. Results from such studies will enable the development of targeted treatment and prevention programs.

RECOMMENDATION

Substantial progress has been made during the past 20 years in our knowledge of drug abuse treatment. Research has shown that drug abuse treatment is both effective and cost-effective in reducing not only drug consumption but also the associated health and social consequences. Continued research on drug abuse treatment is needed in many priority areas.

The committee recommends that the appropriate federal and private agencies continue to support research to improve and evaluate the effectiveness of drug abuse treatment. This includes studies on optimal strategies for matching patients to the most appropriate treatment modalities; development of medications for the treatment of drug abuse and dependence; the efficacy of pharmacotherapies and psychosocial therapies to treat individuals with co-occurring psychiatric disorders and drug abuse; the natural history of HIV infection among drug users and effective models of health care delivery for HIV-infected drug abusers; and the efficacy of treatment programs designed toward addressing the needs of special populations (i.e., women, adolescents, and prisoners).

REFERENCES

Alterman AI, O'Brien CP, McLellan AT, August DS, Snider EC, Droba M, Cornish JW, Hall CP, Raphaelson AH, Schrade FX. 1994. Effectiveness and costs of inpatient versus day hospital cocaine rehabilitation. *Journal of Nervous and Mental Disease* 182:157–163.

Alterman AI, Snider EC, Cacciola JS, May DJ, Parikh G, Maany I, Rosenbaum PR. 1996. Treatments for cocaine dependence. *Journal of Nervous and Mental Disease* 184(1):54–56.

APA (American Psychiatric Association). 1994. *Diagnostic and Statistical Manual of Mental Disorders. Fourth Edition*. Washington, DC: APA.

Ball JC, Ross A. 1991. *The Effectiveness of Methadone Maintenance Treatment*. New York: Springer-Verlag.

Bayer R, Wilkinson D. 1995. Directly observed therapy for tuberculosis: History of an idea. *Lancet* 345(8964):1545–1548.

Beck AT, Wright FD, Newman CF. 1990. *Cognitive Therapy of Cocaine Abuse.* Philadelphia: Center for Cognitive Therapy.

Beckman LJ. 1994. Treatment needs of women with alcohol problems. *Alcohol Health and Research World* 18(3):206–211.

Beral V, Peterman TA, Berkelman RL, Jaffe HW. 1990. Kaposi's sarcoma among persons with AIDS: A sexually transmitted infection? *Lancet* 335(8682):123–128.

Bicket WK, Amass L. 1995. Buprehorphine treatment of opioid dependence: A review. *Experimental and Clinical Psychopharmacology* 3:477–489.

Blume SB. 1992. Alcohol and other drug problems in women. In: Lowinson JH, Ruiz P, Millman RB, eds. *Substance Abuse: A Comprehensive Textbook.* Baltimore: Williams & Wilkins. Pp. 794–807.

Brahen LS, Capone T, Bloom S, et al. 1978. An alternative to methadone for probationer addicts: Narcotic antagonist treatment. *Contemporary Drug Issues* 13:117–132.

Breitbart V, Chavkin W, Wise PH. 1994. The accessibility of drug treatment for pregnant women: A survey of programs in five cities. *American Journal of Public Health* 84(10):1658–1661.

Center of Alcohol Studies, Rutgers University. 1993. *Socioeconomic Evaluations of Addictions Treatment.* Prepared for the President's Commission on Model State Drug Laws by the Center of Alcohol Studies, Rutgers University, Piscataway, NJ.

Chaulk CP, Moore-Rice K, Rizzo R, Chaisson RE. 1995. Eleven years of community-based directly observed therapy for tuberculosis. *Journal of the American Medical Association* 274(12):945–951.

Chavaria FR. 1992. Successful drug treatment in a criminal justice setting: A case study. *Federal Probation* 56:48–52.

Cowan A, Lewis J, eds. 1995. *Buprenorphine: Combatting Drug Abuse with a Unique Opioid.* New York: John Wiley & Sons.

Czechowicz D. 1991. Adolescent alcohol and drug addiction and its consequences: An overview. In: Miller NS, ed. *Comprehensive Handbook of Drug and Alcohol Addiction.* New York: Marcel Dekker. Pp. 205–210.

Des Jarlais DC. 1991. Potential cofactors in the outcomes of HIV infection in intravenous drug users. *NIDA Research Monograph* 109:115–124.

Dusenbury L, Khuri E, Millman RB. 1992. Adolescent substance abuse: A sociodevelopmental perspective. In: Lowinson JH, Ruiz P, Millman RB, Langrod JG, eds. *Substance Abuse: A Comprehensive Textbook.* Baltimore: Williams & Wilkins. Pp. 832–842.

Everingham S, Rydell C. 1994. *Modeling the Demand for Cocaine.* MR-332-ONDCP/A/DPRC. Santa Monica, CA: RAND Drug Policy Research Center.

Farizo K, Buehler J, Chamberland M, Whyte BM, Froelicher ES, Hopkins SG, Reed CM, Mokotoff ED, Cohn DL, Troxler S, et al. 1992. Spectrum of disease in persons with human immunodeficiency virus infection in the United States. *Journal of the American Medical Association* 267:1798–1805.

Finnegan LP. 1991. Treatment issues for opioid-dependent women during the perinatal period. *Journal of Psychoactive Drugs* 23:191–199.

Garnick DW, Hendricks AM, Drainoni ML, Horgan CM, Comstock C. In press. Private sector coverage of people with dual diagnoses. *Journal of Mental Health Administration.*

Gerstein DR, Johnson RA, Harwood HJ, Fountain D, Suter N, Malloy K. 1994. *Evaluating Recovery Services: The California Drug and Alcohol Treatment Assessment (CALDATA).* Sacramento, CA: California Department of Alcohol and Drug Programs.

Goldstein A, Kalant H. 1990. Drug policy: Striking the right balance. *Science* 249:1513–1521.

Haverkos H. 1991. Infectious diseases and drug abuse. *Journal of Substance Abuse Treatment* 8:269–275.

Hayashida M, Alterman AI, O'Brien CP, McLellan AT. 1989. Comparative effectiveness of inpatient and outpatient detoxification of patients with mild-to-moderate alcohol withdrawal syndrome. *New England Journal of Medicine* 320:358–365.

Higgins ST, Budney AJ, Bickel WK, Hughes JR, Foerg F, Badger G. 1993. Achieving cocaine abstinence with a behavioral approach. *American Journal of Psychiatry* 150:763–769.

Higgins ST, Budney AJ, Bickel WK, Foerg FE, Donham R, Badger GJ. 1994. Incentives improve outcome in outpatient behavioral treatment of cocaine dependence. *Archives of General Psychiatry* 51:568–576.

Holmberg SD. 1996. The estimated prevalence and incidence of HIV in 96 large U.S. metropolitan areas. *American Journal of Public Health* 86(5):642–654.

Hser Y. 1995. A referral system that matches drug users to treatment programs: Existing research and relevant Issues. *Journal of Drug Issues* 25(1):209–224.

Hubbard RL, Marsden ME, Rachal JV, Harwood HJ, Cavanaugh ER, Ginzburg HM. 1989. *Drug Abuse Treatment: A National Study of Effectiveness*. Chapel Hill, NC: University of North Carolina Press.

Inciardi JA, McBride DC. 1991. *Treatment Alternatives to Street Crime (TASC): History, Experiences, and Issues*. Rockville, MD: NIDA.

IOM (Institute of Medicine). 1990a. *Broadening the Base for Alcohol Problems*. Washington, DC: National Academy Press.

IOM (Institute of Medicine). 1990b. *Treating Drug Problems*. Washington, DC: National Academy Press.

IOM (Institute of Medicine) 1994. *AIDS and Behavior: An Integrated Approach*. Washington, DC: National Academy Press.

IOM (Institute of Medicine). 1995a. *Federal Regulation of Methadone Treatment*. Washington, DC: National Academy Press.

IOM (Institute of Medicine). 1995b. *The Development of Medications for the Treatment of Opiate and Cocaine Addictions*. Washington, DC: National Academy Press.

Johnson RE, Jaffe JH, Fudala PJ. 1992. A controlled trial of buprenorphine treatment for opioid dependence. *Journal of the American Medical Association* 267(20):2750–2755.

Kaminer Y. 1994. Adolescent substance abuse. In: Galanter M, Kleber HD, eds. *The American Psychiatric Press Textbook of Substance Abuse Treatment*. Washington, DC: American Psychiatric Press.

Kessler R, McGonagle K, Zhao S, Nelson CB, Hughes M, Eshleman S, Wittchen HU, Kendler KS. 1994. Lifetime and 12-month prevalence of DSM-IIIR psychiatric disorders in the United States: Results from the National Comorbidity Survey. *Archives of General Psychiatry* 51:8–19.

Kidorf M, Stitzer ML, Brooner RK, Goldberg J. 1994. Contingent methadone take-home doses reinforce adjunct therapy attendance of methadone maintenance patients. *Drug and Alcohol Dependence* 36:221–226.

Kleber HD. 1992. Treatment of cocaine abuse: Pharmacotherapy. *CIBA Foundation Symposium* 166:195–206.

Kosten TR, Schottenfeld R, Ziedonis D, Falcioni J. 1993. Buprenorphine versus methadone maintenance for opioid dependence. *Journal of Nervous and Mental Disease* 181(6):358–364.

Kreek MJ. 1992. Rationale for maintenance pharmacotherapy of opiate dependence. In: O'Brien CP, Jaffe JH, eds. *Addictive States*. New York: Raven Press. Pp. 205–230.

Luborsky L. 1984. *Principles of Psychoanalytic Psychotherapy: A Manual for Supportive-Expressive Treatment*. New York: Basic Books.

Luborsky L, Woody GE, Hole A, Velleco A. 1995. Supportive-expressive dynamic psychotherapy for treatment of opiate drug dependence. In: Barber JP, Crits-Christoph P, eds. *Dynamic Therapies for Psychiatric Disorders (Axis I)*. New York: Basic Books. Pp. 131–160.

Mammo A, Weinbaum DF. 1993. Some factors that influence dropping out from outpatient treatment facilities. *Journal of Studies on Alcohol* 54:92–101.

Mason BJ, Ritvo EC, Morgan RO, Salvato FR, Goldberg G, Welch B, Mantero-Atienza E. 1994. A double-blind, placebo-controlled pilot study to evaluate the efficacy and safety of oral nalmefene HCl for alcohol dependence. *Alcoholism: Clinical and Experimental Research* 18:1162–1167.

Mason BJ, Kocsis JH, Ritvo EC, Cutler RB. 1996. A double-blind, placebo-controlled trial of desipramine for primary alcohol dependence stratified on the presence or absence of major depression. *Journal of the American Medical Association* 275(10):761–767.

Mattick RP, Hall W. 1996. Are detoxification programmes effective? *Lancet* 347:97–100.

McKay JR, McLellan AT, Alterman AI. 1992. An evaluation of the Cleveland Criteria for inpatient substance abuse treatment. *American Journal of Psychiatry* 149:1212–1218.

McKay JR, Alterman AI, McLellan AT, Snider EC. 1994. Treatment goals, continuity of care, and outcome in a day hospital substance abuse rehabilitation program. *American Journal of Psychiatry* 151:254–259.

McLellan AT, Luborsky L, O'Brien CP, Woody GE. 1980. An improved evaluation instrument for substance abuse patients: The Addiction Severity Index. *Journal of Nervous and Mental Disease* 168:26–33.

McLellan AT, Luborsky L, O'Brien CP, Woody GE, Druley KA. 1982. Is substance abuse treatment effective? *Journal of the American Medical Association* 247:1423–1428.

McLellan AT, Woody G, Luborsky L, O'Brien C, Druley K. 1983. Increased effectiveness of substance abuse treatment: A prospective study of patient treatment "matching." *Journal of Nervous and Mental Disease* 171:597–605.

McLellan AT, Woody GE, Luborsky L, Goehl L. 1988. Is the counsellor an "active ingredient" in methadone treatment? An examination of treatment success among four counselors. *Journal of Nervous and Mental Disease* 176:423–430.

McLellan AT, Alterman AI, Woody GE, Metzger D. 1992. A quantitative measure of substance abuse treatments: The Treatment Services Review. *Journal of Nervous and Mental Disease* 180:101–110.

McLellan AT, Arndt IO, Metzger DS, Woody GE, O'Brien CP. 1993. The effects of psychosocial services in substance abuse treatment. *Journal of the American Medical Association* 269(15):1953–1959.

McLellan AT, Alterman AI, Metzger DS, Grissom GR, Woody GE, Luborsky L, O'Brien CP. 1994. Similarity of outcome predictors across opiate, cocaine, and alcohol treatments: Role of treatment services. *Journal of Consulting and Clinical Psychology* 62:1141–1158.

McLellan AT, Metzger DS, Alterman AI, Woody GE, Durell J, O'Brien CP. In press, a. Is addiction treatment "worth it"? Public health expectations, policy-based comparisons. *Milbank Quarterly*.

McLellan AT, Grissom GR, Zanis D, Randall M, Brill P, O'Brien CP. In press, b. Improved outcomes from problem-service "matching" in substance abuse patients: A controlled study in a four-program, EAP network. *Archives of General Psychiatry*.

Metzger DS, Woody GE, McLellan T, O'Brien CP, Druley P, Navaline H, DePhilippis D, Stolley P, Abrutyn E. 1993. Human immunodeficiency virus seroconversion among in- and out-of-treatment intravenous drug users: An 18-month prospective follow-up. *Journal of Acquired Immune Deficiency Syndromes* 6:1049–1056.

Mientjes G, van Ameijden E, van den Hoeck A, Coutinho RA. 1992. Increasing morbidity without rise in non-AIDS mortality among HIV-infected intravenous drug users in Amsterdam. *AIDS* 6:207–212.

National Commission on AIDS. 1991. *The Twin Epidemics of Substance Use and HIV*. Washington, DC: U.S. Government Printing Office.

NRC (National Research Council). 1989. *AIDS, Sexual Behavior and Intravenous Drug Abuse.* Washington, DC: National Academy Press.

NRC (National Research Council). 1990. *AIDS: The Second Decade.* Washington, DC: National Academy Press.

NRC (National Research Council). 1993. *The Social Impact of AIDS in the United States.* Washington, DC: National Academy Press.

NRC (National Research Council). 1995. *Preventing HIV Transmission: The Role of Sterile Needles and Bleach.* Washington, DC: National Academy Press.

Nunes EV, McGrath PJ, Quitkin FM, Ocepek-Welikson K, Stewart JW, Koenig T, Wager S, Klein DF. 1995. Imipramine treatment of cocaine abuse: Possible boundaries of efficacy. *Drug and Alcohol Dependence* 39:185–195.

O'Brien CP, McLellan AT. 1996. Myths about the treatment of addiction. *Lancet* 347:237–240.

O'Connor P, Molde S, Henry S, Shockcor WT, Schottenfeld RS. 1992. Human immunodeficiency virus infection in intravenous drug users: A model for primary care. *American Journal of Medicine* 93:382–386.

O'Connor PG, Selwyn PA, Schottenfeld RS. 1994. Medical care for injection-drug users with human immunodeficiency virus infection. *New England Journal of Medicine* 331(7):450–459.

ONDCP (Office of National Drug Control Policy). 1996. *National Drug Control Strategy, 1996.* Washington, DC: ONDCP.

Prendergast ML, Anglin MD, Maugh TH, Hser Y. In press. *The Effectiveness of Treatment for Drug Abuse.* Draft manuscript prepared April 7, 1994 for NIDA Treatment Services Research Branch. Los Angeles: UCLA Drug Abuse Research Center.

Prochaska JO, DiClemente CC. 1983. Stages and processes of self-change: Toward an integrative model of change. *Journal of Consulting and Clinical Psychology* 51:390–395.

Prochaska JO, DiClemente CC. 1986. Toward a comprehensive model of change. In: Miller WR, Heather N, eds. *Treating Addictive Behaviors: Process of Changes.* New York: Plenum Press.

Rawson RA, Obert JL, McCann MJ, Marinelli-Casey P. 1993. Relapse prevention strategies in outpatient substance abuse treatment. *Psychology of Addictive Behaviors* 7:85–95.

Regier D, Farmer M, Rae D, Locke BZ, Keith SJ, Judd LL, Goodwin FK. 1990. Comorbidity of mental disorders with alcohol and other drug abuse: Results from the Epidemiologic Catchment Area (ECA) Study. *Journal of the American Medical Association* 264:2511–2518.

Rhodes W, Scheiman P, Pittayathikhun T, Collins L, Tsarfaty V. 1995. *What America's Users Spend on Illegal Drugs, 1988–1993.* Prepared for the Office of National Drug Control Policy, Washington, DC.

Rounsaville BJ, Weissman MM, Kleber HD. 1982. Heterogeneity of psychiatric diagnoses in treated opiate addicts. *Archives of General Psychiatry* 39:161–166.

Rydell C, Everingham S. 1994. *Controlling Cocaine: Supply Versus Demand Programs.* MR-3331-ONDCP/A/DPRC. Santa Monica, CA: RAND Drug Policy Research Center.

SAMHSA (Substance Abuse and Mental Health Services Administration). 1993. *State Methadone Treatment Guidelines.* Treatment Improvement Protocol (TIP) Series 1. Rockville, MD: SAMHSA.

SAMHSA (Substance Abuse and Mental Health Services Administration). 1994a. *Client Data System FY 1992: Opiate and Cocaine/Crack Admissions to Treatment.* Prepared under contract for the Office of Applied Studies.

SAMHSA (Substance Abuse and Mental Health Services Administration). 1994b. *Practical Approaches in the Treatment of Women Who Abuse Alcohol and Other Drugs.* DHHS Publication No. (SMA)94-3006. Rockville, MD: SAMHSA.

SAMHSA (Substance Abuse and Mental Health Services Administration). 1995a. *Overview of the FY94 National Drug and Alcoholism Treatment Unit Survey (NDATUS): Data from 1993 and 1980–1993.* Advance Report Number 9A, August 1995. Rockville, MD: SAMHSA.

SAMHSA (Substance Abuse and Mental Health Services Administration). 1995b. *The Role and Current Status of Patient Placement Criteria in the Treatment of Substance Use Disorders.* Treatment Improvement Protocol (TIP) Series 13. DHHS Publication No. (SMA) 95-3021. Rockville, MD: SAMHSA.

SAMHSA (Substance Abuse and Mental Health Services Administration). 1995c. *LAAM and the Treatment of Opiate Addiction.* Treatment Improvement Protocol (TIP) Series 22. Rockville, MD: SAMHSA.

Sanchez-Craig M, Leigh G, Spivak K, Lei H. 1989. Superior outcome of females over males after brief treatment for the reduction of heavy drinking. *British Journal of Addiction* 84:395–404.

Schmidt L, Weisner C. 1995. The emergence of problem-drinking women as a special population in need of treatment. *Recent Developments in Alcoholism* 12:309–334.

Schuckit MA. 1994. The relationship between alcohol problems, substance abuse, and psychiatric syndromes. In: Widiger TA, Frances AJ, Pincus HA, eds. *DSM-IV Sourcebook, Vol. 1.* Washington, DC: American Psychiatric Association Press. Pp. 45–66.

Sellers EM, Ciraulo DA, DuPont Rl, Griffiths RR, Kosten TR, Romach MK, Woody GE. 1993. Alprazolam and benzodiazepine dependence. *Journal of Clinical Psychiatry* 54(10 Suppl.):64–77.

Selwyn PA, O'Connor PG. 1992. Diagnosis and treatment of substance users with HIV infection. *Primary Care* 19(1):119–156.

Selwyn PA, Feingold AR, Iezza A, Satyadeo M, Colley J, Torres R, Shaw JF. 1989a. Primary care for patients with human immunodeficiency virus (HIV) infection in a methadone maintenance treatment program. *Annals of Internal Medicine* 111:761–763.

Selwyn PA, Hartel D, Wasserman W, Drucker E. 1989b. Impact of the AIDS epidemic on morbidity and mortality among intravenous drug users in a New York City methadone maintenance program. *American Journal of Public Health* 79(10):1358–1362.

Selwyn PA, Alcabes P, Hartel D, Buono D, Schoenbaum EE, Klein RS, Davenny K, Friedland GH. 1992. Clinical manifestations and predictors of disease progression in drug users with human immunodeficiency virus infection. *New England Journal of Medicine* 327:1697–1703.

Shopshaw S, Frosch D, Rawson R, Ling W. 1995. *Reduction in Risky Behavior Associated with Treatment for Cocaine Dependence.* Presented at the Third Science Symposium on HIV Prevention: Current Status and Future Directions. Northern Arizona University, Flagstaff, AZ.

Simpson DD, Sells SB. 1982. Effectiveness of treatment for drug abuse: An overview of the DARP Research Program. *Advances in Alcohol and Substance Abuse* 2:7–29.

Simpson DD, Sells SB, eds. 1990. *Opioid Addiction and Treatment: A 12-Year Follow-Up.* Malabar, FL: Krieger Publishing.

Sorensen JL, Batki SL. 1992. Management of the psychosocial sequelae of HIV infection among drug abusers. In: Lowinson JH, Ruiz P, Millman RB, eds. *Substance Abuse: A Comprehensive Textbook.* Baltimore: Williams & Wilkins. Pp. 788–793.

Stitzer ML, Iguchi MY, Felch LJ. 1992. Contingent take-home incentive: Effects on drug use of methadone patients. *Journal of Consulting and Clinical Psychology* 60:927–934.

Tyrer P. 1984. Benzodiazepines on trial. *British Medical Journal* 288:1101–1102.

Umbricht-Schneiter A, Ginn DH, Pabst KM, Bigelow GE. 1994. Providing medical care to methadone clinic patients: Referral vs. on-site care. *American Journal of Public Health* 84(2):207–210.

Van Stelle KR, Mauser E, Moberg DP. 1994. Recidivism to the criminal justice system of substance-abusing offenders diverted into treatment. *Crime and Delinquency* 40:175–196.

Volpicelli JR, Alterman AI, Hayashida M, O'Brien CP. 1992. Naltrexone in the treatment of alcohol dependence. *Archives of General Psychiatry* 46:876–880.

Washton AM. 1989. *Cocaine Addiction: Treatment, Recovery and Relapse Prevention*. New York: W. W. Norton.

Weisner C, Schmidt L. 1992. Gender disparities in treatment for alcohol problems. *Journal of the American Medical Association* 268(14):1872–1876.

WHO (World Health Organization). 1992. *International Statistical Classification of Diseases and Related Health Problems*. 10th Revision. Geneva: WHO.

Woody G, Cacciola J. 1994. Review of remission criteria. In: Widiger T, Frances A, Pincus H, First M, Ross R, Davis W, eds. *DSM-IV Sourcebook, Vol. 1*. Washington, DC: American Psychiatric Association Press. Pp. 81–92.

Woody GE, Luborsky L, McLellan AT, O'Brien CP, Beck AT, Blaine J, Herman I, Hole A. 1983. Psychotherapy for opiate addicts: Does it help? *Archives of General Psychiatry* 40:639–645.

Woody GE, McLellan AT, Luborsky L, O'Brien CP, Blaine J, Fox S, Herman I, Beck AT. 1984. Psychiatric severity as a predictor of benefits from psychotherapy: The Penn-VA study. *American Journal of Psychiatry* 141:1172–1177.

Woody GE, McLellan AT, Bedrick J. 1995a. Dual diagnosis. *Annual Review of Psychiatry* 14:83–104.

Woody GE, McLellan AT, Luborsky L, O'Brien CP. 1995b. Psychotherapy in community methadone programs: A validation study. *American Journal of Psychiatry* 159:1302–1308.

Woody GE, McNicholas LF, Vocci F, eds. 1996. *Guidelines for Research Involving Medications for the Treatment of Drug Addiction*. Accepted by the Pilot Drug Evaluation Program and under review by the Food and Drug Administration.

9

Managed Care

Managed care has become an important trend in drug abuse treatment. In response to the escalating costs of treatment, managed care proposes to contain costs, increase access, and ensure quality. It entails many changes from traditional fee-for-service coverage, including changes in the organization, financing, and delivery of services—most recognizably through case management, which seeks to match patients to the most appropriate, yet least restrictive, treatment setting.

Despite its enormous growth, there is a dearth of peer-reviewed research about whether managed drug abuse care is achieving these goals. Due to the proprietary nature of data collected by private managed care organizations and the competitive managed care market, most of the studies conducted to date are from Medicaid or other publicly subsidized programs. Further, research has not addressed concerns about patients being denied treatment or being undertreated; the quality of care being reduced; or the cost of care being shifted to families, public health and welfare agencies, and the criminal justice system (Mechanic et al., 1995). Evaluations of the performance of managed care are largely in the form of anecdotal reports, proprietary evaluations, and studies published in journals that are not peer reviewed. The paucity of independent, peer-reviewed research on a topic of such pervasive importance presents health services researchers with an opportunity to provide crucial information to policymakers, payers, providers, and consumers.

This chapter describes the modest body of research on the topic, relying exclusively on government-sponsored or peer-reviewed, published research. It identifies significant research opportunities in areas such as access, costs, utilization, and treatment outcomes, including quality of care. It also examines the formidable barriers to research and the need to ensure the rapid translation of research results into clinical practice. This chapter uses the term "managed drug abuse care" to refer to the drug abuse component of managed *behavioral* health care, the branch of managed care that administratively combines the traditionally separate areas of drug abuse and mental health.

OVERVIEW

Managed behavioral health care is characterized by a variety of approaches designed to control the cost of services by altering the treatment decisions of both patients and providers (IOM, 1989; Mechanic et al., 1995). There is no single model of managed behavioral health care, and the various approaches are evolving rapidly in a dynamic and highly competitive market, thereby hampering research efforts to characterize them and to evaluate their impact. The overall goal is to alter the orientation and restrain the costs of behavioral health care through changes in the organization, financing, and delivery of services. By incorporating the elements of managed care, which are described later in this section, projected costs can be reduced by up to 30 or 40 percent, according to some industry estimates (Geraty et al., 1994).

Virtually unheard of a decade ago, the burgeoning industry of managed behavioral health care is estimated to cover more than 102 million people across the United States, most of whom are insured under employer-sponsored private health insurance (Oss, 1994). This estimate represents the majority of those covered under employer health care plans, given that 143 million people in the U.S. population have such coverage (CRS, 1994). The figure of 120 million enrollees refers to those eligible individuals whose private or public insurance covers managed behavioral health care, not to those who receive treatment. According to a recent, nationally representative survey, about 50 percent of specialty drug abuse providers, both publicly and privately owned, report that an average of 23 percent of their clients have their treatment paid for by managed care (T. D'Aunno, University of Chicago, personal communication, 1995).

Managed behavioral health care is offered most commonly through one of two general types of managed care organizations: health maintenance organizations (HMOs) or carve-out vendors (also known as managed behavioral health care organizations or MBHCOs) (Table 9.1). These organizations are under contract mostly to employers and public agencies, which pay for some or all of the cost of care. Carve-out vendors are fiscal and management intermediaries that typically contract with pro-

TABLE 9.1 Managed Behavioral Health Care

Organization	Access	Providers[a]
Carve-out vendor →	EAP, 24-hour toll-free number or primary care professional →	Networks
↑ Carve-out of behavioral health care		
HMOs →	Primary care professional or mental health staff →	Staff or IPA[b]

NOTE: EAP = Employee assistance program.

[a]Institutions, programs, and practitioners.
[b] Independent practice association, a group of office-based practitioners who operate on a fixed budget under contract to an HMO.

SOURCES: Freeman and Trabin (1994); Suzanne Gelber, Brandeis University, personal communication (1996).

viders for the actual delivery of mental health and drug abuse services through groups of preferred providers organized as networks. Access to the network is controlled by a "gatekeeper" (typically a primary care physician, an evaluation counselor, or a professional with an employee assistance program) who assesses the need for treatment and is responsible for referrals; it is critical that the gatekeeper function be performed by someone credentialed in drug abuse treatment. Carve-out vendors may be specialized units within larger managed care organizations, or they may function independently. It would appear that at each stage in the contracting and subcontracting of treatment there would be additional administrative costs that are not being put into treatment.

Staff model HMOs (those HMOs with salaried staff on-site) have traditionally provided managed behavioral health care through their own staff. Increasingly, however, both staff model HMOs and independent practice association (IPA) HMOs[1] are entering into contracts or joint ventures with carve-out vendors to administer and deliver behavioral health

[1]These are groups of office-based practitioners that operate on a fixed budget and contain many elements of managed care.

care. Likewise, a traditional fee-for-service (or indemnity) medical insurer may "carve out" behavioral health care through a contract with a carve-out vendor. In such a plan, which accounts for almost 30 percent of managed behavioral plans, the behavioral health care benefit is managed via a network even though other health care benefits in the same plan are not (Foster Higgins, Inc., 1994).

Despite the diversity of managed behavioral health care models, they share four common elements that derive from broader managed care principles (Shueman and Troy, 1994): (1) selective contracting, (2) mechanisms for monitoring or managing services, (3) financing structure, and (4) benefit structure (described below).

Selective Contracting

Managed care organizations refer drug abuse patients to selected individual and institutional providers with whom the companies have negotiated set fees for service, either at a discount from standard rates or on a capitated basis (see below). Patients are penalized financially for using providers outside the network, and the in-network benefits package and provider network tend to be more inclusive and comprehensive. In addition to establishing fees, the contracts between organizations and providers stipulate the providers' roles in adhering to the organization's protocols and procedures for managing patient care, reporting results, and allowing the organization to audit care on a confidential basis.

Mechanisms for Monitoring or Managing Services

These procedures ensure the necessity, appropriateness, and quality of care. They typically involve readmission review; utilization management to refer patients to the most appropriate providers and medically necessary services; utilization management prior to, during, and after discharge from inpatient or 24-hour care; and intensive case management of complex or high-risk cases.

Financing Structure

Managed care organizations commonly operate on a fixed administrative fee basis, on a budget referred to as "capitation" (a flat dollar fee per covered beneficiary), or on a flat fee per case. Rates are negotiated in advance with the employer or entity that hires the managed behavioral health care organization. When the expected rate is exceeded, the managed care organization assumes some or all of the financial risk. This financial risk is sometimes shared "downward" with network practitioners. Risk sharing is intended to provide incentives to deliver cost-effective and innovative services.

Benefit Structure

A benefit plan outlines the services and providers that are covered and the terms of coverage (e.g., beneficiary deductibles or copayments; service duration or limits). Under managed care, the benefit plan usually is designed to give incentives to both patients and providers for early intervention (although this often has not been the case for illicit drug and alcohol dependence), the use of network providers, and the use of services consistent with medical efficacy.

An important element is whether drug abuse benefits are offered as part of an integrated medical plan—a "carve-in" policy—or whether they are separated (like dental care) from other medical services in a "carve-out" policy. Carve-in policies, most common in staff model HMOs, offer the potential advantages of increased provider communication and coordination, destigmatization, and accounting for cost offsets (reduced medical costs stemming from treatment of the drug abuse).[2] Carve-in policies are potentially advantageous for drug-abusing patients with medical or psychiatric problems (e.g., compliance with antituberculosis therapy has been shown to be most effective when patients' daily medication is directly observed by a health care provider in the context of a treatment program) (Chaulk et al., 1995). It is less burdensome on the patient and more fruitful for public health, because of better compliance, when patients can obtain their primary care and drug abuse treatment at the same site.

On the other hand, carve-out vendors offer the advantages of linkage with employee assistance programs, more specialized medical staff (e.g., medical directors and clinical case managers), more elaborate protocols, more specialized quality management, more extensive customer services and comprehensive network, and the ability to offer a consistent benefit plan anywhere in the United States (S. Gelber, Brandeis University, personal communication, 1996). They also offer a cost-saving alternative for employers who want to retain traditional indemnity medical insurance for employees but feel they cannot afford the expense of unmanaged behavioral health care. One disadvantage is that carve-out vendors may have incentives for cost-shifting,[3] because they usually have no responsi-

---

[2]This assumes that the behavioral health component of care is integrated with the medical component and is not contracted out through a carve-out vendor.

[3]Cost-shifting occurs when the costs of care are transferred from the treatment provider to other health care providers, families, schools, public health and welfare agencies, or the criminal justice system.

bility for the provision and/or funding of patients' medical services (Mechanic et al., 1995). This is also true to a lesser extent for carve-in vendors, because they are generally responsible for all health care services. Another disadvantage is fragmentation of the sites of service delivery, which may prove problematic, especially in emergency situations with suicidal patients, since drug abusers often have co-occurring psychiatric disorders (see Chapter 8) (Regier et al., 1990). Data from the National Comorbidity Study revealed that 41–66 percent of those with a lifetime addictive disorder also have a lifetime history of at least one psychiatric disorder (Kessler et al., 1996). Patients with co-occurring addictive and psychiatric disorders are thought to be treated most effectively in integrated systems of care (Osher, 1996).

Drug abuse practitioners and treatment facilities have not fully embraced managed behavioral health care. Their reasons are varied but likely emanate from concerns about decreased professional autonomy, lower fees, the potential for decreased confidentiality of patient records, and enhanced supervision by individuals who may not be credentialed in drug abuse treatment.

Growth of Drug Abuse Treatment Benefits

By the early 1990s, almost 100 percent of employer health plans in medium and large corporations covered some type of drug abuse benefits, either managed or unmanaged. That was in stark contrast to 1983, when only about 43 percent of employers made such provisions (BLS, 1992, 1994). The growth in drug abuse coverage stemmed from rising employee demand, state mandates, and awareness by employers and clinicians that untreated drug abuse reduces productivity and contributes to absenteeism, health problems, theft, and accidents (IOM, 1995). Drug abuse benefits in conventional, unmanaged indemnity policies were usually subject to special limitations that were more restrictive than general health benefits. The limitations usually pertained to the total number of days of care available per year or to the total dollar amount that could be spent per year, per confinement, or per lifetime. For example, a typical policy restricted inpatient drug abuse care to 30 days per year, restricted outpatient care to 20 to 30 visits per year, and/or contained maximum dollar amounts such as $50,000 per lifetime for all treatment modalities (BLS, 1992, 1994).

By the mid-1980s, managed behavioral health care began to take hold, particularly due to employer pressures for cost containment and the availability of venture capital financing for new carve-out providers (Freeman and Trabin, 1994). Another impetus came from studies showing that many, but not all, drug abuse patients could be treated just as cost-effectively in outpatient settings as they could in more costly inpatient settings (Center of Alcohol Studies, 1993; Alterman et al., 1994). Managed care promised the attractive alternative of lower costs, increased access, and more clinically appropriate treatment. It became so alluring that by the mid-1990s, industry surveys showed private managed behavioral health care enrollment to have increased from 48 million to 60 million over a two-year period (Geraty et al., 1994). Instead of relying on previous benefit plan limitations in treatment dollars or days of coverage, managed care organizations stressed benefit flexibility and patient matching to the most appropriate level of care through individual case management, utilization review, and provider networks. Patient placements were dictated by placement criteria that typically were developed internally but were not made available publicly.

One important means of referral into managed drug abuse care has been through employee assistance programs (EAPs). These are workplace programs, usually paid for by employers, designed to help employees address problems that affect their performance, including drug abuse problems. EAPs began in the 1950s as internal occupational alcohol programs run by recovering alcoholics. They often referred alcohol-dependent employees to self-help groups such as Alcoholics Anonymous (Mucnick-Baku and Traw, 1992). Since then, EAPs have proliferated nationwide and have expanded to address other employee problems. With respect to employee drug use, EAPs typically perform a brief assessment or crisis intervention and make referrals to treatment programs. They may also monitor treatment and provide follow-up counseling as part of continuing care. EAPs generally do not provide treatment services (although some offer short-term counseling); rather, they help to ensure that employees receive the treatment they need and return to productive employment. Some EAPs are internal or external stand-alone programs, whereas others are integrated into a treatment network organized through a carve-out vendor and serve as a gateway to treatment (Freeman and Trabin, 1994). A review of EAPs has been performed by the National Research Council (NRC, 1994).

Public Versus Private Systems

The initial growth in managed behavioral health care originally took place in the private sector, through employer-sponsored health insurance, but this trend is changing rapidly. State and local agencies, which pay for the majority of drug abuse clients in treatment, have been forced by budget pressures to turn to carve-out vendors or HMOs to oversee their programs for low-income drug abusers. In other words, state and local authorities are beginning to purchase services from some of the same organizations under contract to private employers. While it is not known how many Medicaid recipients or other publicly subsidized clients are covered by managed behavioral health care, about 7.8 million (25 percent) Medicaid recipients are enrolled in managed care in general (Rowland et al., 1995). A number of states—including Massachusetts, Ohio, and Minnesota—have developed managed drug abuse care for their Medicaid patients through special waivers from the agency that oversees the Medicaid program, the Health Care Financing Administration (HCFA).[4] About 30 states have waivers approved or pending (Kushner, 1995).

Greater reliance on carve-out vendors and HMOs to manage public and private drug abuse patients may have the potential to reverse the historic separation between privately and publicly funded drug abuse treatment providers. An earlier Institute of Medicine (IOM) report described the drug abuse treatment system as a "two-tiered system" (IOM, 1990). A private tier of providers serves clients who have private health insurance or sufficient resources to pay for expensive treatment out of pocket. The public tier—which accounts for the majority of clients and treatment expenditures (Batten et al., 1992)—serves mostly indigent clients and is made up of publicly owned programs or private not-for-profit programs whose revenues are largely from public agencies. Publicly funded clients are heavier users of drug abuse services than privately funded clients, in part because they enter treatment with a greater degree of impairment and more associated psychiatric and medical problems. They also often lack the financial, social, and emotional resources available to private populations. Among public sector patients, disabled clients who receive Supplemental Security Income use services with far greater intensity than other publicly subsidized clients (Callahan et al., 1994), thus underscoring the importance of associated problems in contributing to the complexity and expense of treatment. It will be important to monitor the outcome of treatment provided to both public and private clients if these sectors are integrated under managed care.

The major stakeholders in managed drug abuse treatment are regulators, payers, managed care organizations, providers, advocates, and clients (Figure 9.1). In a typical example, an employer or public purchaser hires a managed care organization, which in turn contracts with mental health and drug abuse practitioners to offer services to enrollees. In 1992,

[4]Under the Omnibus Budget Reconciliation Act of 1981, states can apply for special waivers exempting them from requirements to give patients their choice of providers. The waivers have enabled states to restrict provider choice in order to develop innovative managed care demonstration programs for Medicaid recipients (CRS, 1993).

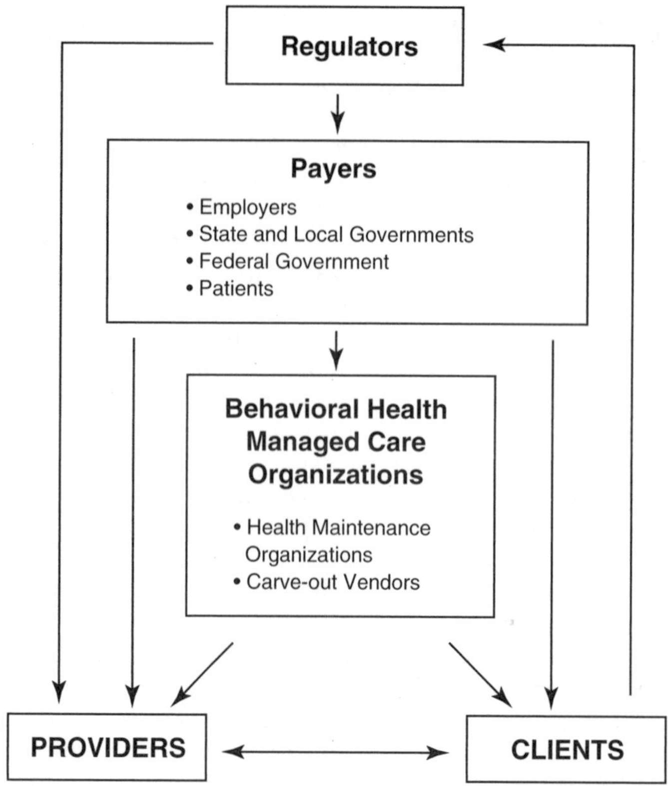

FIGURE 9.1 Stakeholders in behavioral health managed care.

Massachusetts was the first state to transfer all of its non-HMO Medicaid patients to a private carve-out vendor, which established a network of mental health and drug abuse providers. In contrast, the Department of Veterans Affairs (VA) medical centers still function as both the payer for and the provider of a range of drug abuse, psychiatric, and medical treatments in a capitated arrangement. These medical centers operate somewhat like HMOs, but without many of the managed care elements described earlier.

Until there is a solid body of independent research evaluating managed drug abuse care, both the putative benefits and the risks remain unsubstantiated. Thus far, managed drug abuse care has largely eluded scrutiny by the health services research community for reasons described at the end of this chapter. The models of managed drug abuse care are best developed for employed, middle- to upper-class patients. These patients are much less disabled than lower-income, publicly subsidized patients who are likely to have greater treatment needs. However, there is little published information about the most elementary characteristics of managed drug abuse treatment, such as staff–client ratios, staff training, and frequency and duration of services. Even less is known about the impact on patient care of financial incentives to curtail costs. Finally, although managed behavioral health care organizations appear to be increasingly willing to publish their patient placement criteria, little is known about whether these criteria are actually adhered to by those responsible for making placements. Thus, there is a need to undertake studies of the organization, financing, and characteristics of managed drug abuse care.

The committee recommends that the appropriate federal agencies (e.g., the Substance Abuse and Mental Health Services Administration [SAMHSA], the Health Care Financing Administration [HCFA], the National Institute on Drug Abuse [NIDA], and the National Institute on Alcohol Abuse and Alcoholism [NIAAA]) and private organizations undertake studies of the organization, financing, and characteristics of drug abuse treatment in the managed care setting, including variations in the content, intensity, continuum of care, and duration of treatment as they relate to patient needs.

Particular attention needs to be given to well-controlled studies of patient outcomes for private and public sector patients, credentials of gatekeepers, accountability systems, and patient placement criteria.

ACCOMPLISHMENTS AND RESEARCH OPPORTUNITIES

Access, Costs, and Utilization

Four major studies have examined the impact of managed care on access to drug abuse treatment, cost of treatment, and utilization of services. All four were conducted in naturalistic, nonexperimental settings, and three of the four examined Medicaid populations (Table 9.2). These studies were methodologically diverse and examined various models of managed care, but all four compared managed care with unmanaged care and/or alternative models of managed care—the kinds of comparisons that are most compelling for those responsible for choosing among different managed and unmanaged plans for their beneficiaries.

In 1992, Massachusetts instituted a privately contracted managed care program for Medicaid patients. Research on this program documented a 48 percent reduction in drug abuse treatment expenditures per enrollee in the first year of the program, compared with the prior year's fee-for-

TABLE 9.2 Access, Cost, and Utilization Comparisons Between Managed Substance Abuse Treatment and Fee-for-Service Treatment

Study	Comparison Groups	Client Types	Number of Clients	Access	Cost per Enrollee	Utilization
Callahan et al., 1994[a]	Before vs. after	Public	375,000	5%	–48%	IP –69% OP[c] –4% MM[c] 20%
Ellis, 1992[a]	Before vs. after	Private	140,000	–43%	–72%	IP –41% OP 19% OC 54%
Asher et al., 1995[b]	County vs. PPO vs. HMO vs. FFS	Public	10,000	County 4.9% PPO 3.9% HMO 2.0% FFS N/A	County $4,553[c] PPO $5,397 HMO $7,720 FFS $4,840	County 36.7 units PPO 11.7 units HMO 11.8 units FFS 18.6 units
Minnesota Department of Human Services, 1995[b]	Fund (FFS) vs. prepaid	Public	740[d]	N/A	N/A	Fund IP 48% Fund OP 52% Prepaid IP 27% Prepaid OP 73%

IP = inpatient; N/A= not applicable; OC = office claims; OP = outpatient; PPO = preferred provider organization.

[a]These studies were before- and after-comparisons; data are presented in relative values.
[b]These studies compared several plans during one time period; data are presented in absolute values.
[c]Cost per client instead of cost per enrollee.
[d]1994 clients only.

service (FFS) system (Callahan et al., 1994). This average decrease reflected a 67 percent reduction in expenditures for 24-hour care and an 8 percent increase in outpatient expenditures per enrollee. Access, as measured by the number of service users for every 1,000 enrollees, increased by 4.6 percent.[5] Inpatient length of stay declined by 25.4 percent. Inpatient admissions for drug abuse treatment declined by 69 percent from the prior year, much of which was attributed to the program's provision for detoxification in nonhospital settings (where utilization surged). Denial of request for 24-hour care was about 7 percent at the beginning of the program but declined to about 3 percent by the end of the first year. Because of the absence of data from the prior year, there was no basis for comparison with denials in the earlier FFS program, which was also the case with quality of care. Nevertheless, providers perceived quality improvements relative to the FFS system, according to a provider survey included in the analysis.

Some of those same trends were found in the second year of the managed care program. Enrollment increased by 3 percent, and there was a gain in access of 5 percent (in terms of the number of users per 1,000 enrollees) compared with the first year (Beinecke et al., 1995). Inpatient utilization continued to decline, but acute residential days increased by 72 percent. Expenditures for inpatient and outpatient drug abuse care declined by 32 and 9 percent, respectively. Surveys of providers and patients reinforced the earlier year's perception of improved access and quality.

A study of privately insured patients found some similar results (Ellis, 1992). This study took advantage of a natural experiment by a private employer whose health coverage extended to 140,000 employees, retirees, and dependents. The employer mandated managed drug abuse and mental health benefits through a preferred provider organization (PPO) at the beginning of the third year of this four-year study (1986–1990). Access, cost, and utilization were compared between year two and year four. For drug abuse treatment, the study found that access—as measured by the number of patients per 1,000 enrollees—declined by 43 percent. This dramatic decline was most likely the result of an increase in the average charge per inpatient episode of treatment, leading fewer to seek treatment, rather than to patients' being denied treatment. The average charges per enrollee declined by 72 percent over the two-year period, from $778 to $216. The decrease was attributed to reductions in the number of patients seeking treatment, the number of episodes per patient, and the average

[5]The study authors point out, however, that the access figures might be skewed because of an increase in the proportion of disabled enrollees, who tend to use more services.

charges per episode. Correspondingly, inpatient episodes per patient declined by 41 percent, outpatient episodes increased by 19 percent, and office visit claims increased by 54 percent. Clearly, the paramount finding of the study was the significant decline in drug abuse treatment costs per enrollee.

A third study examined the Minnesota Consolidated Chemical Dependency Treatment Fund, which pooled different funding streams for publicly subsidized drug abuse clients who had previously been treated in a patchwork of programs with varying requirements for eligibility and service delivery. The Minnesota fund operated on a FFS basis but incorporated standardized assessment and treatment placement criteria, features of managed care. The fund increased access by about 30 percent and was associated with lower costs per treated client relative to prior years (Minnesota Department of Human Services, 1993).

Because of perceived opportunities for further cost savings, the Minnesota fund is being phased out in favor of legally mandated prepaid plans. This transition was examined in a study comparing a sample of prepaid plan admissions with a matched, randomly selected sample of fund admissions; both plans have the same patient placement criteria (Minnesota Department of Human Services, 1995). The study examined treatment placement, completion, and length of stay each year over a three-year period. In 1994, prepaid clients were far less likely to be placed in inpatient settings (27 percent for prepaid plan clients versus 48 percent for fund clients). Correspondingly, 73 percent of prepaid admissions were to the outpatient setting, compared with 52 percent of fund admissions. There were no differences in severity of inpatient admissions, treatment completion rate, or outpatient length of stay. Neither access, cost, nor outcome comparisons were made between the two programs in this study.

The fourth study is the only one thus far to compare several different models of managed care with a FFS model (Figure 9.2; Asher et al., 1995). The study was the outgrowth of a Pennsylvania law, passed in 1988, that was designed to provide Medicaid patients with a broader continuum of drug abuse care. Before passage of the legislation, Medicaid clients were restricted to costly hospital-based services, methadone maintenance, and outpatient drug-free services; they were denied access to short- and long-term residential services. When the new statewide system was implemented, Medicaid enrollees were assigned to one of four types of providers: a county agency, an HMO, a PPO, or a FFS.[6] The first three groups

[6]The study referred to the county provider as a "single county authority." This was a local agency responsible for the coordination and monitoring of drug and alcohol services, which were provided under contract by local providers. It received county, state, and federal block grant funds. The PPO was referred to as a "health insuring organization." It functioned as a fiscal intermediary which also contracted with local providers.

had varying features of managed care, whereas the FFS group was considered the "control" group. The county providers used a mix of managed and unmanaged elements; they operated on a fixed budget and used a case manager to assign patients to the most appropriate care, but each service was reimbursed on an FFS basis.

Drug abuse treatment services were provided to 10,000 clients over the course of an 18-month study period from 1990 to 1991. The demographic characteristics of each study group were similar, but the pretreatment level of drug abuse severity was unknown (except for county clients). Measures of access, cost, and utilization were examined retrospectively (see next section for discussion of outcome findings), and on all of these measures, county clients fared the best and HMO clients fared the worst.

County clients experienced the highest degree of access (4.9 percent of eligible recipients), followed by PPO clients (3.9 percent) and then by HMO clients (2 percent); the degree of access was not documented for FFS clients. County patients also received the greatest average number of units of service for the lowest average cost per client, followed by FFS patients and then by PPO patients; the HMO provided the least amount of services for the greatest cost per patient (Figure 9.2). A unit of service was calculated by a special formula that created comparability across different service modalities. The FFS group received the most inpatient care, whereas the HMO group received the least. HMO patients with the greatest need for services were given intensive outpatient treatment almost exclusively, an option not available to the four other groups of patients.

The four studies described in this section allow some tentative conclusions. All of the studies reported lower costs in managed drug abuse care relative to traditional FFS plans. In almost all of the studies, there appeared to be a shift in the delivery of treatment from inpatient to outpatient settings. These findings are consistent with those of a comprehensive literature analysis of managed care plan performance since 1980 for all medical services (Miller and Luft, 1994).

Nevertheless, the studies described in this section were not rigorous from an experimental point of view. All were performed in naturalistic settings in which random assignment was not possible, and there were no controls for patient severity. Furthermore, the types of managed care plan under study varied widely. In light of those limitations, it is difficult to draw firm conclusions—or to extrapolate findings—about access, cost, and utilization. There also are virtually no data on the extent of denial of treatment and its impact, a topic discussed later in this chapter.

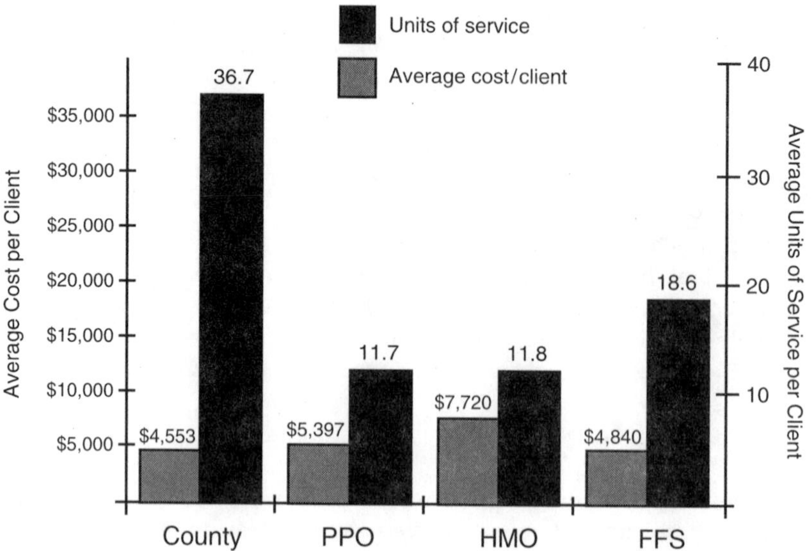

FIGURE 9.2 Cost and utilization comparisons of three managed care models and a fee-for-service model for Pennsylvania Medicaid patients. The county model had the lowest average cost per client for the highest average number of units of service. The second best performer was the fee-for-service model, which had the second lowest cost and the second highest units of service. SOURCE: Asher et al. (1995).

The committee recommends that the appropriate federal agencies (e.g., SAMHSA, NIDA, NIAAA) and private organizations support research on the impact of drug abuse treatment in the managed care setting, including studies on: client access, costs, and utilization; effectiveness and cost-effectiveness of drug abuse treatment under managed care; quality of drug abuse treatment in the managed care setting and its impact on treatment outcomes; development of uniformly accepted patient placement criteria that have predictive validity; and denial of treatment, undertreatment, and cost-shifting practices by providers of managed care (including comparisons between carve-in and carve-out vendors).

Outcomes

Policymakers and employers are placing increasing emphasis on monitoring treatment outcomes under all health care delivery systems, both managed and unmanaged. The purposes of studying outcomes are

TABLE 9.3 Measures of Treatment Effectiveness

Reduction in drug use
Abstinence from drug use
Completion of drug treatment
Readmission to drug treatment
Time until readmission to treatment
Client satisfaction with treatment
Improvement in health status and well-being
Improvement in employment and productivity
Reduction in criminal activity

to determine treatment effectiveness and cost-effectiveness, to improve program performance on the basis of quality, and to improve resource allocation. With those purposes in mind, this section discusses research on the most important outcomes of managed drug abuse care, namely, effectiveness, cost-effectiveness, quality of care, cost offsets, and cost-shifting.

Effectiveness

A universal question asked of managed care is, Does it work? However, the more appropriate questions facing employers and policymakers are slightly different. They need to decide, from among many competing plans, which plan offers the most effective services for their beneficiaries. The key questions are, Does managed care work compared to fee-for-service care? and What models of managed care are more effective than others? Measures of the effectiveness of drug abuse treatment, which are used in one or more of the studies cited in this chapter, are listed in Table 9.3.

The first evidence of the effectiveness of managed behavioral health care came from the mental health field. The Medical Outcome Study, a large two-year observational study, compared prepaid care with FFS care for a variety of chronic medical illnesses, including depression.[7] The depression component of the study, which evaluated treatment outcomes for 617 depressed patients, found no differences in treatment effectiveness between the two payment systems when patients were treated by

[7]There were no baseline differences in psychological and physical sicknesses between patients in prepaid care and FFS care. FFS care was provided by solo practitioners and by large, multispecialty groups. Prepaid care was provided by group practice HMOs, large multispecialty groups, and IPAs.

psychologists and general medical clinicians (Rogers et al., 1993). However, patients with more severe psychiatric disorders, who tended to be treated by psychiatrists, fared worse under prepaid care; those patients used less antidepressant medication over time and had greater limitations in role and physical functioning. Because there was no difference in the baseline degree of impairment between FFS and prepaid patients seen by psychiatrists, the investigators concluded that the differences in outcomes were based on the care received. This conclusion prompted investigators to recommend that policymakers focus attention on patients with the highest levels of impairment.

Two published studies have addressed the effectiveness of managed drug abuse care. The first, described earlier, examined treatment effectiveness in relation to treatment modality in Pennsylvania Medicaid clients (Asher et al., 1995). Treatment modality was a proxy for different types of managed care providers because each provider relied more heavily on one type of modality. The outcome measures covered criminal activity, economic status, medical care, and readmission to drug and alcohol treatment. Comparing the post- with the pretreatment period, the study found that intensive outpatient treatment (which was provided only by HMOs) was the least effective modality, whereas 24-hour long-term residential treatment—a combination of case management techniques and FFS reimbursement—was the most effective modality.

Another study examined the relative effectiveness of managed care and unmanaged care models provided at a single facility for drug abuse treatment, the Castle Medical Center in Hawaii (Renz et al., 1995). Researchers undertook a retrospective review of 1,594 patient records in order to examine treatment outcome and length of stay. Treatment outcome was defined in this study in terms of recidivism (i.e., the return to treatment at the same or higher level of care at any time within the two-year study period [January 1, 1990, through December 31, 1991]). Castle Medical Center afforded the opportunity to study the impact of managed care because it provided treatment to four separate groups of patients that were distinguished on the basis of reimbursement mechanisms: intensive managed care, traditional managed care, private pay, and state funded.

The study found that, with respect to recidivism, there were no differences among the four groups in spite of significant baseline differences in age, gender, marital status, and ethnicity. The analysis revealed no significant interactions between these demographic variables and the study findings. In fact, the highest degree of recidivism was dictated not by method of payment but by patient severity (i.e., a high number of ICD-9 [International Classification of Diseases] diagnoses at baseline). With respect to length of stay (defined as the total number of days spent in treatment converted into weighted hours by a special formula), significant differences among the four groups emerged. The state-funded group had the shortest length of stay, followed by the intensive managed care group and then the traditional managed care group. This suggested to the authors that the state-funded and intensive managed care patients could be treated at lower cost than the traditional managed care patients without compromising treatment effectiveness, although they noted that other outcome measures should be studied besides recidivism.

One of the greatest problems in using client records is the lack of measures of treatment effectiveness. Relapse is a common measure used in research because it is one of the few objective outcome measures for which data are readily available. The Addiction Severity Index, which is one of the most comprehensive and commonly used research instruments for measuring effectiveness, takes about 45–60 minutes to administer at baseline and about 20 minutes at follow-up. It requires administration by a trained technician. Due to the length of time and cost, this type of research instrument would not be feasible in routine clinical use for a variety of reasons. One new outcome instrument, which is being developed to assess the effectiveness of alcoholism treatment, requires only 5 minutes for the average clinician to complete and 20 minutes for the average patient (Rost et al., 1996). There is a critical need for similar, easy-to-administer instruments that measure the effectiveness of drug abuse treatment in clinical settings.

One outcome study that did use the Addiction Severity Index, but has not yet been published, compared the effectiveness of FFS drug abuse treatment with that of HMOs. In 1991, when the study began, 75 percent of the study population—Philadelphia Medicaid patients treated by 11 separate programs—were FFS patients; by 1995, 70 percent were treated by HMOs. Each year randomly selected samples of patients were followed through treatment and for six months postdischarge. Since the dramatic shift to managed care was not foreseen at the start of this study, comparisons between FFS and HMO treatment were considered to be inadvertent findings. Patients treated in 1995 received fewer services and experienced worse outcomes relative to those treated in the first year of the study, which suggests superior treatment under FFS (T. McLellan, University of Pennsylvania, personal communication, 1996).

Cost-Effectiveness

The cost-effectiveness outcome measure provides an economic evaluation by comparing alternative treatments to determine which produces a desired outcome for the lowest cost (Center of Alcohol Studies, 1993). There have been only two studies of cost-effectiveness of managed drug abuse care, both performed at the VA medical center in Philadelphia (Alterman et al., 1994, 1996). VA medical centers operate somewhat like HMOs insofar as they have a fixed annual budget, but they do not incorporate many of the other features of managed care presented earlier. Therefore, the studies described below might be characterized as comparisons between different treatment modalities or intensities, rather than between different models of managed care. They are included here primarily because of their methodological value for future research and the absence of other published cost-effectiveness studies.

The first study compared the costs and effectiveness of day-hospital and inpatient treatment for cocaine dependence. Day-hospital treatment, which consisted of 27 hours per week of treatment, was far less costly than inpatient treatment, which consisted of 48 hours per week. The subjects, 111 male veterans, were assigned randomly to one of the two treatments, after excluding subjects who refused to be randomized and those with the most severe dependence and associated problems (because it would have been unethical and inappropriate to randomize them). This study is unusual because it is the only one described in this chapter to have used random assignment.

The study found no significant differences between day-hospital and inpatient treatment in terms of effectiveness; both were effective at reducing drug use and improving psychological functioning and health status for mildly and moderately impaired patients (Alterman et al., 1994). For example, six months after the one month of treatment, 53 percent of day-hospital and 47 percent of inpatient clients were abstinent from cocaine usage, as determined by the follow-up Addiction Severity Index and urinalysis. There were no significant differences between the two groups on entry into the study, including measures of drug use and social functioning. The most profound difference was the cost. The one-month episode of day-hospital treatment cost providers $2,260, whereas the episode of inpatient treatment cost $6,146. Researchers concluded that day-hospital treatment was more cost-effective, although they still viewed inpatient treatment as best for patients with serious physical, psychiatric, and/or motivational problems, since day-hospital clients were found to be less likely to complete the recommended course of treatment.

A follow-up study compared a scaled-down version of day-hospital treatment (12 hours per week) with an even less intensive outpatient regimen of 6 hours per week (Alterman et al., 1996). The treatments lasted four weeks and the follow-up took place three months after treatment entry. The 50 cocaine-dependent subjects were not assigned randomly, but a random assignment study is now in progress. Contrary to expectations, both groups had similar outcomes on measures of drug use, psychological functioning, and health status. In addition, there were no differences between the two groups in program attendance, treatment completion, or baseline demographic and drug use measures. Given its lower cost and similar effectiveness, outpatient treatment offered at this lower level of intensity was clearly more cost-effective, but without random assignment and a longer follow-up period, the investigators did not view the results as generalizable.

Quality of Care

Another fundamental question about managed care models is whether they increase or decrease the quality of care relative to FFS care. The answer is likely to depend on what indicator of quality is used, how it is measured, and the model of managed care that is studied. Some of the major indicators of quality relate to patient satisfaction, time to relapse, and severity of relapse. Other quality indicators relate to the process of care delivery, such as the credentials of providers, the appropriateness of placement, and adherence to practice guidelines (Shueman and Troy, 1994).

Very few studies have examined the quality of managed drug abuse care; some have been cited earlier in this chapter. In the study of managed care versus FFS coverage for the Massachusetts Medicaid population, researchers used readmission rates to 24-hour care as a proxy measure for quality, under the assumption that inadequate treatment would necessitate readmission in a short period (Callahan et al., 1994). No significant differences in quality were found, because readmission rates within 30, 60, and 90 days of discharge were similar under both systems (the data were combined for mental health and drug abuse patients). However, this period of time may not have been sufficient to capture the extent of readmission, because a significant number of relapses occur between three and six months after treatment completion (Woody and Cacciola, 1994). Renz and coworkers (1995) also defined quality in terms of recidivism rates, finding no differences between managed and unmanaged patients.

A study by independent researchers in 1990 found the content of managed care practices to vary considerably (Garnick et al., 1994b). This telephone survey of 31 managed behavioral health care firms found a broad range of professionals to be responsible for case management. Researchers were not able to identify the percentage of cases to which a case manager with specialized qualifications in drug abuse or mental health treatment was assigned. The study found large variations in utilization review programs. In terms of clinical criteria for authorizing admissions, all firms had requirements for timeliness in responding to patient and practitioner requests, but many held their actual criteria confidential. In the time since this survey was done, however, managed behavioral health care firms have become more forthcoming about the release of their placement criteria (SAMHSA, 1995).

In one of the few studies of patient placements in a mental health setting, Thompson and coworkers (1992) studied the level of care to which 9,055 patients were assigned by one carve-out vendor. This 30-month study found that over time, more and more patients were being referred away from inpatient care without regard to severity, reflecting a policy decision to limit the use of inpatient services. This finding prompted the authors to question the quality of the care provided by the vendor.

Appropriate placement criteria are viewed as an important measure of quality and an important predictor of treatment outcome (SAMHSA, 1995). That is why there is a major emphasis on identifying placement criteria that could be adopted uniformly by all drug abuse treatment providers, including managed care organizations. One set of criteria, prepared by the American Society of Addiction Medicine and used by many managed care organizations, addresses a broad continuum of care. These criteria were developed by a consensus group, and although they are not universally accepted, they are viewed by the drug abuse field as a stepping stone to the creation of a new generation of uniform placement criteria (SAMHSA, 1995). Currently there is a large randomized trial to determine their predictive validity (D. Gastfriend, Massachusetts General Hospital, personal communication, 1995). However, placement criteria alone do not ensure quality placements. The experience, judgment, and credentials of those who make placement decisions, as well as the fiscal incentives under which they operate, are likely to play important roles. These factors have not been investigated thus far.

Accrediting organizations and the managed behavioral health care industry itself are becoming more active in quality assurance. Initiatives are under way by the National Committee on Quality Assurance and by the Joint Commission on Accreditation of Health Care Organizations. Through its member association, the American Managed Behavioral Healthcare Association, the industry has announced plans to release its first standardized "report card" on access, consumer satisfaction, and preliminary indicators of quality. Member companies have agreed to collect data on up to 30 distinct measures, thus enabling comparisons to be made about their performance.

Medical Cost Offsets

Medical cost offsets are defined as reductions in other areas of medical care utilization as a result of treatment in a given area. The opportunities for cost offsets with drug abuse treatment are potentially vast because of the array of medical conditions associated with untreated dependence, including AIDS, tuberculosis, and fetal effects (see Chapter 7). At least 60 medical conditions can be caused, in whole or in part, by alcohol, tobacco, and illicit drugs (Fox et al., 1995).

Research reveals that treatment for psychiatric disorders and alcoholism significantly lowers medical care utilization for patients covered by both HMOs and traditional FFS arrangements (Jones and Vischi, 1979; Holder and Blose, 1992; Hoffman et al., 1993). Families of treated alcoholics also experience lower medical care utilization (Holder and Hallan, 1986; Spear and Mason, 1991). Drug abuse treatment is associated with lower subsequent medical costs, but there are fewer studies and they often do not separate the impact of alcohol versus illicit drug dependence and treatment. Yu and coworkers (1991) found reductions in medical costs for one group of privately insured patients treated for illicit drug and/or alcohol problems. A large study of publicly funded drug abuse treatment programs in California found reductions in health care costs of 23.5 percent following treatment (Gerstein et al., 1994). This study also found large offsets in criminal justice system costs due to reductions in illegal behavior.

With the advent of managed care, there is greater potential for realizing cost offsets. The reason for this possibility is managed care's emphasis on accountability and the appropriateness of treatment (i.e., tailoring treatments to each individual client's needs [Mechanic et al., 1995]). Capturing cost offsets is more likely for carve-in policies, in which the provider covers drug abuse, mental health, and medical treatment. The provider stands to realize significant reductions in overall medical care utilization by treated patients and their families. Carve-out vendors do not realize these savings themselves and, thus, may have financial incentives to shift health care costs to other health care providers, a topic discussed in more detail in the next section.

Cost-Shifting

Cost-shifting occurs when the costs of care are transferred from the treatment provider to other health care providers, families, schools, public health and welfare agencies, or the criminal justice system. If, for example, a patient is denied coverage for treatment or is covered insufficiently, the patient or family may have to pay for treatment costs. If the patient and the family are unable to pay for treatment and no financial assistance is offered, the dependence can go untreated. Untreated drug abuse places a great burden on society in terms of lost productivity and additional criminal activity, as well as health care costs (IOM, 1995). Involuntary discharge of opioid-dependent clients from methadone programs, which were publicly financed and unmanaged, resulted in higher rates of readdiction and higher arrests and incarceration rates, according to several studies (Prendergast et al., in press).

It is simply not known whether some types of managed care contribute to, reduce, or have no effect on cost-shifting. Carve-out firms may have incentives for cost-shifting because they do not bear the consequences (Mechanic et al., 1995). The extent of cost-shifting is difficult to identify and track because the costs can appear in many different areas. One of the many problems is that untreated drug dependence can lead to loss of jobs and loss of private health benefits, at which point the paper trail ceases.

BARRIERS TO RESEARCH

Problems abound in conducting research on the impact of managed care on drug abuse treatment. The problems fall under two general areas: (1) access to and utility of data and (2) variations in coverage. These problems are so intractable, and research funding is so competitive, that academic researchers face hurdles in securing research grants from NIDA, NIAAA, and SAMHSA, all of which are under fiscal constraints. Consequently, little research has been undertaken, as demonstrated throughout this chapter.

In terms of data access, one problem is the proprietary nature of data collected by managed care organizations treating privately insured patients. It is for this reason that most of the studies cited in this chapter are from Medicaid or other publicly subsidized programs. Managed care organizations offering private coverage are reluctant to grant researchers access to their data, given the highly competitive market in which they operate and their concerns about protecting patient confidentiality. The records of public providers can also be difficult to access at times because of the fragmentation in sources of payment. For example, records for a facility's Medicaid patients are kept separate from those for patients funded by local, state, and federal block grants. Loss of coverage from one source of payment means that patients must be switched to different payment systems that often carry different eligibility and benefit structures. It becomes very difficult to follow public patients during a treatment episode or through repeated episodes. The fragmentation of payment systems and the desultory impact on treatment propelled the State of Minnesota to create a special consolidated fund that was described earlier in this chapter.

Even if researchers gain access to patient data, problems do not cease. Administrative data sets containing claims and utilization information are often separate from medical records. The records may be incomplete, sometimes lacking important information—such as whether a drug abuse diagnosis refers to alcohol, other drugs, or both. Records often lack information about whether the patient has a co-occurring psychiatric disorder. Since people with co-occurring psychiatric disorders and drug abuse account for a sizable proportion of the mental health and drug abuse populations in treatment—and for much higher than average utilization and charges—their inclusion in a sample of drug abusers might skew findings (Garnick et al., in press). Some of the additional problems faced by researchers are the failure to capture and detail utilization; missing information about deductibles and prescription drug claim data (usually handled by a separate data system); sparse demographic data; and lack of information about benefits (Garnick et al., 1994a).

Variations in benefit plans pose other problems. Coverage may change over time under the same plan, leading to different patterns of utilization. There are variations in benefits and in placement criteria across different plans, thus making it difficult to aggregate patients from different plans, even in the same treatment facility. This compromises the ability to carry out large-scale studies.

There is some cause for optimism, however, as managed behavioral health care organizations become more receptive to uniform patient placement criteria (SAMHSA, 1995). Uniformity will enable greater ease in comparing disparate patient populations. Employers and policymakers are requiring more attention to tracking of patient outcomes in contracts with managed care organizations. Additionally, managed behavioral health care organizations are expanding their use of information technology, a trend that is expected to improve large-scale data collection and electronic interchange (Freeman and Trabin, 1994). The industry's member association has embarked on the design of a common data set. Finally, as the public sector moves toward greater reliance on private managed behavioral health care organizations to administer treatment for publicly subsidized patients, there are likely to be heightened requirements for data collection, analysis, and dissemination. These changes may provide a more favorable environment in which to conduct research.

One innovative strategy for research is greater reliance on modeling, by using strategies analogous to those used to predict prevalence or health costs of other diseases such as AIDS. Modeling would obviate the need for access to all medical records. Modeling might be particularly useful in comparing the costs of patient care in different types of managed care. For example, patient assessment could be used to yield diagnoses and needs for care. The costs for treatment of drug abuse and associated psychiatric and medical problems could then be estimated under different scenarios, such as carve-in versus carve-out care.

Managed care organizations may also become interested in forming partnerships with the public sector in data collection and analysis. Both public and private agencies appear to be eager to use the fruits of research in more rational program design and to promote managed care as a means of improving access, preserving quality, and lowering costs. Once these improved data sets are in place, researchers will for the first time be in a position to confirm or refute the allegations of cost-shifting, denial of treatment, and undertreatment under managed drug abuse care.

In light of the formidable barriers to the conduct of research, the committee recommends that the appropriate federal agencies (e.g., SAMHSA, NIDA, NIAAA) and private organizations work together to develop innovative research strategies and funding mechanisms to ensure that research proceeds on the impact of drug abuse treatment in the managed care setting. Innovative funding mechanisms may include contracts, memoranda of understanding, and public–private partnerships.

CONCLUSION

The only definitive conclusion to be reached on the pivotal claims of managed health care—that it enhances access, lowers cost, and ensures quality—is that there are insufficient data. The modest body of research does point to lower costs and less reliance on inpatient care. However, treatment outcomes are still unknown due to the current lack of research on the effectiveness and cost-effectiveness of managed care treatment. Additionally, there is no research on what could potentially be inadequacies in managed drug abuse care: denial of treatment; undertreatment; and cost shifting to other providers, public health and welfare agencies, and the criminal justice system. The committee urges appropriate federal and private agencies to undertake the studies recommended throughout this chapter.

REFERENCES

Alterman AI, O'Brien CP, McLellan AT, August DS, Snider EC, Droba M, Cornish JW, Hall CP, Raphaelson AH, Schrade FX. 1994. Effectiveness and costs of inpatient versus day hospital cocaine rehabilitation. *Journal of Nervous and Mental Disease* 182(3):157–163.

Alterman AI, Snider EC, Cacciola JS, May DJ, Parikh G, Maâny I, Rosenbaum PR. 1996. A quasi experimental comparison of the effectiveness of 6- versus 12-hour per week outpatient treatments for cocaine dependence. *Journal of Nervous and Mental Disease* 184(1):54–56.

Asher M, Friedman N, Lysionek C, Peters C. 1995. *Evaluation of the Implementation of Pennsylvania's Act 152. 1988. The Quantitative Findings*. Villanova, PA: Human Organization Science Institute, Villanova University.

Batten H, Prottas J, Horgan CM, Simon LJ, Larson MJ, Elliott EA, Marsden ME. 1992. *Drug Services Research Survey Final Report: Phase II*. Contract number 271-90-8319/1. Submitted to the National Institute of Drug Abuse, February 12, 1992. Waltham, MA: Bigel Institute for Health Policy, Brandeis University.

Beinecke RH, Goodman M, Rivera M. 1995. *An Assessment of the Massachusetts Managed Mental Health/Substance Abuse Program: Year Three*. Boston: Suffolk University, Department of Public Management.

BLS (Bureau of Labor Statistics). 1992. *Substance Abuse Provisions in Employee Benefit Plans*. Bulletin 2412. Washington, DC: Department of Labor, Bureau of Labor Statistics.

BLS (Bureau of Labor Statistics). 1994. *Employee Benefits in Small Private Establishments, 1992*. Bulletin 2441, Tables 50–52. Washington, DC: Department of Labor, Bureau of Labor Statistics.

Callahan JJ, Shepard DS, Beinecke RH, Larson M, Cavanaugh D. 1994. *Evaluation of the Massachusetts Medicaid Mental Health/Substance Abuse Program*. Submitted to the Massachusetts Division of Medical Assistance, Mental Health Substance Abuse Program. Waltham, MA: Institute for Health Policy, Brandeis University.

Center of Alcohol Studies, Rutgers University. 1993. *Socioeconomic Evaluations of Addictions Treatment*. Prepared for the President's Commission on Model State Drug Laws. Piscataway, NJ: Rutgers University.

Chaulk CP, Moore-Rice K, Rizzo R, Chaisson RE. 1995. Eleven years of community-based directly observed therapy for tuberculosis. *Journal of the American Medical Association* 275:945–951.

CRS (Congressional Research Service). 1993. *Medicaid: An Overview*. 93-144 EPW. Washington, DC: Library of Congress, CRS.

CRS (Congressional Research Service). 1994. *Health Insurance*. Report No. IB91093. Washington, DC: Library of Congress, CRS.

Ellis RP. 1992. *Drug Abuse Treatment Patterns Before and After Managed Care*. Prepared under contract #271-89-8516 for the Third Annual Advisory Committee Meeting. Washington, DC, April 27–29, 1992. Boston, MA: Boston University.

Foster Higgins, Inc. 1994. *Managed Behavioral Healthcare Quality and Access Survey Report*. Prepared for the American Managed Behavioral Healthcare Association. Washington, DC: AMBHA.

Fox K, Merril JC, Chang HH, Califano JA Jr. 1995. Estimating the costs of substance abuse to the Medicaid hospital care program. *American Journal of Public Health* 85(1):48–54.

Freeman MA, Trabin T. 1994. *Managed Behavioral Healthcare: History, Models, Key Issues, and Future Course*. Prepared for the Center for Mental Health Services, SAMHSA.

Garnick DW, Hendricks AM, Comstock CB. 1994a. Measuring quality of care: Fundamental information from administrative datasets. *International Journal for Quality in Health Care* 6(2):163–177.

Garnick DW, Hendricks AM, Dulski JD, Thorpe KE, Horgan C. 1994b. Characteristics of private-sector managed care for mental health and substance abuse treatment. *Hospital and Community Psychiatry* 45(12):1201–1205.

Garnick DW, Hendricks AM, Drainoni ML, Horgan CM, Comstock C. In press. Private sector coverage of people with dual diagnoses. *Journal of Mental Health Administration*.

Geraty R, Bartlett J, Hill E, Lee F, Shusterman A, Waxman A. 1994. The impact of managed behavioral healthcare on the costs of psychiatric and chemical dependency treatment. *Behavioral Healthcare Tomorrow* March/April:18–30.

Gerstein DR, Johnson RA, Harwood HJ, Fountain D, Suter N, Malloy K. 1994. *Evaluating Recovery Services: The California Drug and Alcohol Treatment Assessment (CALDATA)*. Sacramento, CA: California Department of Alcohol and Drug Programs.

Hoffmann NG, DeHart SS, Fulkerson JA. 1993. Medical care utilization as a function of recovery status following chemical addictions treatment. *Journal of Addictive Diseases* 12:97–108.

Holder HD, Blose JO. 1992. The reduction of health care costs associated with alcoholism treatment: A 14-year longitudinal study. *Journal of Studies on Alcohol* 53(4):293–302.

Holder HD, Hallan JD. 1986. Impact of alcoholism treatment on total health care costs: A six-year study. *Advances in Alcohol and Substance Abuse* 6(1):1–15.

IOM (Institute of Medicine). 1989. *Controlling Costs and Changing Patient Care? The Role of Utilization Management*. Washington, DC: National Academy Press.

IOM (Institute of Medicine). 1990. *Treating Drug Problems*. Washington, DC: National Academy Press.

IOM (Institute of Medicine). 1995. *Development of Medications for the Treatment of Opiate and Cocaine Addictions: Issues for the Government and Private Sector*. Washington, DC: National Academy Press.

Jones KR, Vischi T. 1979. Impact of alcohol, drug abuse and mental health treatment on medical care utilization: A review of the research literature. *Medical Care* 17(12):1–82.

Kessler RC, Nelson CB, McGonagle KA, Edlund MJ, Frank RG, Leaf PJ. 1996. The epidemiology of co-occurring addictive and mental disorders in the National Comorbidity Survey: Implications for prevention and service utilization. *American Journal of Orthopsychiatry* 66(1):17–31.

Kushner JN. 1995. *Managing State Managed Care Contracts. Treatment Improvement Exchange Communique*. Rockville, MD: Center for Substance Abuse Treatment, SAMHSA.

Mechanic D, Schlesinger M, McAlpine DD. 1995. Management of mental health and substance abuse services: State of the art and early results. *Milbank Quarterly* 73(1):19–55.

Miller RH, Luft HS. 1994. Managed care plan performance since 1980. *Journal of the American Medical Association* 271(19):1512–1519.

Minnesota Department of Human Services. 1993. *1993 Status Report on the Minnesota Consolidated Chemical Dependency Treatment Fund, Report to the Minnesota Legislature from the Chemical Dependency Program Division*. St. Paul, MN: Minnesota Department of Human Services.

Minnesota Department of Human Services. 1995. *Research News*. St. Paul, MN: Minnesota Department of Human Services, Chemical Dependency Division.

Mucnick-Baku S, Traw KL. 1992. *Employee Assistance Programs: An Evolving Human Resource Management Strategy*. Washington, DC: Washington Business Group on Health.

NRC (National Research Council). 1994. *Under the Influence? Drugs and the American Work Force*. Washington, DC: National Academy Press.

Osher FG. 1996. A vision for the future: Toward a service system responsive to those with co-occurring addictive and mental disorders. *American Journal of Orthopsychiatry* 66(1):71–76.

Oss ME. 1994. Managed behavioral health programs widespread among insured Americans. *Open Minds Newsletter* 8(3). Gettysburg, PA: Behavioral Health Industry News, Inc.

Prendergast ML, Anglin MD, Maugh TH, Hser Y. In press. *The Effectiveness of Treatment for Drug Abuse*. Draft manuscript prepared April 7, 1994 for NIDA Treatment Services Research Branch. Los Angeles: UCLA Drug Abuse Research Center.

Regier DA, Farmer ME, Rae DS, Locke BZ, Keith SJ, Judd LL, Goodwin FK. 1990. Comorbidity of mental disorders with alcohol and other drug abuse: Results from the Epidemiologic Catchment Area (ECA) Study. *Journal of the American Medical Association* 264(19):2511–2518.

Renz EA, Chung R, Fillman TO, Mee-Lee D, Sayama M. 1995. The effect of managed care on the treatment outcome of substance use disorders. *General Hospital Psychiatry* 17:287–292.

Rogers WH, Wells KB, Meredith LS, Sturm R, Burnam A. 1993. Outcomes for adult outpatients with depression under prepaid or fee-for-service financing. *Archives of General Psychiatry* 50:517–525.

Rost KM, Ross RL, Humphrey J, Frank S, Smith J, Smith GR. 1996. Does this treatment work? Validation of an outcomes module for alcohol dependence. *Medical Care* 34(4):283–294.

Rowland D, Rosenbaum S, Simon L, Chait E. 1995. *Medicaid and Managed Care: Lessons from the Literature.* Report of the Kaiser Commission on the Future of Medicaid. Menlo Park, CA: Kaiser Foundation.

SAMHSA (Substance Abuse and Mental Health Services Administration). 1995. *The Role and Current Status of Patient Placement Criteria in the Treatment of Substance Use Disorders.* Treatment Improvement Protocol Series. Rockville, MD: Center for Substance Abuse Treatment.

Shueman SA, Troy WG. 1994. *Managed Behavioral Health Care: An Industry Perspective.* Springfield, IL: Charles C Thomas.

Spear SF, Mason M. 1991. Impact of chemical dependency on family health status. *International Journal of the Addictions* 26(2):79–87.

Thompson JW, Burns BJ, Goldman HH, Smith J. 1992. Initial level of care and clinical status in a managed mental health program. *Hospital and Community Psychiatry* 43(6):599–603.

Woody G, Cacciola J. 1994. Review of remission criteria. In: Widiger T, Frances A, Pincus H, First M, Ross R, Davis W, eds. *DSM-IV Sourcebook, Vol. 1.* Washington, DC: American Psychiatric Association Press. Pp. 81–92.

Yu J, Chen PJ, Harshman EJ. 1991. An analysis of substance abuse patterns, medical expenses and effectiveness of treatment in the workplace. *Employer Benefits Journal* September:26–30.

10

Drug Control

For almost a century, the central component of U.S. illicit drug policy has been a legal structure under which the medical and scientific uses of opiates, cocaine, and other controlled drugs are tightly restricted and the production and distribution of these drugs for nonmedical and nonscientific uses are prohibited. Violations of those prohibitions are punishable by severe criminal sanctions under both federal and state laws. Additionally, federal and state penalties against commercial drug offenses are supplemented by criminal sanctions against users (i.e., for possessing drugs for one's own use).

The effects of drug control usually are not included within the ambit of "drug abuse research" and are assumed to lie instead within the purview of criminal justice research. In the committee's view, however, the effects of legal controls, and of different strategies for implementing and enforcing them, should be seen as an important component of a comprehensive drug abuse research strategy. Conceived broadly, policy-relevant effects encompass all the benefits of legal controls (in reducing use, abuse, and dependence on illicit drugs and the associated adverse consequences) and the costs, or side-effects, of those controls (ranging from violence associated with the illicit drug trade to the costs of imprisonment). On many of these questions, there is no dearth of opinion but little in the way of systematic, rigorous research (Tonry, 1990). Any effort to explore the wide range of issues relating to the effects (benefits or costs) of drug control would far exceed the scope of this report and the committee's expertise. Instead, the committee discusses several areas of inquiry that relate most directly to the public health and to the other fields of investigation explored in previous chapters.

An integrated perspective that encompasses interventions aimed at both supply and demand can yield important advances by overcoming disciplinary and bureaucratic boundaries. Many aspects of drug control and its enforcement are inescapably related to mainstream fields of drug abuse research, especially etiology, prevention, and treatment. Because the law and its enforcement affect the price and accessibility of illicit drugs, drug control policies can affect many aspects of drug-using behavior, including which drugs are used and how they are ingested. A full understanding of factors relating to initiation or intensification of drug use might usefully encompass measures of perceived availability and the perceived likelihood that sanctions (both legal and social) will be imposed. Treatment outcome studies might take into account the impact of variations in drug availability on entry and retention, as well as the coercive "leverage" produced by the threat of prosecution or punishment. The design of community prevention programs might encompass measures of drug availability (e.g., price and access) as well as other variables relating to the intensity of law enforcement in the communities being studied. As noted in Chapter 7, the consequences of drug abuse (e.g., violence) are often intertwined with the sequelae of illicit drug markets and drug law enforcement.

An important trend in public health research is the inclusion of legal controls and interventions within a single model of drug abuse research. A prime example is injury control. For example, the field of highway safety encompasses studies of the effects of mandatory seatbelt laws, mandatory helmet laws, speed limits, and various types of licensing restrictions. In recent years, injury control researchers have also focused on the effects of gun controls on firearms injuries. The compelling need to bring legal controls within a comprehensive public health research model has recently been recognized in the field of tobacco research, where studies are being conducted on the design and enforcement of youth access restrictions, the effects of advertising restrictions, and the effects of a significant increase in tobacco excise taxes (IOM, 1994). In fact, some public health officials and tobacco research funding agencies have come to believe that "policy research" is an essential component of a tobacco research program (Davis, 1995).

RECURRENT ISSUES IN DRUG ABUSE CONTROL

Arguments about drug control policy proceed too often on the basis of intuition and supposition rather than empirical data. Even though some of the disputed issues defy scientific investigation, many of the controversies that have recurred throughout the history of drug control can be informed by systematic empirical research. Following a brief survey of potentially researchable issues, four specific opportunities for policy research are explored in some depth.

Prohibition Versus Regulatory Discouragement

At the broadest level, drug control policy requires a choice between a system of prohibition (under which drugs are not legally available for nonmedical use) and a strategy of regulatory containment or management (under which drugs are legally available for nonmedical use by adults). Each of these models can be implemented in a variety of ways. Within the prohibitory model, varying strategies of enforcement will differentially affect the price and accessibility of the prohibited drugs and the patterns and consequences of their use. Within the regulatory model, the channels of authorized access can be more or less tightly restricted, and the product and its marketing can be more or less heavily regulated, depending on whether and in what ways policymakers aim to affect the prevalence and circumstances of consumption.

The basic choice between prohibitory and regulatory approaches has been a subject of ongoing dispute in the field of drug control. Although most commentators assess these choices within a cost–benefit framework (e.g., Nadelmann, 1989; Goldstein and Kalant, 1990), they tend to disagree about the consequences of adopting a regulatory approach in lieu of the existing prohibition. To what extent would the incidence and prevalence of drug use, abuse, and dependence, and the associated social costs, increase under a regulatory regime? To what extent would the costs incurred under the current prohibitory strategy be avoided under an alternative approach? What new costs would be incurred?

Efforts to address these questions often draw on the experience of other countries that have adopted different approaches toward drug control (e.g., Reuter and MacCoun, 1995). However, meaningful comparisons are impeded by numerous cross-cultural differences and by inadequate or dissimilar data; the ongoing argument about the consequences and significance of de facto legalization of cannabis in some Amsterdam coffee houses (compare Kleber, 1996, with Ossebaard, 1996, and Sifanek and Kaplan, 1995) is illustrative. It should be noted, however, that cross-national studies of the effects of tobacco advertising restrictions have made a significant contribution to policy debate in this country (IOM, 1994). "Noisy data" on the epidemiology of illicit drug use and on the effects of drug control policies may be superior to anecdotes, but opportunities for significant advances in knowledge based on cross-national research will have to await improvements in data systems and in the conceptualization of policy-relevant variables (MacCoun et al., 1993, 1995).

Another set of comparisons relates to this country's own evolving regulatory policies toward tobacco and alcohol. Tobacco policy has recently entered an intriguing period of transition from a laissez-faire approach to a tightened regulatory model explicitly aiming to discourage the use of tobacco products without prohibiting them. This use of legal tools to discourage consumption (advertising limitations, pricing policy, product regulation, public use restrictions) provides a model of public health regulation formerly absent in the drug abuse field (IOM, 1994). The effects of these new initiatives in tobacco regulation should be carefully studied, not only because reducing the toll of tobacco-related disease is a major public health priority, but also because these new regulatory initiatives in tobacco control may yield useful lessons for controlled substance regulation. Similarly, the public health effects of alcoholic beverage regulation should be carefully studied. A growing body of research on the relationship between density of retail outlets and alcohol consumption (Gruenwald et al., 1993) and on access to alcohol by underage drinkers (Waagenar et al., 1996) highlights methods of restricting availability within a regulatory framework and may also yield important insights regarding fundamental behavioral relationships between availability and consumption of psychoactive drugs.

All of these issues are interesting and relevant to a broad understanding of the public health effects of legal controls on psychoactive drugs. Of more immediate relevance to the current research agenda, however, are questions regarding potential improvements in the implementation of the nation's prohibitory drug control strategy.

Abuse Reduction Versus Medical Use

Within a few years after enactment of the Harrison Narcotics Act in 1914, the difficulty of reducing illicit (nonmedical) use of narcotic drugs without interfering with legitimate medical use became evident. Federal enforcement authorities decided that maintenance treatment of persons already dependent on opiates, by private physicians or by local clinics, was incompatible with the goal of reducing drug dependence (see Musto, 1987). When methadone maintenance became a recognized treatment for heroin dependence in the 1960s, the debate resurfaced. The proper balance between therapeutic discretion and law enforcement efforts to suppress drug abuse and minimize diversion has been a source of continuing controversy (IOM, 1995b). Arguments about methadone maintenance often turn on empirical disputes about the magnitude of diversion associated with various treatment protocols and the "chilling effect" of enforcement practices on medical care, particularly in preventing or discouraging physicians from prescribing methadone treatment and from utilizing other therapeutically indicated procedures (IOM, 1995b).

Another source of continuing conflict has been the inhibiting effect of controlled substance regulation on other medical uses of the regulated drugs. Beginning with the Harrison Act, regulatory structures have been established to restrict the manufacture and distribution of regulated drugs (as a means of reducing nonmedical use) while allowing the continued use of such drugs in legitimate medical practice. The Controlled Substances Act, enacted by the Congress in 1970, established a hierarchy of regulatory controls purporting to balance abuse reduction and medical need. This act has served as a model for parallel controlled substance statutes in every state. Again, however, the preventive effect of those legal controls on abuse and their inhibiting effect on medical practice have been sources of continuing dispute (IOM, 1995a). These issues will be explored in greater detail below.

Penalties for Users

A legal strategy of prohibiting availability of controlled drugs for nonmedical use does not necessarily entail criminal penalties against users. (Possession of alcohol for personal use was an offense in only a few states during Prohibition.) Whether criminal sanctions should be prescribed for alcohol or tobacco possession by underage users or for possession of controlled substances or drug paraphernalia, depends at least in part on an assessment of the social benefits of these sanctions (in reducing use and, ultimately, in reducing abuse and dependence) and the social costs of enforcing them.

In 1972, the National Commission on Marihuana and Drug Abuse recommended that criminal sanctions for possession of marijuana for personal use be repealed. The commission concluded that sporadic enforcement of criminal penalties for marijuana use did not achieve a substantial preventive effect and that whatever preventive effect such enforcement did achieve was outweighed by the social and individual costs of enforcing the prohibition. Although 11 states repealed criminal penalties for marijuana possession in the wake of the commission's report and most other states ameliorated the impact of criminal sanctions (Bonnie, 1977), this trend ended in the late 1970s in response to a substantial rise in adolescent marijuana use. Interestingly, there has not yet been a definitive study of the behavioral effects of decriminalization of marijuana use (compare Maloff, 1981, with Cuskey, 1981). Such a study faces two substantial methodological problems: (1) measuring and controlling for enforcement of the prescribed sanctions, and (2) disentangling the "declarative" or moralizing effect of the sanction from the other social forces influencing people's beliefs and attitudes about marijuana use (Bonnie, 1986).

The debate about criminalization of drug users has intensified in recent years, partly in response to European developments (Reuter et al., 1993). Although criminal penalties have been ameliorated in Italy, Spain, Switzerland, and Germany, decriminalization in Italy and Spain has been associated with substantially higher rates of opiate dependence (CASA, 1995; Reuter and MacCoun, 1995). Because of the absence of reliable data and the relatively passive enforcement of sanctions against users in most Western European countries (outside Scandinavia), it is impossible to assess the impact of decriminalization through comparative studies.

Perhaps the most significant policy-relevant research on the effects of criminalization in recent years pertains to the effects of needle exchange programs. Two important empirical questions lie at the center of the policy debate about these programs and about the enforcement of existing prohibitions against possessing needles for purposes of illicit drug use: whether and to what extent needle sharing (and therefore the risk of transmitting HIV disease) is reduced, and whether and to what extent the legal availability of clean needles increases illicit drug use. As noted in a recent National Research Council report (NRC, 1995), research has shown that needle exchange programs have the ability to retard the spread of HIV infection among participating injection drug users, do not affect the level of self-reported drug use among the participants, and do not appear to recruit new users to injection drugs, at least in the short term. The public health imperative of containing HIV transmission argues for continued research on the long-term impact of these programs and on ways to improve their effectiveness along the lines recommended in the NRC report. In light of well-established methods of monitoring the incidence and prevalence of HIV infection, this area may be ripe for cross-national policy research.

Strategies of Enforcement

Not surprisingly, criminal justice specialists have often disagreed about the relative utility of various strategies employed to suppress the availability of illicit drugs. These strategies include an international effort to eradicate naturally growing sources of illicit drugs; interdiction of shipments intended for the U.S. market; investigation, penetration, and disruption of trafficking networks; and state and local police actions directed at street-level retail dealing and use. From a public health perspective, the central question is how the contending strategies might be deployed most effectively to reduce consumption and its adverse consequences, while also avoiding increases in crime and violence. These important empirical questions should be amenable to systematic investigation (Moore, 1990). Research in this area is explored further below.

Severity of Penalties

Over the course of the twentieth century, criminal penalties for drug offenses have escalated, de-escalated, and re-escalated. The differential impact on drug trafficking and consumption is difficult to assess, in large part because the behavioral effects of threatened sanctions are mediated by many factors, including the probability of punishment, the strength of other social deterrents to offending, and the strength of peoples' incentives to offend. However, substantial resources have been allocated to the apprehension, prosecution, and incarceration of drug offenders, often at the expense of other potentially useful interventions, particularly treatment. For this reason, it is important to assess the behavioral effects of various types of criminal punishment in reducing drug abuse and dependence. This subject is explored below.

Conflicting Aims of Treatment and Punishment

One of the most puzzling features of drug control policy is the inherent tension between two public attitudes about drugs—that illicit drug use should be penalized, while people with drug problems should be helped. These divergent inclinations produce numerous contradictions in legal policy. For example, the desire to facilitate treatment of drug users sometimes leads to policies that insulate illicit drug use from discovery and ameliorate its punishment in favor of therapeutic dispositions. Drug offenses are not the only context in which criminal law is used as a device for achieving therapeutic effects—therapeutic referrals are not uncommon following charges of family violence, for example. However, the practice has become more formalized and more routinized in drug cases than in other contexts.

The empirical issues here are important and numerous. Does the availability of a therapeutic disposition erode the deterrent effect of the criminal sanction? Alternatively, does the perceived threat of punishment undermine the effort to recruit people into treatment? Does the use of criminal sanction as therapeutic leverage produce better treatment outcomes than would be achieved by either erasing the threat of punishment or relying on punishment alone? These questions, too, are further explored below.

The remainder of this chapter discusses in greater detail four opportunities for research on the public health effects of drug control: (1) the effects of controlled substance regulation on legitimate medical use (including medical modalities of drug abuse treatment); (2) the effects of supply reduction on drug consumption; (3) the effects of criminal sanctions against users (including coerced treatment) on drug consumption; and (4) the effects of beliefs about confidentiality (or the lack of it) on participation in treatment.

EFFECTS OF REGULATION ON LEGITIMATE MEDICAL USE AND SCIENTIFIC RESEARCH

In 1970, Congress enacted the Controlled Substances Act (CSA), which places drugs in control schedules according to their abuse potential, ranging from Schedule I, including drugs (such as heroin and LSD) that have high abuse potential and no established medical use, to Schedule V, including drugs (such as nonprescription codeine elixirs) that have low abuse potential and are legally marketed as cough remedies. CSA controls the production and distribution of scheduled drugs by, among other things, requiring manufacturers and distributors to maintain records of their production and transportation, limiting refills of prescriptions, placing production quotas (limits) on such drugs, and requiring the use of special order forms to transfer these drugs to the retail level.

Although enacted in an effort to curtail drug abuse, its legislative history makes it clear that CSA was not intended to interfere either with medical practice or with the availability of controlled substances for legitimate medical or scientific use. However, that has not been an easy balance to strike. The Drug Enforcement Administration (DEA) and most state drug control bodies generally favor more extensive regulations on any drugs with the potential for abuse, so that they can reduce drug diversion.[1] Unfortunately, the measures they advocate, including government-issued multiple-copy prescription forms, elaborate measures for record keeping and for storing drugs, and stricter scheduling of substances, tend to increase the difficulty associated with prescribing such medications or making them available for scientific study. Many physicians and medical organizations perceive that these measures discourage physicians from prescribing the best drugs for conditions such as chronic pain, anxiety, attention deficit–hyperactivity disorder, epilepsy, obesity,

[1]This is not to say that drug law enforcement officials are indifferent to the impact of controlled substance regulation on medical use. For example, the DEA Administrator recently ruled that the long-term prescribing of opioid analgesics for a patient with chronic nonmalignant pain is a legitimate medical use for these drugs and, if appropriately supervised, is not grounds for sanctions against the prescribing physician.

and narcolepsy. The medical and drug enforcement communities are therefore frequently at odds in debates on public policy, particularly during the development of legislation, and the gap between their perspectives has been growing wider (IOM, 1995a,b). Furthermore, federal and state regulatory obstacles act as a disincentive to the pharmaceutical industry in developing anti-addiction medications (Chapter 1; IOM, 1995b).

As the controversy grows, the need for better data has become increasingly evident. Very little systematic research has been conducted on the actual effects of specific regulations or enforcement practices on either illicit drug use or medical use. To begin examining these issues, the National Institute on Drug Abuse (NIDA) recently conducted a technical review (Cooper et al., 1993). The resulting publication, *Impact of Prescription Drug Diversion Control Systems on Medical Practice and Patient Care,* presents preliminary evidence that drug control regulations have adverse effects on the treatment of a number of diseases. For example, DEA has been encouraging states to introduce multiple-copy prescription programs for certain controlled substances. When New York applied this regulation to the benzodiazepines, prescriptions of these drugs for anxiety and insomnia declined and were replaced, in some cases, by increased prescribing of outmoded and more dangerous sedative hypnotics (Weintraub et al., 1991). Introduction of multiple-copy prescriptions in Texas led to a halving in the number of prescriptions of controlled opioids for pain (Sigler et al., 1984).

Drug control agencies assert that reductions in the number of prescriptions written for controlled substances indicate that multiple-copy prescription programs are a success. However, a reduction in the number of prescriptions does not automatically translate into a reduction in the illicit use and abuse of that drug, nor does it indicate that the prior level of prescriptions reflected overprescribing. On the contrary, reductions in the number of prescriptions may reflect a reluctance on the part of physicians to prescribe, and pharmacists to dispense or even stock, such drugs for legitimate medical use. The primary sources of amphetamines and similar psychostimulants appear to be illicit manufacturers rather than legitimate sources such as pharmacists and physicians (Angarola and Minsk, 1994). Existing research simply does not include enough direct measurement of prescribing patterns and patient outcomes to give a definitive picture of the risks or benefits of government-issued prescription programs.

There are other examples of ways in which drug control regulations and enforcement practices appear to interfere with the physician's ability to treat patients, including the threat of criminal prosecution.[2] A few

[2]Under 21 C.F.R. section 291.505, failure "to abide by all the requirements" of the methadone regulations (which contain many specific provisions relating to inventory control as

additional examples include restricting the prescribing of opioids to patients with pain and a history of substance abuse (e.g., AIDS patients) (Joranson and Gilson, 1994a,b); as well as the cumbersome procedures, forms, and fees that must be fulfilled before a hospital or physician can use methadone to detoxify heroin-dependent patients (SAMHSA, 1992).

The committee recommends additional research on the effects of controlled substance regulations on medical use and scientific research. Specifically, these studies should encompass the impact of such regulations and their enforcement on prescribing practices and patient outcomes in relation to conditions such as pain, anxiety, attention deficit disorder, obesity, and narcolepsy and on the availability of treatment and outcomes for patients with addictive disorders.

EFFECTS OF SUPPLY REDUCTION ON CONSUMPTION

Approximately 64 percent ($8.5 billion) of federal expenditures for drug control ($13.3 billion) in FY 1995 was allocated to law enforcement efforts to control the supply of drugs to illicit markets in the United States (ONDCP, 1996). Such "supply-reduction efforts" include (1) international efforts such as crop eradication, crop substitution, the negotiation of mutual legal-assistance treaties, and cooperative international enforcement efforts; (2) interdiction, for example, border inspections and patrols conducted by the U.S. Customs Service and the U.S. Immigration and Naturalization Service and the interdiction of ships and planes suspected of carrying contraband by the U.S. Coast Guard and the U.S. Armed Forces; (3) investigations, such as efforts by DEA, the Federal Bureau of Investigation (FBI), and U.S. attorneys to investigate and prosecute drug trafficking organizations; and (4) state and local drug enforcement efforts, for example, the enforcement activities of the nation's 4,000 municipal police departments directed at street-level traffickers and users (Moore, 1990).

The primary goal of supply-reduction efforts is to decrease the availability and increase the cost of obtaining illicit drugs and thereby reduce their consumption and associated adverse consequences. There can be little doubt that a prohibitory system of drug control, if enforced, does suppress consumption and otherwise affect patterns of drug use, compared to a system under which these drugs are legally available for nonmedical use through authorized channels (Goldstein and Kalant, 1990).

---

well as clinical practice) can subject the service provider to criminal prosecution. In no other area of health care, with the possible exception of some abortion procedures, is the threat of criminal prosecution used as a tool for enforcing requirements of clinical practice.

What is less clear, however, is the extent to which particular strategies of supply reduction (such as interdiction and street-level enforcement) affect accessibility and price and, in turn, affect consumption (Moore, 1990).

The total cost of illicit drugs includes both their dollar price and the nonmonetary costs of acquiring them (e.g., how long it takes to find them and how risky it is to purchase or sell them) (Moore, 1973). Those two elements of total cost are the mediating variables between enforcement and consumption. Due to the nature of illicit drug markets, the availability of drugs may be reduced more often by uncertainty than by actual physical scarcity. Dealer inventories and the presence of many suppliers in the market make it possible, albeit less convenient, to acquire drugs even when import, wholesale, or retail markets have been temporarily disrupted.[3]

Existing evidence is mixed as to whether specific enforcement-generated changes in the availability and cost of illicit drugs reduce consumption. Some studies have found no evidence that cocaine consumption responds to enforcement-induced price increases (Dinardo, 1993). Others, using Drug Abuse Warning Network (DAWN) data, have observed that the number of cocaine mentions for emergency room patients varies inversely with the price of cocaine at both national and city levels (ONDCP, 1992).

Among economists it is now generally acknowledged that the demand for drugs is elastic, rising and falling in response to changes in price.[4] Indeed, despite the addictiveness of nicotine, researchers have found that cigarette consumption exhibits surprisingly high elasticity (e.g., Wasserman et al., 1991; Peterson et al., 1992; Hu et al., 1994). Recent work suggests that the demand for both heroin and cocaine may also be highly elastic (Caulkins, 1995). Additional research is needed to establish the relationship between price and consumption and, particularly, to measure variations in elasticity among different categories of users and within different submarkets. For example, teenagers appear to be more sensitive than adults to tobacco price increases (IOM, 1994).

If significant reductions in availability and increases in price do reduce consumption, it is important from a policymaking perspective to understand the extent to which alternative approaches to supply reduction and enforcement can reduce the availability and price of illicit drugs. Interdiction of drugs that have not yet reached retail markets, for ex-

---

[3]An exception can occur with certain synthetic drugs (e.g., methaqualone) which can be produced only with sophisticated technology.

[4]Elasticity is the percentage change in consumption in response to a 1 percent change in price. The demand for a drug is "perfectly inelastic" if there is no change in the consumption of a drug in response to a change in its price.

ample, has been estimated to have a much smaller effect on prices than concentrated efforts by local police to arrest or otherwise harass dealers in street markets (Caulkins, 1994). Unfortunately, however, available data are not adequate to assess the effectiveness of specific supply reduction strategies.

Data relating to arrests, convictions, and imprisonments are available, but reliable data do not now exist concerning the total pools of buyers and sellers or the number of transactions. Thus, even though arrests of drug dealers have increased substantially in recent years, the effect of such enforcement on drug price cannot be established empirically until measures of the quantity of illegal drug transactions (the denominator for measuring the effects of enforcement) have been developed. Much empirical work remains to be accomplished before the relationships among drug control activities, the price and accessibility of the drugs, and consumption are understood well enough to provide an empirical foundation for focused policy interventions (Kleiman and Smith, 1990). Certainly, police have shown that they can at least temporarily disrupt neighborhood drug markets; however, there are no data that correlate a percentage increase in drug price with the increased probability of arrest or imprisonment of dealers. Furthermore, understanding is needed of consumption adjustments relative to price, the elasticities of different user groups, the drug substitutions and behavioral changes that are stimulated, and any shifts in user populations that might result. The call for state and local police to collect data on local drug prices to match the systematic federal price data represented in the STRIDE (System to Retrieve Information from Drug Evidence) data series, is not unwarranted. Evaluations of the epidemiology of drug use, of drug treatment programs, and of law enforcement efforts themselves would be enhanced by solid evidence about the prices and price changes to which people are responding. Thus, research on advancing an understanding of the effects of supply reduction on drug consumption would allow for more focused strategies by law enforcement agencies.

The committee encourages the Department of Justice to support research to determine the relationships between changes in the accessibility and price of illicit drugs and changes in consumption, and to develop adequate measures for assessing the impact of various supply-reduction strategies on the accessibility and price of illicit drugs.

EFFECTS OF CRIMINAL SANCTIONS ON DRUG USE

As noted earlier, a central feature of national drug policy over the past 15 years has been a substantial escalation of criminal penalties for drug offenses. In 1982, Congress lengthened prison sentences, made incarceration mandatory, and placed restrictions on bail for specific federal drug offenses (Wisotsky, 1990). Many states followed suit; by 1990, laws in nearly every state and the federal sentencing guidelines had been amended to prescribe mandatory sentences for specific drug offenses.[5] The most severe penalties were prescribed for offenses and offenders involved in crack cocaine (Belenko, 1993; Fagan, 1995; Tonry, 1995; U.S. Sentencing Commission, 1995). Additionally, enforcement efforts have been strengthened. Police crackdowns on street-level drug trafficking, such as Operation Pressure Point (Zimmer, 1987) and the Tactical Narcotics Teams (Sviridoff et al., 1992), have been widely implemented (Moore, 1977; Chaiken, 1988; Sherman, 1989). In order to process the growing volume of arrests, court capacities have been increased, and special narcotics courts and prosecution teams have been created (Belenko et al., 1990, 1991).

As a result of this mobilization of legal institutions, arrests, prosecutions, convictions, prison sentences, and parole revocations all have increased sharply in a relatively short time (Goerdt and Martin, 1989; Zimring and Hawkins, 1992; Tonry, 1995). Sharp increases in drug arrests, both for possession and selling and escalated sentences, including mandatory minimum terms, have created dramatic changes in the composition of defendant and prison populations. According to FBI data, there were 1,066,400 state and local arrests for drug offenses in 1992, an increase of 61 percent from 1983. Approximately 68 percent of these arrests were for possession offenses. (Of the possession arrests, 47 percent were for opiate or cocaine offenses and 38 percent were for marijuana offenses.) The trends in major cities have been striking. For example, drug arrests in New York City increased from 18,521 in 1980 (40 percent for heroin or other opiates) to 88,641 in 1988 (44 percent for crack) (Belenko et al., 1991). In New York City, the proportion of drug arrestees increased from 11 percent of the arrestee population in 1980 to 31 percent in 1989 (New York City Police Department, 1990).

Since 1983, drug offenders in New York City have had a higher probability of felony charges at arrest, have been less likely to make bail, and have been more likely to be held in pretrial detention without bail (Belenko et al., 1991). In the courts, drug caseloads increased by 56 percent between 1983 and 1987 in a sample of 26 cities nationwide (Goerdt

---

[5] For example, in 1988, New York legislators reduced the threshold for a felony cocaine possession charge from one-eighth ounce (3.5 grams) to approximately 1 gram, or six vials of crack. Penalties for felony sale convictions were set at the same level as mandatory minimum sentences for armed robbery, aggravated assault, and first-degree manslaughter.

and Martin, 1989). By 1989, felony drug probationers made up 39 percent of all felony probationers in New York State (Greenstein, 1990).

In the New York, California, and federal prison systems, drug offenders are now the largest inmate group. In federal correctional facilities, drug offenders accounted for 61 percent of the population in 1993, up from 16 percent in 1970, 25 percent in 1980, and 52 percent in 1990 (BJS, 1994). In state prisons, drug offenders represented 22 percent of the population in 1991, up from 6 percent in 1979 (BJS, 1994); almost one-third of all new court commitments to state prisons were for drug offenses (BJS, 1993). Drug offenders made up 35 percent of all New York State inmates in 1992, compared to 16 percent in 1987 (BJS, 1993). Analyses of prison commitments show similar trends. From 1983 to 1992, commitments resulting from drug offenses rose from 12.5 to 44.5 percent of all new commitments in New York State.

Whether the escalation of criminal punishment for drug offenses has been a prudent and effective social policy is a matter of intense debate (Reuter, 1992). The costs of this policy are well known. What is lacking is a systematic assessment of the benefits. In addressing the benefits of severe sanctions for drug offenses, it is important to distinguish between trafficking offenses and consumption-related offenses, notwithstanding the overlap in some cases. From a preventive standpoint, by threatening and imposing sanctions against drug trafficking, the law aims to increase the "cost" of selling and, ultimately, to increase the cost to consumers of finding and buying drugs. By threatening and imposing sanctions against users, the law aims to deter consumption directly.

The deterrent effect of criminal sanctions on drug dealing is bound up with the more general issues, addressed earlier in this chapter, regarding the effects of supply reduction on consumption. The existing body of research raises substantial doubts about the deterrent and incapacitative effects of heightened punishment on retail drug dealing during the 1980s. Ethnographic research in inner city drug markets reveals that drug selling expanded dramatically in the 1980s and that the cocaine economy is a major employer of unemployed youths (Johnson et al., 1990). Studies of arrestees tend to show a substantial increase in the number of young males participating in drug dealing at precisely the time that penalties were being raised and enforcement was being intensified (MacCoun et al., 1993; Saner et al., 1994). Even among punished drug offenders, increasing the severity of punishment apparently did not significantly reduce the likelihood of future offending (through "specific deterrence"). Comparing recidivism rates for more than 6,000 cocaine and crack offenders in New York City during the 1980s, Fagan (1994) found evidence of a criminogenic effect rather that a deterrent effect. All of these findings suggest that removing retail drug sellers from the market has little impact on overall supply because the powerful economic incentives for drug dealing will entice others to replace the incapacitated offenders (Blumstein et al., 1983).

In this section of the report, the committee focuses on the impact of criminal sanctions for use-related offenses on the demand for drugs[6] with the primary goal of connecting research on the effects of criminal sanctions to the bodies of research on prevention and treatment reviewed in Chapters 6 and 8. The two main ways in which criminal sanctions might be used to reduce drug use are explored in this section. First, general deterrence is considered: To what extent and under what conditions does threatened punishment depress consumption by reducing initiation, or by reducing frequency or intensity of use? This is followed by consideration of the use of threatened sanctions for therapeutic leverage: To what extent does criminal justice control facilitate successful treatment interventions?[7]

General Deterrence

Efforts to test the general deterrent effects of criminal sanctions on drug use have been limited in several ways. First, deterrence studies typically rely on general population surveys to provide measures of undeterred drug use (e.g., Meier and Johnson, 1977). However, the actual probability that sanctions will be imposed on law violators differs widely across demographic groups, and there are substantial differences in the characteristics of persons who use drugs and those who are arrested and punished for using drugs (Husak, 1992; Kleiman and Smith, 1992; Zimring and Hawkins, 1992; Tonry, 1995). Since social "position" may interact with punishment effects, this selection bias can limit or even invalidate empirical research on the deterrent effects of law for drug users (Berk et al., 1992; Sherman, 1992).

Second, very few of these studies have included the use of opiates or cocaine as the dependent variable. Most have tested the deterrent effects of punishment and social control on alcohol or marijuana use, drunk

---

[6]As already noted, disruption of retail drug markets (by enforcing sanctions against dealers) can also reduce demand by increasing "search costs" for potential users. It therefore bears repeated emphasis that the dichotomy between supply reduction and demand reduction is an imperfect one.

[7]This section does not address the declarative or moralizing effects of criminal sanctions (i.e., the impact of prohibition and punishments on attitudes and beliefs about drug use independent of the direct motivational effect of threatened apprehension and punishment). Nor is the "specific deterrent effect" of punishing users, aside from facilitating treatment, addressed (e.g., Erickson, 1976).

driving, or other crimes that have higher base rates (e.g., Meier and Johnson, 1977; Ross, 1984). Since both social and legal sanctions for these crimes are relatively less severe than the penalties for opiate or cocaine offenses, the findings have limited generalizability. Deterrence research on opiate and cocaine offenses must also take account of the significant overlap between use offenses and distribution offenses. Many users are not dealers, but many become involved in dealing to support their habits.

Finally, most empirical studies on the general deterrent effects of law and social control have proceeded on a separate track from studies on the specific deterrent effects of punishment experiences. This bifurcation of the empirical literature has led some researchers to suggest a revised, "perceptual deterrence" framework that incorporates both direct (arrests, incarceration) and indirect (friends' and acquaintances' experiences) punishment experiences within the conceptual model (Stafford and Warr, 1993).

A new generation of research on the deterrence of drug use should be based on a theoretical model that integrates legal deterrence in a social control framework. This model would encompass a broad range of elements relating to the perceived costs and benefits of drug use. These elements include: personal costs (e.g., risks of dependence, disease, and violence); social, physiological, and psychological returns (e.g., pleasures, status, life-style); actual and perceived direct costs of punishment (e.g., arrest, incarceration, loss of income or drugs); social costs of punishment (e.g., job or relationship loss; see Williams and Hawkins, 1989); and motivational components (e.g., risk taking and sensation seeking; see Chapter 2).

A research agenda on deterrence should also recognize the distinctions in deterrent effects across populations of drug users and in different sectors of society. Research should also take adequate account of the balance of motivations and restraints on drug use, including both external restraints from threatened legal sanctions and internal restraints reflecting social and moral inhibitions. The threat of punishment carries different weight for different people, depending on their personal circumstances.

Differences in the effects of legal controls on illegal behaviors may reflect not only individual factors, but also the effects of contextual variables that either strengthen or neutralize the effects of legal controls—for example, by increasing the returns from drug use (or drug dealing) or by discounting the social costs of arrest and punishment. Many of these factors reflect the structure of opportunities and controls at the neighborhood or community level. In some cases, neighborhood effects powerfully reinforce legal deterrents to drug use. In other cases, neighborhood effects can delegitimize law and reinforce involvement with drugs (Tonry,

1995). At the community level, the deterrent effects of legal sanctions and other social controls on drug use and drug dealing are confounded. Several studies have shown, for example, that incomes from illicit drug dealing were significantly higher than legal wages in inner cities (see Fagan, 1995, for a review). In areas of high unemployment, an active economic incentive also shapes the opportunities for social status and roles, and provides a source of social control that reinforces illegal activity. Thus, strong institutionalized drug markets themselves become sources of social control that compete with legal norms and sanctions. In addition, the social and economic isolation of neighborhoods with active drug markets can disrupt the intergenerational job networks that in the past eased the entry of unskilled workers into stable (although low-wage) jobs.

A research agenda is needed to assess the effects of legal controls on drug use and dealing. Furthermore, there is a need to understand how the informal social controls that compete with punishment costs influence compliance with the law. Such factors are likely to explain neighborhood variation in the effects of legal controls on drug use and may suggest effective community-based prevention intervention efforts.

Therapeutic Leverage

Apprehension of drug users provides an opportunity to reduce drug use (and future offending) through treatment, by using the threat of sanctions as a form of leverage for inducing satisfactory compliance with therapeutic requirements (see Chapter 8). In 1973, the National Commission on Marihuana and Drug Abuse concluded that the primary utility of criminal sanctions for consumption-related drug offenses lies in their use as means of therapeutic leverage (NCMDA, 1973). The commission endorsed a multistage linkage between the criminal justice system and community-based treatment systems, under which favorable dispositions would be conditioned on participation in treatment.[8] During the ensuing decade, the White House Special Action Office for Drug Abuse Prevention (SAODAP) and NIDA joined hands with the Department of Justice to implement this strategy through a variety of initiatives, the most important of which was Treatment Alternatives for Street Crime (TASC). Although federal funding for TASC and related initiatives was reduced during the 1980s, most states retained their TASC programs, albeit on a

[8]The commission also endorsed a parallel structure of short-term community-based civil commitment, as an alternative to criminal justice intervention, together with model legislation to implement this approach (Bonnie and Sonnenreich, 1975).

reduced scale. In 1991, there were 178 TASC programs in 32 states (Weinman, 1992).

In recent years, new initiatives linking criminal justice intervention to drug abuse treatment have begun to emerge, largely on an ad hoc basis. One important example is the proliferation of so-called drug courts—a generic term for several different types of initiatives designed to cope with the growing number of drug cases. These initiatives include distinctive case management systems and/or pretrial diversion programs. Many of the new drug courts hear evidence and adjudicate guilt, whereas others serve as special "plea bargaining" forums. Some drug courts handle only first offenders; others have no such limitations. Since all of the drug court initiatives are relatively new, outcome data are limited, and their efficacy remains open to question. The renascent interest in drug treatment-criminal justice linkages heightens the need for rigorous studies of the therapeutic utility (and cost-effectiveness) of these coercive legal strategies: To what extent, and under what circumstances, does coerced treatment through the criminal justice system achieve beneficial effects as compared with voluntary treatment, with nontherapeutic criminal justice intervention, or with no intervention at all?

Legal strategies to coerce drug users into treatment have been used both at the "front end" in diversionary programs and among parole and probation populations. As noted in Chapter 8, however, experimental designs are rare, and it is difficult to disentangle the effects of treatment from the effects of coercion. Also, many studies have been concerned primarily with treatment retention or length of stay, rather than treatment outcome or posttreatment involvement in drug use or criminal behavior.

Future research regarding the effects of coerced treatment for drug abuse should compare outcomes (drug use and criminal behavior) for treatment groups under criminal justice supervision with the behavior of groups of matched offenders subjected to similar criminal justice supervision without treatment and of matched drug treatment clients who are not under criminal justice supervision. These studies should focus on coerced treatment at both the front and the back ends of the criminal process and should pay special attention to variations in offender characteristics (e.g., criminal and treatment histories) that bear on risk of recidivism and the risk of relapse. Use of coerced treatment for women offenders, especially those with children, also deserves attention. Many treatment programs are ill equipped to respond to the unique needs of this population, and the effects on treatment and legal outcomes should be evaluated.

Special attention should be paid to the behavioral contingencies used in various criminal justice linkage programs (see generally Winick, 1991). Three important variables in the dynamics of "soft" coercion are whether participation in the program is contractual (the defendant can decline to participate) or mandatory; the nature of the prescribed conditions (e.g., frequency of appointments and of urine testing); and the nature of the sanctions for violating the specified conditions. An important innovation in recent years has been frequent testing combined with the use of graduated sanctions, a scheme that utilizes escalating, though not catastrophic, penalties in response to predictable relapses. Examples of graduated sanctions used in the Washington, D.C., pretrial release program include three days in the jury box observing drug court, three days in jail, seven days in residential detoxification, or seven days in jail (Carver, 1996).

Another important feature of the new generation of programs is the use of inducements to elicit voluntary participation, even within the coercive context of criminal justice control. Lessons about the subjective aspects of coercion can be drawn from recent research on coercion in mental health treatment, which tends to show that, even in objectively coercive situations, people feel less "coerced" if they feel that they have had a "voice" and that they have been treated fairly (Lidz et al., 1995; Monahan et al., 1996). Careful study of the dynamics of therapeutic leverage represents an important new frontier in drug abuse research.

The committee recommends a strategic research initiative to determine the conditions under which threatened criminal sanctions deter drug use and the ways in which criminal sanctions can be used most effectively, in the context of other social controls and in conjunction with other initiatives such as treatment programs, to maximize their beneficial effects while minimizing their deleterious effects.

CONFIDENTIALITY AND FEAR OF PUNISHMENT

In 1972, in response to the increasing incidence of drug abuse in the United States, Congress passed the Drug Abuse Office and Treatment Act of 1972 (86 U.S. Stat. 65; 21 U.S. Code 1175, 1972). The act was intended to increase the number of drug users who would willingly seek treatment by guaranteeing the confidentiality of the clinical records of all drug patients in federal drug treatment programs, based on the assumption that a guarantee of confidentiality is a necessary prerequisite to the success of any voluntary drug treatment program. The act also was intended as a minimum requisite for confidentiality in drug treatment programs; it was expected that state laws governing confidentiality would go beyond the federal model. In fact, however, the rules governing confidentiality in federal drug treatment programs offer a greater degree of protection than do the laws of many states that govern confidentiality in state drug treatment programs and in the physician–patient or therapist–client relationship.

Little research has been conducted to assess the effect that a guarantee of confidentiality, or the real or perceived lack thereof, has on the treatment-seeking behavior of drug users. The research that has been conducted has focused primarily on pregnant women and adolescents, who often are not protected by confidentiality laws at the state level. As discussed in more detail below, anecdotal reports and existing research indicate that laws denying confidentiality to pregnant women and adolescents may have unintended deleterious health effects. Additional research on the effects of various laws governing confidentiality would enable policymakers to make informed judgments when considering such laws. Moreover, research on the effects of confidentiality, and fear of disclosure, on treatment-seeking behavior has been given heightened importance in the era of managed care with its erosion of confidentiality on many levels.

Pregnant Women

As state courts and legislatures have become more aware of the risks of drug use during pregnancy, they have responded with a variety of both rehabilitative and punitive measures. Many courts have permitted the prosecution of women, under general child abuse and neglect statutes, if they have been found to use drugs while pregnant. State legislatures have enacted a variety of laws, ranging from statutes mandating the creation of counseling programs for pregnant drug abusers, to those requiring physicians (under certain circumstances) to test women and/or their newborns for the presence of controlled substances and to report positive test results to appropriate state agencies. There also has been an increasing trend toward imposing criminal sanctions on women who use drugs while pregnant.

Proponents of these requirements and sanctions argue that such measures will deter women from using drugs while they are pregnant and will prompt pregnant drug abusers to seek drug treatment. Opponents, including many representatives of the medical profession, counter that such measures will cause pregnant drug abusers to avoid prenatal or medical care in order to avoid detection of their drug use. In addition, researchers protest that mandatory reporting laws, requiring them to report pregnant women who admit drug use, often prevent them from gathering any meaningful data from that population. Little empirical evidence exists regarding the effects of mandatory reporting laws and the imposition of civil and criminal penalties on pregnant drug abusers (Berlin et al., 1991; Poland et al., 1993). To assist policymakers and the courts in developing effective approaches for the reduction of drug use during pregnancy, studies should be undertaken to examine the attitudes and actions of women both before and after a variety of laws are implemented so as to better understand the impact of such laws on drug use and prenatal care.

Adolescents

Adolescents also may be deterred from seeking treatment for drug use due to a lack of confidentiality in the physician–patient relationship. Although many states currently allow for confidential medical evaluation and treatment of minors for alcohol and other drug abuse problems, the extent to which physicians confidentiality is respected is unclear (Marks et al., 1990). Moreover, researchers have found that uncertainty about confidentiality may cause adolescents to suppress relevant information or to delay or avoid medical visits (Resnick et al., 1980; Cheng et al., 1993). There is also evidence that some pediatricians are not comfortable providing care to adolescents for such problems (Marks et al., 1990). Additional studies of adolescent confidentiality and its effect on care-seeking behavior would provide an important guide to policymakers and health care service providers who are trying to encourage adolescents to enter drug abuse treatment.

The committee urges research on confidentiality and disclosure laws to determine their impact on treatment-seeking behaviors among adolescents and pregnant women.

CONCLUSION AND RECOMMENDATION

In this chapter, the committee has presented a menu of policy-relevant issues pertaining to the effects of drug control and has identified four specific topics for future research. In the course of its deliberation on these questions, the committee noted, with considerable uneasiness, that some readers of this report might regard the very raising of these questions, and the use of a "public health" framework, as a declaration of dissent from current policies. This is not the committee's intention. Its aim is simply to include the public health effects of drug control within the field of drug abuse research and, thereby, to strengthen the empirical foundation of drug policymaking.

The committee recognizes that drug policy debate has become highly polarized. Committee members are convinced, however, that the empirical issues bearing on drug policy can be usefully organized within a public health framework, that the use of this framework is compatible with the entire range of positions on drug policy, and that it represents a commitment to none of them. The committee is also convinced that a common understanding of the current state of knowledge and of the questions that should be addressed would clarify the areas of dispute and thereby promote rational and informed debate.

The committee encourages NIDA, the National Institute of Justice (NIJ), and other public and private sponsors of drug abuse research to incorporate policy-relevant studies of drug control within a comprehensive scientific agenda.

The committee is aware that this recommendation raises important questions about the relative priority of drug control research and the proper locus of responsibility for funding it. NIDA's current budget could not feasibly be stretched to include a broad new realm of investigation, and the NIJ budget is not now adequate to fund a rigorous new initiative. For the present, the committee recommends that NIDA, the Department of Justice, and other public and private agencies review the substantive suggestions made in this chapter and consider the most sensible ways to encourage and support research on the public health effects of drug control.

REFERENCES

Angarola RT, Minsk AG, 1994. Regulation of psychostimulants: How much is too much? In: Schwartz HI, ed. *Psychiatric Practice Under Fire: The Influence of Government, the Media and Special Interests on Somatic Therapies*. Washington, DC: American Psychiatric Press.

Belenko S. 1993. *Crack and the Evolution of Anti-Drug Policy*. Greenwich CT: Greenwood Press.

Belenko S, Nickerson G, Rubinstein T. 1990. *Crack and the New York City Courts: A Study of Judicial Responses and Attitudes*. Final Report, Grant No. SJI-88-14X-E-050. New York: State Justice Institute.

Belenko S, Fagan J, Chin K. 1991. Criminal justice responses to crack. *Journal of Research in Crime and Delinquency* 28(1):55–74.

Berk RA, Campbell A, Klap R, Western B. 1992. The deterrent effect of arrest in incidents of domestic violence: A Bayesian analysis of four field experiments. *American Sociological Review*. 57:698–708.

Berlin F, Malin M, Dean S. 1991. Effects of statutes requiring psychiatrists to report suspected sexual abuse of children. *American Journal of Psychiatry* 148(4):449–453.

BJS (Bureau of Justice Statistics). 1993. *Prisoners in 1992*. BJS Bulletin NCJ-141874. Washington, DC: U.S. Department of Justice.

BJS (Bureau of Justice Statistics). 1994. *Fact Sheet: Drug Data Summary*. NCJ-148213. Washington, DC: U.S. Department of Justice.

Blumstein A, Cohen J, Martin SE, Tonry ME. 1983. *Research on Sentencing: The Search for Reform, Vol. 1*. Washington DC: National Academy Press.

Bonnie RJ. 1977. Decriminalizing the marijuana user: A drafter's guide. *University of Michigan Journal of Law Reform* 11:3–50.

Bonnie RJ. 1986. The efficacy of law as a paternalistic instrument. In: Melton G, ed. *Nebraska Symposium on Human Motivation, 1985*. Lincoln, NE: University of Nebraska. Pp. 131–211.

Bonnie RJ, Sonnenreich MR. 1975. *Legal Aspects of Drug Dependence*. Cleveland, OH: CRC Press.

Carver JA. 1996. Pretrial urine testing: Implications for drug courts from a decade's positive experience. *On Balance* Spring:2–3.

CASA (Center on Addiction and Substance Abuse, Columbia University). 1995. *Legalization: Panacea or Pandora's Box*. White Paper 1. New York: CASA.

Caulkins JP. 1994. What is the average price of an illicit drug? *Addiction* 89(7):815–819.

Caulkins JP. 1995. *Estimating Elasticities of Demand for Cocaine and Heroin with DUF Data*. Carnegie Mellon University, Heinz School Working Paper 95-13. Under review in *Marketing Science*.

Chaiken M, ed. 1988. *Street-Level Drug Enforcement: Examining The Issues*. Washington, DC: National Institute of Justice.

Cheng T, Savageau J, Sattler A, DeWitt T. 1993. Confidentiality in health care: A survey of knowledge, perceptions, and attitudes among high school students. *Journal of the American Medical Association* 269(11):1404–1407.

Cooper JR, Czechowicz DJ, Molinari SP, eds. 1993. *Impact of Prescription Drug Diversion Control Systems on Medical Practice and Patient Care*. NIDA Research Monograph 131. Rockville, MD: NIDA.

Cuskey WR. 1981. Critique of marijuana decriminalization research. *Contemporary Drug Problems* 10:323–334.

Davis R. 1995. Tobacco policy research comes of age. *Tobacco Control* 4:6.

Dinardo J. 1993. Law enforcement, the price of cocaine, and cocaine use. *Mathematical Modelling* 17(2):53–64.

Erickson PG. 1976. Deterrence and deviance: The example of cannabis prohibition. *Journal of Criminal Law and Criminology* 67(2):222–232.

Fagan J. 1994. Do criminal sanctions deter drug offenders. In: MacKenzie DL, Uchida CD, eds. *Drugs and Crime: Evaluating Public Policy Initiatives*. Thousand Oaks, CA: Sage.

Fagan J. 1995. *Cocaine and Federal Sentencing Policy*. Testimony to the Subcommittee on Crime, Committee on the Judiciary, U.S. House of Representatives, Washington DC. June 29, 1995.

Goerdt JA, Martin JA. 1989. The impact of drug cases on case processing in urban trial courts. *State Court Journal* 13(4):4–12.

Goldstein A, Kalant H. 1990. Drug policy: Striking the right balance. *Science* 249:1513–1521.

Greenstein SC. 1990. *Trends in Recidivism Among Felons Sentenced to Probation*. New York: New York State Division of Criminal Justice Services, Office of Justice Systems Analysis.

Gruenwald P, Ponicki W, Holder H. 1993. The relationship of outlet densities to alcohol consumption: A time series cross-sectional analysis. *Alcoholism: Clinical and Experimental Research* 17:38–47.

Hu TW, Bai J, Keeler TE, Barnett PG, Sung HY. 1994. The impact of California Proposition 99, a major anti-smoking law, on cigarette consumption. *Journal of Public Health Policy* 15(1):26–36.

Husak D. 1992. *Drugs and Rights*. New York: Cambridge University Press.

IOM (Institute of Medicine). 1994. *Growing Up Tobacco Free*. Washington, DC: National Academy Press.

IOM (Institute of Medicine). 1995a. *The Development of Medications for the Treatment of Opiate and Cocaine Addictions*. Washington, DC: National Academy Press.

IOM (Institute of Medicine). 1995b. *Federal Regulation of Methadone Treatment*. Washington, DC: National Academy Press.

Johnson BD, Williams T, Kei KA, Sanabria H. 1990. Drug abuse in the inner city: Impact on hard-drug users and the community. In: Morris N, Tonry M, eds. *Drugs and Crime, Vol. 13*. Chicago: University of Chicago Press. Pp. 9–68.

Joranson DE, Gilson AM. 1994a. Controlled substances, medical practice, and the law. In: Schwartz HI, ed. *Psychiatric Practice Under Fire: The Influence of Government, the Media, and Special Interests on Somatic Therapies*. Washington, DC: American Psychiatric Press. Pp. 173–194.

Joranson DE, Gilson AM. 1994b. Policy issues and imperatives in the use of opioids to treat pain in substance abusers. *Journal of Law, Medicine, and Ethics*. 22:215–223.

Kleber H. 1996. Decriminalization of cannabis. *Lancet* 346:1708.

Kleiman MR, Smith KD. 1990. State and local drug enforcement: In search of a strategy. In: Morris N, Tonry M, eds. *Drugs and Crime, Vol. 13*. Chicago: University of Chicago Press. Pp. 69–108.

Kleiman MR, Smith KD. 1992. *Against Excess: Drug Policy for Results*. New York: Basic Books.

Lidz C, Hoge S, Gardner W, Bennett N, Monahan J, Mulvey E, Roth L. 1995. Perceived coercion in mental health admission: Pressures and process. *Archives of General Psychiatry* 52:1034–1039.

MacCoun R, Saiger AJ, Kahan JP, Reuter P. 1993. Drug policies and problems: The promise and pitfalls of cross-national comparisons. In: Heather N, Wodak A, Nadelmann E, O'Hare P, eds. *Psychoactive Drugs and Harm Reduction: From Faith to Science*. London: Whurr Publishers. Pp. 103–117.

MacCoun R, Model K, Phillips-Shockley H, Reuter P. 1995. Comparing drug policies in North America and Western Europe. In: Estienenart G, ed. *Policies and Strategies to Combat Drugs in Europe*. Netherlands: Kluwer Academic.

Maloff D. 1981. A review of the effects of the decriminalization of marijuana. *Contemporary Drug Problems* 10:307–322.

Marks A, Fisher M, Lasker S. 1990. Adolescent medicine in pediatric practice. *Journal of Adolescent Health Care* 11(2):149–153.

Meier R, Johnson W. 1977. Deterrence as social control: The legal and extralegal production of conformity. *American Sociological Review* 42:292–304.

Monahan J, Hoge S, Lidz C, Roth L, Bennett N, Gardner W, Mulvey E, Roth L. 1996. Coercion to inpatient treatment: Initial results and implications for assertive treatment in the community. In: Dennis D, Monahan J, eds. *Coercion and Aggressive Community Treatment: A New Frontier in Mental Health Law*. New York: Plenum.

Moore MH. 1973. Achieving discrimination in the effective price of heroin. *American Economic Review* 63.

Moore MH. 1977. *Buy and Bust*. Lexington, MA: Lexington Books.

Moore MH. 1990. Supply reduction and drug law enforcement. In: Morris N, Tonry M, eds. *Drugs and Crime, Vol. 13*. Chicago: University of Chicago Press. Pp. 109–158.

Musto D. 1987. *The American Disease: Origins of Narcotic Control*. New York: Oxford University Press.

Nadelmann EA. 1989. Drug prohibition in the United States: Costs, consequences, and alternatives. *Science* 245:939–946.

NCMDA (National Commission on Marihuana and Drug Abuse). 1973. *Drug Use in America: Problem in Perspective*. Washington, DC: U.S. Government Printing Office.

New York City Police Department. 1990. *Statistical Report: Complaints and Arrests, 1989*. New York: Office of Management Analysis and Planning.

NRC (National Research Council). 1995. *Preventing HIV Transmission: The Role of Sterile Needles and Bleach*. Washington, DC: National Academy Press.

ONDCP (Office of National Drug Control Policy). 1992. *Price and Purity of Cocaine: The Relationship to Emergency Room Visits and Deaths, and to Drug Use Among Arrestees.* Washington, DC: ONDCP.

ONDCP (Office of National Drug Control Policy). 1996. *National Drug Control Strategy: Budget Summary.* Washington, DC: ONDCP.

Ossebaard HC. 1996. Netherlands' cannabis policy (letter). *Lancet* 347:7676–7678.

Peterson DE, Zeger SL, Remington PL, Anderson HA. 1992. The effect of state cigarette tax increases on cigarette sales, 1955 to 1988. *American Journal of Public Health* 82(1):94–96.

Poland M, Dombrowski M, Ager J, Sokol R. 1993. Punishing pregnant drug users: Enhancing the flight from care. *Drug and Alcohol Dependence* 31(3):199–203.

Resnick M, Blum R, Hedin D. 1980. The appropriateness of health services for adolescents: Youth's opinions and attitudes. *Journal of Adolescent Health Care* 1(2):137–141.

Reuter P. 1992. Hawks ascendant: The punitive trend of drug policy. *Daedalus* 121:15–52.

Reuter P, MacCoun R. 1995. Assessing the legalization debate. In: Estienenart G, ed. *Policies and Strategies to Combat Drugs in Europe.* Netherlands: Kluwer Academic.

Reuter P, Falco M, MacCoun R. 1993. *Comparing Western European and North American Drug Policies: An International Conference Report.* RAND MR-287-GMF/SF. Santa Monica, CA: RAND.

Ross HL. 1984. Social control through deterrence: Drinking and driving laws. *Annual Review of Sociology* 10:21–35.

SAMHSA (Substance Abuse and Mental Health Services Administration). 1992. *Approval and Monitoring of Narcotic Treatment Programs: A Guide on the Roles of Federal and State Agencies (Draft).* Rockville, MD: SAMHSA.

Saner H, MacCoun R, Reuter P. 1994. *On the Ubiquity of Drug Selling Among Youthful Offenders, 1985–1991: Age, Period, or Cohort Effect?* Working Paper #213. University of California, Graduate School of Public Policy.

Sherman LW. 1989. Police crackdowns: Initial and residual deterrence. In: Morris N, Tonry M, eds. *Crime and Justice: An Annual Review of Research, Vol. 12.* Chicago: University of Chicago Press.

Sherman LW. 1992. The influence of criminology on criminal law: Evaluating arrests for misdemeanor domestic violence. *Journal of Criminal Law and Criminology* 83: 1–45.

Sifanek SJ, Kaplan CD. 1995. Keeping off, stepping on, and stepping off: The Steppingstone theory reevaluated in the context of the Dutch cannabis experience. *Contemporary Drug Problems* 22(3):483–512.

Sigler KA, Guernsey BG, Ingrim NB, Buesing AA. 1984. Effect of a triplicate prescription law on the prescribing of schedule II drugs. *American Journal of Hospital Pharmacy* 41:108–111.

Stafford M, Warr M. 1993. A reconceptualization of general and specific deterrence. *Journal of Research in Crime and Delinquency* 30(2):123–135.

Sviridoff M, Sadd S, Curtis R, Grinc R. 1992. *The Neighborhood Effects of Street-Level Drug Enforcement: Tactical Narcotics Teams in New York.* Final Report to the National Institute of Justice. New York: Vera Institute of Justice.

Tonry M. 1990. Research on drugs and crime. In: Morris N, Tonry M, eds. *Drugs and Crime, Vol. 13.* Chicago: University of Chicago Press. Pp. 1–8.

Tonry M. 1995. *Malign Neglect: Race, Crime and Punishment in America.* New York: Oxford University Press.

U.S. Sentencing Commission. 1995. *Special Report to Congress: Cocaine and Federal Sentencing Policy.* Washington DC: U.S. Sentencing Commission.

Waagenar AC, Toomey T, Murray D, Short B, Wolfson M, Jones-Webbr M. 1996. Sources of alcohol for underage drinkers. *Journal of Studies on Alcohol* 57:325–333.

Wasserman J, Manning WG, Newhouse JP, Winkler JD. 1991. The effects of excise taxes and regulations on cigarette smoking. *Journal of Health Economics* 10:43–64.

Weinman B. 1992. A coordinated approach for drug-abusing offenders: TASC and parole. *NIDA Research Monograph* 118:232–245.

Weintraub M, Singh S, Byrne L, Maharaj K, Guttmacher L. 1991. Consequences of the 1989 New York State benzodiazepine prescription regulations. *Journal of the American Medical Association*. 266:2392–2397.

Williams K, Hawkins R. 1989. Controlling male aggression in intimate relationships. *Law & Society Review* 23:591–612.

Winick BJ. 1991. Harnessing the power of the bet: Wagering with the government for social and individual change. In: Wexler DB, Winick BJ, eds. *Essays in Therapeutic Jurisprudence*. Durham, NC: Carolina Academic Press.

Wisotsky S. 1990. *Beyond the War on Drugs*. 2nd ed. Buffalo NY: Prometheus Books.

Zimmer L. 1987. *Operation Pressure Point*. Occasional paper of the Center for Crime and Justice, New York University School of Law. New York: New York University School of Law.

Zimring FE, Hawkins G. 1992. *The Search for Rational Drug Control*. Cambridge, England: Cambridge University Press.

Appendixes

A

Acknowledgments

Huda Akil
Mental Health Research Institute
University of Michigan

Douglas Anglin
Drug Abuse Research Center
University of California, Los Angeles

Robert Balster
Medical College of Virginia

Albert Bandura
Stanford University

Guardia Bannister
Providence Hospital
Washington, DC

Deborah Beck
Drug and Alcohol Service Providers Organization of Pennsylvania
Harrisburg, PA

Jack Bergman
Harvard University

Warren Bickel
University of Vermont

Floyd Bloom
The Scripps Research Institute
La Jolla, CA

Joseph Brady
Johns Hopkins University School of Medicine

Barry Brown
Consultant
Carolina Beach, NC

William E. Bunney
California College of Medicine
University of California, Irvine

Marilyn Carroll
University of Minnesota School of Medicine

Marsha Chaiken
LINC
Alexandria, VA

Laurie Chassin
Arizona State University

Anna Rose Childress
University of Pennsylvania School of Medicine

Alec Christoff
D.C. Pretrial Services Agency
Washington, DC

Linda Collins
Center for Developmental and Health Research Methodology
Pennsylvania State University

R. Lorraine Collins
Research Institute on Addictions
Buffalo, NY

Jean Comolli
National Institute on Drug Abuse
Rockville, MD

Tim Condon
National Institute on Drug Abuse
Rockville, MD

Linda Cottler
Washington University School of Medicine

Joseph T. Coyle
Harvard Medical School

Thomas J. Crowley
University of Colorado School of Medicine

Thomas D'Aunno
University of Chicago

Miriam Davis
Science and Health Policy Consultant
Silver Spring, MD

Nancy Day
University of Pittsburgh School of Medicine

Don Des Jarlais
Chemical Dependency Institute
National Development and Research Institutes, Inc.
New York City

Glen Elliott
University of California, San Francisco

Margaret Ensminger
Johns Hopkins University School of Medicine

Jeffrey Fagan
Columbia University

John Falk
Rutgers University

Ronald A. Feldman
The Columbia University School of Social Work

Loretta P. Finnegan
National Institutes of Health
Rockville, MD

Joanna S. Fowler
Brookhaven National Laboratory
Upton, NY

Deborah Frank
Boston University School of Medicine

Ellen Frank
University of Pittsburgh School of Medicine

Alfred Friedman
Belmont Medical Center
Philadelphia

Saunji Fyffe
National Institute of Justice
Rockville, MD

Suzanne Gelber
Brandeis University

Barry Glick
Fighting Back
Washington, DC

Avram Goldstein
Stanford University

Denise C. Gottfredson
University of Maryland
College Park

Elizabeth Griffin
Baltimore Coalition Against Substance Abuse
Baltimore, MD

Beatrix A. Hamburg
William T. Grant Foundation
New York City

Roger Hartman
Office of the Assistant Secretary of Defense (Health Affairs)
Washington, DC

Jimmie C.B. Holland
Memorial Sloan-Kettering Cancer Center
New York City

Philip S. Holzman
Harvard University

Connie Horgan
Institute for Health Policy
Brandeis University

Steven Hyman
National Institute of Mental Health
Rockville, MD

Chris-Ellyn Johanson
Wayne State University School of Medicine

David E. Joranson
University of Wisconsin Medical School

Yifrah Kaminer
University of Connecticut Health Center

Stephen R. Kandall
Beth Israel Medical Center
New York City

Denise Kandel
Columbia University

Eric Kandel
Columbia University

Howard B. Kaplan
Texas A & M University

Herbert D. Kleber
Center on Addiction and Substance Abuse
New York City

Thomas R. Kosten
Yale University

Alan Leshner
National Institute on Drug Abuse
Rockville, MD

David Lewis
Brown University

Richard Lopez
D.C. General Hospital
Washington, DC

Spero Manson
University of Colorado Health Sciences Center

G. Alan Marlatt
University of Washington

Linda Mayes
Yale University School of Medicine

Duane McBride
Andrews University

Nancy A. McLauglin
Hunton and Williams
Richmond, VA

Nancy Mello
Alcohol and Drug Abuse Research Center
McLean Hospital
Belmont, MA

Kathleen Merikangas
Yale University School of Medicine

Robert Michels
Cornell University Medical College

Klaus Miczek
Tufts University

Mark Moore
Harvard University School of Medicine

David Musto
Yale University School of Medicine

Kenrad Nelson
The Johns Hopkins University

Charles P. O'Brien
University of Pennsylvania School of Medicine

Eugene R. Oetting
Colorado State University

Perry Renshaw
McLean Hospital
Belmont, MA

Peter Reuter
University of Maryland
College Park

Dorothy Rice
Institute for Health and Aging
University of California, San Francisco

Cynthia Robbins
University of Delaware

Lee N. Robins
Washington University School of Medicine

Terry Robinson
University of Michigan

David Rosenbloom
Join Together
Boston

Sally Satel
Consultant
Washington, DC

Marc Schuckit
San Diego, CA

Charles Schuster
Wayne State University School of Medicine

Steven S. Sharfstein
The Sheppard and Enoch Pratt Hospital
Baltimore, MD

D. Wayne Simpson
Texas Christian University

Maxine Stitzer
Johns Hopkins University

Jeffrey Swanson
Psychiatric Epidemiology and Health Services Research Program
Duke University Medical Center

Ralph E. Tarter
University of Pittsburgh School of Medicine

Gary Tischler
The Neuropsychiatric Institute
University of California School of Medicine, Los Angeles

William Vodra
Arnold and Porter
Washington, DC

Nora Volkow
Brookhaven National Laboratory
Upton, NY

Stephen Waxman
Yale University School of Medicine

Ellen A. Wortella
University of Texas at Austin

B

Drug Abuse Research in Historical Perspective

David F. Musto, M.D.

Attempts to understand the nature of illicit drug abuse and addiction can be traced back for centuries, however, the search has always been limited by the scientific theories and social attitudes available or dominant at any one time. Dr. Benjamin Rush, a founder of the first medical school in the United States and a signer of the Declaration of Independence, was one of the pioneers of U.S. drug abuse research. However, he had few scientific resources available to attack the problem. The intricacies of cellular response to a drug could not be understood until tools were developed to measure the response and to integrate this knowledge with complex cellular biochemistry—a technology that has been developed only in the past decade. One can compare this situation with that of pneumonia. A myriad of treatments and partially effective remedies were used until the discovery of penicillin, when the old treatments became a part of medical history. It is now possible, however, to be optimistic that the tools needed to resolve the addiction problem are at hand.

BEGINNINGS OF MODERN DRUG ABUSE RESEARCH

Although the funding of drug abuse research has increased substantially since the 1960s—largely due to grants by the National Institute on Drug Abuse (NIDA) and the National Institute of Mental Health (NIMH)—significant research began much earlier. The vicissitudes of this research illustrate changing popular and professional attitudes toward illicit drugs and drug users and also provide insights into the relationship between scientific findings and drug policy.

Most of the modern problems, as well as the benefits, resulting from drug use are the outcome of scientific and technological progress. Excluding distilled spirits, the first addictive ingredient isolated from a natural product was morphine, which was extracted from crude opium by F.W.A. Serturner, a German pharmacist, in 1806. Increasingly widespread use of morphine, which constitutes roughly 10 percent of crude opium, revolutionized pain control.

One of the first careful studies of morphine addiction was made in 1875 by Levinstein, who identified key elements in opiate addiction that would interest researchers: the fixation on the drug that made it the highest priority even when the user's life situation was deteriorating, and the curious phenomenon of withdrawal that could be reversed quickly by giving more opiate (Levinstein, 1878).

Around the turn of the century, several new medical research issues attracted investigators: communicable diseases, bacteria, and viruses; the immune system, with its antibodies and antigens; autointoxication, or the body poisoning itself; the endocrine glands and their production of hormones; and the rapidly developing fields of biochemistry and pharmacology. A number of researchers in the United States and abroad attempted to apply those contemporary approaches to the study of illicit drug abuse, addiction (specifically, opiate addiction), and its treatment.

A particularly popular line of research related to discoveries about the immune system and concerned the possible creation in the user's body of either antibodies or a toxin to morphine. This research attempted to parallel the success of antitoxins to diphtheria and tetanus. Gioffredi reported in 1897 that serum from addicted dogs could be injected into kittens, who were then protected against large doses of morphine (Gioffredi, 1897). In 1914, Valenti stated that he had extracted serum from dogs undergoing the abstinence reaction and was able to produce similar effects by injecting the serum into normal animals—giving support for the hypothesis that a toxin produced abstinence effects (Valenti, 1914).

Application of the concept of "autointoxication" to research on narcotic dependence emerged from the theories of Elie Metchnikoff, who won a Nobel Prize in medicine in 1908 for his work on toxins thought to be the product of fermentation in the large intestine (Metchnikoff, 1901). Other theories applied to drug addiction in the early 1900s included the blockage of endocrine gland passages (Sollier, 1898), changes in cell protoplasm (Cloetta, 1903), degenerative changes in brain cells (Wilcox, 1923), or changes in cell permeability (Fauser and Ottenstein, 1924). One other approach, exemplified by the New York physician Dr. Ernest S. Bishop, led to the claim that as long as the toxin or antibodies were balanced by a dose of morphine, the person would feel and function normally—a theory similar to that proposed for methadone treatment today (Bishop, 1920).

This early and active stage of research was characterized by optimism for medical research and the success of medical treatment. Estimates of cure ranged as high as 75–99 percent (Musto, 1987). Hope was great that the key to addiction had been found and that eventually a treatment as effective as that against diphtheria would be developed.

END OF MEDICAL OPTIMISM

Soon, however, this situation changed dramatically. Around the time of World War I, extensive drug use in the United States—a combination of morphine, heroin, opium, and cocaine—created a growing fear of drug abuse. The association of opium with Chinese immigrants, cocaine with African Americans, and morphine addiction with careless physicians prompted more and more restrictive legislation and an antagonism to easy access to those drugs. A six-year federal effort to control the distribution of opiates and cocaine led to the Harrison Anti-Narcotics Act of 1914.

Regulations associated with the Harrison Act and promulgated by the U.S. Treasury Department in 1915 indicated that the maintenance of nonmedical addicts on narcotics to avoid withdrawal would not be considered legitimate medical practice. The federal government then began to use the act to prosecute doctors who issued prescriptions for that purpose. In 1919, the Supreme Court ratified the federal government's interpretation of the laws. The position against maintenance was controversial, however, not only because it seemed to represent an intrusion into medical practice, but also because the Gioffredi and Valenti hypotheses—that opiate use causes permanent physiological changes through creation of antibodies or a toxin—seemed to give support to those who considered addiction a medical disease.

E.J. Pellini, the Assistant City Chemist of New York, actively examined the Gioffredi and Valenti claims and, in the early 1920s, published a refutation of their hypotheses (Pellini and Greenfield, 1920, 1924). The general conclusion drawn from this debate over antibodies and toxins was that there was no organic basis for addiction and withdrawal and that these phenomena were "functional" or "psychological." Thus, research into addiction and withdrawal became a controversial field after 1919 due to the fact such that research might find evidence supporting a medical model and thereby possibly challenge established government policy.

RESEARCH IN THE 1920s

Drug abuse research in the 1920s seems to have been at a relatively low level of activity. The Public Health Service (PHS) produced some estimates of the number of addicts and general statements on the nature and treatment of drug users. Perhaps the chief scientific contribution of that decade was the demonstration of morphine dependence in monkeys.

In addition to PHS, the Rockefeller Institute supported drug research. In 1913, the institute created the Bureau of Social Hygiene to study social problems generally and criminology in particular, and by the time the bureau was disbanded in 1933, 32 papers and books on addiction had been published with its support (Eddy, 1973). The vast majority described studies at Iowa State University of the effect of morphine on the gastrointestinal system and its fate in the body, as well as clinical efforts in Philadelphia to cure addicts and monitor morphine in the bodies of the patients. The foundation also supported the compendium *The Opium Problem*, a large anthology of information that is still in use (Terry and Pellens, 1928).

NATIONAL RESEARCH COUNCIL COMMITTEE ON DRUG ADDICTION

At the close of the 1920s, the Bureau of Social Hygiene decided to transfer its support of research to the National Research Council (NRC), where it was hoped greater central direction could be achieved. In 1929, the Committee on Drug Addiction was established by the NRC's Chair of the Medical Sciences Division (May and Jacobson, 1989). Its members included medical school researchers and key government scientists and administrators, including the head of the Federal Bureau of Narcotics, H. J. Anslinger. Their first task was to decide the direction of research, and their reasoning is quite instructive as to the state of research around 1930. The committee considered that further sociological studies were unlikely to help the drug situation. Given its resources, the committee felt that one drug should be targeted. Cocaine was considered but was dropped because it was no longer much of an abuse problem. Codeine appeared to be less addictive, thus posing less danger, so morphine was chosen as the target of this new research effort.

The goal of studying morphine was to find substitutes that were not habit forming. Scientists were well aware that they worked in a framework of law and policy that precluded maintenance and in an atmosphere of extreme antagonism to narcotic drugs. In addition to seeking safe substitutes, the NRC committee approved three more tasks: (1) synopses of the literature on morphine and other addictive drugs were to be prepared; (2) based on the literature search, rules and regulations governing the legitimate use of morphine and other habit-forming drugs were to be established; and (3) a determination of where gaps existed in biological knowledge was to be made.

The committee proceeded to attack the problem by working in three settings—chemical laboratories that would create possible substitutes, a pharmacology lab where these would be tested, and a clinical setting in which human subjects could be studied. New substances for trial were created first at Yale and then at Dr. L.F. Small's laboratory at the University of Virginia. The substances were then sent to a new pharmacology unit at the University of Michigan headed by Dr. Nathan Eddy, where they were tested on laboratory animals.

Clinical facilities were meager until the "narcotic farms" opened in Lexington, Kentucky, in 1935 and Ft. Worth, Texas, in 1938. These institutions, dubbed farms by the sponsor of the legislation that established them, Representative Stephen G. Porter of Pennsylvania, were in fact special prisons for drug addicts, complete with cells and bars. They were officially under the control of the Treasury Department, which was charged with the enforcement of narcotic laws but were staffed by PHS officers. It was not until the late 1960s that the facility at Lexington became a true PHS hospital (Musto, 1987). Eventually the Addiction Research Center, under the leadership of C.K. Himmelsbach, was established at Lexington to determine the addictive liability of various compounds. Pharmacological research at the Lexington facility provided major contributions to the understanding of opiate and alcohol dependence and withdrawal, and included research on the quantification of opiate dependence as a physical or physiological phenomenon and on the effect of methadone on opiate withdrawal.

When it became apparent that the Rockefeller funding would not be continued, the chemical and pharmacological work was transferred to the PHS. At that time—in 1941—a non-habit-forming analgesic to replace morphine had not been found. However, many drugs had been tested, and experts were hopeful that compounds with a more salutary balance of effects, although still habit forming, might be developed. Certainly, many of the pitfalls of drug testing had been recognized. Judged by today's sophisticated research, the methods were simple. Addiction liability was typically tested by substituting the test drug for a regular dose of morphine in a morphine-dependent person and observing the results. The relation of molecular composition to effect was considered but at a level that could not take into account the actual shape of the molecule or the site on which it acted. These early studies illustrate the limitations of knowledge at the molecular level, where pain relief and dependence actually occurs.

FROM THE CLOSE OF WORLD WAR II TO THE 1960s

In 1947, the National Research Council established a successor body, the Committee on Drug Addiction and Narcotics. Prominent among the reasons for this renewed activity was the appearance of methadone from German laboratories. Methadone had been substituted for morphine to meet German needs during World War II. Researchers' considerable interest in methadone's possibilities, together with other unfunded ideas for scientific studies in the field, prompted the group to consider asking pharmaceutical manufacturers for contributions to a research fund that the committee would administer. NRC approved, and by the end of 1949, eight firms had contributed a total of $18,500. This episode reveals the paucity of funding sources and the extremely modest amounts with which basic and practical research on pain relief was conducted immediately after World War II.

There were other supports for research in this area. University science departments contributed some of their own funds to these studies. Furthermore, pharmaceutical companies themselves conducted research on analgesics, although their practice of sending new drugs for testing under the committee's auspices suggests that their programs in this area were not comprehensive.

In addition to its funding from pharmaceutical companies, NRC's Committee on Drug Addiction and Narcotics began to receive small annual amounts from the Veterans Administration (VA) and the World Health Organization (WHO) in 1961. Research sponsored by the committee was varied and included studies of methadone as well as the opiate antagonists nalorphine, naloxone, and naltrexone. Additionally, the committee advised the Federal Bureau of Narcotics and the Food and Drug Administration on the potential abuse liability of marketable drugs. The committee changed its name to the Committee on Problems of Drug Dependence (CPDD) in 1965 to meet the new definition of "addiction" promulgated by WHO. By 1977, CPDD had incorporated as an independent organization; it continued to grow as a locus of scientific interchange, later changing its name to the College of Problems of Drug Dependence.

NATIONAL COMMISSION ON MARIHUANA AND DRUG ABUSE

The era from World War I through 1960 had seen a loss of faith in the possibility of successfully treating narcotics addicts. Dr. Alexander Lambert, a leading advocate of addiction treatment since 1909, exemplified this trend with his abandonment in 1920 of the "cure" he had advocated for 11 years. Federal drug policy became concentrated on narcotics control through law enforcement, and prevention and treatment were deemphasized. However, this trend began to decline with time.

During the 1960s, the entrenched commitment to law enforcement confronted an unprecedented rise in the nature and extent of illicit drug use. The transformation, especially in marijuana use, was associated with social and political turmoil, including the deep fissures caused by the Vietnam War, the civil rights movement, and profound demographic changes as the "baby boom" generation approached maturity. The first of several steps toward abandonment of the punitive-deterrent philosophy was the report of the President's Commission on Narcotics and Drug Abuse, which was an outgrowth of the 1962 White House Conference on Drug Abuse. The report advocated adoption of approaches more in keeping with the view of illicit drug abuse as a disease and with theories of social deviance control through medical means. This sort of thinking enjoyed widespread acceptance at that time and was the philosophy behind the establishment of federally funded community mental health centers which began the same year.

Congress responded by enacting the Comprehensive Drug Abuse and Control Act of 1970. This act attempted to deal with the growing wave of drug use in the context of new attitudes and approaches by making penalties, especially for marijuana possession, less severe and more flexible and by creating categories for drugs of varying dangerousness that would allow shifts between classes to be achieved administratively rather than requiring a new statute. One of the most important initiatives of the new law was the establishment of the National Commission on Marihuana and Drug Abuse, which would report over two years (1971–1973) on the whole range of issues linked to drug use.

The commission's first report, *Marihuana: A Signal of Misunderstanding* (NCMDA, 1972), recommended "decriminalization" as a response to the widespread use of marijuana. Although dealing in the drug would be still prohibited under this approach, users would no longer be subject to criminal punishment. This proposal was disavowed by President Nixon but influenced a number of state laws in the 1970s. Furthermore, the report urged substantial studies on marijuana, commissioned many itself, and published them in two large volumes of technical papers.

The commission's second report, *Drug Use in America: Problem in Perspective* (NCMDA, 1973), continued the strong recommendation both for government-sponsored research and for continuation of national surveys on drug use that the commission had begun. The technical papers of the second report include studies on patterns and consequences of drug use, social responses to drug use, the legal system and drug control, and treatment and rehabilitation. The commission conceived a wide range of research relevant to drug issues and set an example for the research programs of NIMH and NIDA.

FOUNDATION SUPPORT

With the exception of studies on alcoholism, foundation support for drug abuse research did not emerge until the 1960s and 1970s, when changing use patterns made drug abuse a subject of national concern. The Ford Foundation had been receiving requests for support for drug abuse research since the 1950s, but not until 1968 did it award its first grant—$17,500 for a conference to discuss the possible role of the foundation.

In 1970, the Ford Foundation initiated the Drug Abuse Survey Project to pinpoint more precisely what should be done to combat drug abuse. Its final report, *Dealing with Drug Abuse* (Wald, 1972), analyzed in detail the great gaps in basic knowledge of drug actions within the body, psychological factors involved in deciding to use drugs, and the role of drugs in contemporary American society; it also made a strong appeal for more research. The report's practical outcome was creation of the Drug Abuse Council (DAC), which funded studies on illicit drug abuse from 1971 until 1978.

General foundation support for drug abuse research increased slightly in the 1980s, rising in the late 1980s as the crack epidemic crystallized national alarm over the drug abuse problem (Renz, 1989).

NIMH AND NIDA: RECENT FUNDING ON DRUG ABUSE

The National Institute of Mental Health was established in 1949 as one of the National Institutes of Health. Its growth was considerable and included funding not only for research but also for training and services. As successor to the PHS Division of Mental Hygiene, concerns with alcohol and narcotics naturally fell under its mantle. For example, the Addiction Research Center (ARC) at Lexington, Kentucky, became part of NIMH. In the late 1960s, a Division of Narcotic Addiction and Drug Abuse (DNADA) was established within NIMH to oversee this responsibility. Eventually, the drug and alcohol divisions of NIMH evolved into the National Institute on Drug Abuse and the National Institute on Alcohol Abuse and Alcoholism (NIAAA).

NIDA had its origins in the Drug Abuse Office and Treatment Act of 1972, which had established the Special Action Office for Drug Abuse Prevention (SAODAP) in the Executive Office of the President. SAODAP provided the first federal funding of drug abuse treatment and was part of an ambitious response to public fears of widespread drug experimentation among youth, the possibility that drug-addicted Vietnam veterans would pose a danger to public order, and the general perception of a link between drug abuse and crime. This SAODAP legislation established an expiration date for the office of June 30, 1975, and mandated devolution of its functions to a new institute of the Department of Health, Education, and Welfare (HEW), which was to come into existence on December 31, 1974. In fact, NIDA came into being over the summer of 1973 when HEW began a reorganization that created the Alcohol, Drug Abuse, and Mental Health Administration (ADAMHA); DNADA and SAODAP were merged under its aegis. (SAODAP had been operating on a lame duck basis since the 1972 presidential election and the resignation of its director in June 1973.) Further reorganization in 1992 divided drug abuse activities between the National Institutes of Health and the Substance Abuse and Mental Health Services Administration and assigned NIDA to the former.

The creation of NIDA was itself an indication that the drug abuse problem was not expected to go away soon and that sustained research into the treatment, prevention, and biology of drug abuse was a national necessity. Over the years, however, NIDA's research budget has undergone unsettling perturbations as seen in changes of its extramural grant funding (Table B.1). The 29 percent drop in 1982 was the most severe to date in NIDA's history. Drug abuse research is supported when the nation is in a state of alarm over a new drug or an escalation in drug use, but it is quickly reduced with changes in perception of drug use or when other issues become a priority. Thus, funding levels may shift significantly and may detrimentally affect research programs that rely on ongoing support both to maintain a specific research project and to keep trained experts employed in the field. Recent expansion of NIDA's budget can be attributed primarily to funds for research on human immunodeficiency virus and AIDS. In FY 1994, $143 million (34 percent of NIDA's $425 million budget appropriation) was designated for AIDS research (NIH, 1995). It is to NIDA's credit, however, and to the credit of drug abuse researchers that even with unstable funding levels, they have sponsored and conducted an extraordinary range of research that has resulted in many of the major accomplishments in the field discussed throughout this report.

TABLE B.1 Annual NIDA Extramural Research Budget, 1974–1994

Fiscal Year	Extramural Research Funding ($ million[a])	Percentage Change from Prior Year
1974	39	–15
1975	42	7
1976	37	–13
1977	36	–1
1978	37	2
1979	40	8
1980	40	1
1981	40	–1
1982	28	–29
1983	42	10
1984	50	27
1985	57	19
1986	51	8
1987	85	67
1988	107	26
1989	158	47
1990	197	25
1991	231[b]	
1992	228[b]	–1
1993	220[b]	–4
1994	224[b]	1

[a]In 1982 constant dollars.
[b]Figures include construction funds.

SOURCE: GAO (1992), NIDA (1994).

REFERENCES

Bishop ES. 1920. *The Narcotic Drug Problem*. New York: Macmillan.

Cloetta M. 1903. Über das verhalten des morphins im organismus und die ursachen der angewöhnung an dasselbe. *Archives of Experimental Pathology and Pharmacology* 50:453–480.

Eddy NB, ed. 1973. *The National Research Council Involvement in the Opiate Problem, 1928–1971*. Washington, DC: National Academy of Sciences.

Fauser A, Ottenstein B. 1924. Chemisches und physikalisch-chemisches aum problem der "Suchten" und "Entziehungserscheinungen," insbesonders des morphinismus und cocainisums. *Ztsch Neurologic Psychiatry* 88:128–133.

GAO (General Accounting Office). 1992. *Drug Abuse Research, Federal Funding and Future Needs*. Washington, DC: U.S. Government Printing Office.

Gioffredi C. 1897. L'immunité artificelle par les alcaloides. *Archives Italiennes de Biologie* 28:402–407.

Levinstein E. 1878. *Morbid Craving for Morphia: A Monograph Founded on Personal Observations*. Translation by Charles Harrer. London: Smith, Elder, and Co.

May EL, Jacobson AE. 1989. The Committee on Problems of Drug Dependence: A legacy of the National Academy of Sciences. A historical account. *Drug and Alcohol Dependence* 23:183–218.

Metchnikoff E. 1901. *L'Immunité dans les Maladies Infestieuses*. Paris: Masson and Cia.

Musto DF. 1987. *The American Disease: Origins of Narcotic Control*. New York: Oxford University Press.

NCMDA (National Commission on Marihuana and Drug Abuse). 1972. *Marihuana: A Signal of Misunderstanding*. Washington, DC: U.S. Government Printing Office.

NCMDA (National Commission on Marihuana and Drug Abuse). 1973. *Drug Use in America: Problem in Perspective*. Washington, DC: U.S. Government Printing Office.

NIDA (National Institute on Drug Abuse). 1994. *1995 Budget Estimate*. Rockville, MD: NIDA.

NIH (National Institutes of Health). 1995. *NIH Data Book 1994*. NIH Publication No. 95-1261. Bethesda, MD: NIH.

Pellini E, Greenfield AD. 1920. Narcotic drug addiction: I. The formation of protective substances against morphine. *Archives of Internal Medicine* 26:279–292.

Pellini E, Greenfield AD. 1924. Narcotic drug addiction: II. The presence of toxic substances in the serum in morphine addiction. *Archives of International Medicine* 33:547–565.

Renz L. 1989. *Alcohol and Drug Abuse Funding: An Analysis of Foundation Grants*. New York: The Foundation Center.

Sollier P. 1898. La démorphinisation. Mécanisme physiologique. Conséquences au point de vue thérapeutique. *Presse Méd* 1(34):201–201; 2(56):9–10.

Terry CD, Pellens M. 1928. *The Opium Problem*. Montclair, NJ: Patterson Smith.

Valenti A. 1914. Experimentelle untersuchungen über den chronischen morphinismus. *Archives of Experimental Pathology and Pharmacology* 75:437–462.

Wald PM. 1972. *Dealing with Drug Abuse: A Report to the Ford Foundation*. New York: Praeger.

Wilcox WH. 1923. Norman Kerr memorial lecture on drug addiction. *British Medical Journal* (Dec.):1013–1018.

C

Diagnostic Criteria

TABLE C.1 Diagnostic Criteria for Substance Abuse and Dependence (DSM-IV)

Substance Abuse:

A. A maladaptive pattern of substance use leading to clinically significant impairment or distress, as manifested by one (or more) of the following, occurring within a 12-month period:

(1) Recurrent substance use resulting in a failure to fulfill major role obligations at work, school, or home (e.g. repeated absences or poor work performance related to substance use; substance-related absences, suspensions, or expulsions from school; neglect of children or household)
(2) Recurrent substance use in situations in which it is physically hazardous (e.g. driving an automobile or operating a machine when impaired by substance use)
(3) Recurrent substance-related legal problems (e.g. arrests for substance-related disorderly conduct)
(4) Continued substance use despite having persistent or recurrent social or interpersonal problems caused or exacerbated by the effects of the substance (e.g. arguments with spouse about consequences of intoxication, physical fights)

B. The symptoms have never met the criteria for Substance Dependence for this class of substance.

Continued on next page

TABLE C.1 Continued

Substance Dependence:

A maladaptive pattern of substance use, leading to clinically significant impairment or distress, as manifested by three (or more) of the following occurring at anytime in the same twelve month period:

(1) Tolerance, as defined by either of the following:

(a) a need for markedly increased amounts of the substance to achieve intoxication or desired effect
(b) markedly diminished effect with continued use of the same amount of the substance

(2) Withdrawal, as manifested by either of the following:

(a) the characteristic withdrawal syndrome for the substance
(b) the same (or closely related) substance is taken to relieve or avoid withdrawal symptoms

(3) The substance is often taken in larger amounts or over a longer period than was intended

(4) There was a persistent desire or unsuccessful efforts to cut down or control substance use

(5) A great deal of time is spent in activities necessary to obtain the substance (e.g., visiting multiple doctors or driving long distances), use the substance (e.g., chain-smoking), or recover from its effects

(6) Important social, occupational, or recreational activities are given up or reduced because of substance use

(7) The substance use is continued despite knowledge of having a persistent or recurrent physical or psychological problem that is likely to be caused or exacerbated by the substance (e.g., current cocaine use despite recognition of cocaine-induced depression, or continued drinking despite recognition that an ulcer was made worse by alcohol consumption)

Specify if:

With Physiological Dependence: Evidence of tolerance or withdrawal (i.e., either item 1 or 2 is present)

Without Physiological Dependence: No evidence of tolerance or withdrawal (i.e., neither item 1 nor 2 is present).

SOURCE: American Psychiatric Association. 1994. *Diagnostic and Statistical Manual of Mental Disorders.* 4th ed. (DSM-IV). Washington, DC: American Psychiatric Association.

TABLE C.2 Diagnostic Criteria for Harmful Use and Dependence (ICD-10)

Harmful Use:

A pattern of psychoactive substance use that is causing damage to health. The damage may be physical (as in cases of hepatitis from the self-administration of injected drugs) or mental (e.g. episodes of depressive disorder secondary to heavy consumption of alcohol).

Diagnostic Guidelines: The diagnosis requires that actual damage should have been caused to the mental or physical health of the user.

Harmful patterns of use are often criticized by others and frequently associated with adverse social consequences of various kinds. The fact that a pattern of use or particular substance is disapproved of by another person or by the culture, or may have led to socially negative consequences such as arrest or marital arguments is not in itself evidence of harmful use.

Acute intoxication or "hangover" is not in itself sufficient evidence of the damage to health required for coding harmful use.

Harmful use should not be diagnosed if dependence syndrome, a psychotic disorder, or another specific form of drug- or alcohol-related disorder is present.

Dependence Syndrome:

Diagnostic Guidelines: A definite diagnosis of dependence should usually only be made if three or more of the following have been experienced or exhibited at some time during the previous year:

(i) A strong desire or sense of compulsion to take the substance.

(ii) Difficulties in controlling substance-taking behavior in terms of its onset, termination, or levels of use.

(iii) A physiological withdrawal state when substance use has ceased or been reduced, as evidenced by: the characteristic withdrawal syndrome for the substance; or use of the same (or closely related) substance with the intention of relieving or avoiding withdrawal symptoms.

(iv) Evidence of tolerance such that increased doses of the substance are required in order to achieve effects originally produced by lower doses. (Clear examples of this are found in alcohol- and opiate-dependent individuals who may take daily doses sufficient to incapacitate or kill nontolerant users.)

(v) Progressive neglect of alternative pleasures or interests because of psychoactive substance use, increased amounts of time necessary to obtain or take the substance or recover from its effects.

(vi) Persisting with substance use despite clear evidence of overtly harmful consequences, such as harm to the liver through excessive drinking, depressive mood states consequent to periods of heavy substance use, or drug-related impairment of

Continued on next page

TABLE C.2 Continued

cognitive functioning; efforts should be made to determine that the user was actually, or could be expected to be, aware of the nature and extent of harm.

Narrowing of the personal repertoire of patterns of psychoactive substance use has also been described as a characteristic feature (e.g. a tendency to drink alcoholic drinks in the same way on weekdays and weekends, regardless of social constraints that determine appropriate drinking behavior).

It is an essential characteristic of the dependence syndrome that either psychoactive substance taking or a desire to take a particular substance should be present; the subjective awareness of compulsion to use drugs is most commonly seen during attempts to stop or control substance use. This diagnostic requirement would exclude, for instance, surgical patients given opioid drugs for the relief of pain, who may show signs of an opiate withdrawal state when drugs are not given, but who have no desire to continue taking drugs.

The dependence syndrome may be present for a specific substance (e.g., tobacco or diazepam), for a class of substances (e.g., opioid drugs); or for a wider range of different substances (as for those individuals who feel a sense of compulsion regularly to use whatever drugs are available and who show distress, agitation, and/or physical signs of a withdrawal state upon abstinence).

The diagnosis of the dependence syndrome may be further specified by the following:

- Currently abstinent
- Currently abstinent, but in a protected environment (e.g., in hospital, in a therapeutic community, in prison, etc.)
- Currently on a clinically supervised maintenance or replacement regime (e.g., with methadone; nicotine-gum or patch)
- Currently abstinent, but receiving treatment with aversive or blocking drugs (e.g. naltrexone or disulfiram)
- Currently using the substance (active dependence)
- Continuous use
- Episodic use (dipsomania)

SOURCE: WHO (World Health Organization). 1992. *International Statistical Classification of Diseases and Related Health Problems.* 10th Revision. Geneva: WHO. WHO. 1990. Draft of chapter V: mental and behavioural disorders. Clinical descriptions and diagnostic guidelines. *International Classification of Diseases.* 10th Revision. Geneva: WHO. As cited in: O'Brien CP, Jaffe JH, eds. *Addictive States.* New York: Raven Press.

Index

A

D

I

L

M

N

O

P

Q

R

S

T